Preface

This study guide has been prepared to complement the eighth edition of *Essentials of Nursing Research: Appraising Evidence for Nursing Practice* and to bridge the gap between the passive reading of abstract materials and the active development of skills needed to critique studies and use the findings in practice. Each section in this guide helps to reinforce these skills.

The learning exercises in each chapter reinforce the acquisition of basic research skills (some of the articles that are mentioned in the exercises appear on thePoint website and are identified by ✲). The appendices include eight research articles in their entirety. We deliberately selected some studies that are directly relevant to evidence-based practice (EBP), such as a study on the results of an EBP implementation project, and two systematic reviews. There are activities in each chapter of this study guide (the Application Exercises) geared around these studies.

This study guide consists of 19 chapters—one chapter corresponding to every chapter in the textbook. Most of the chapters consist of four sections:

- **A. Fill in the Blanks.** Terms and concepts presented in the textbook are reinforced by having you complete each sentence. All answers are in the Answer Key at the back of the book (Appendix I) for easy reference and cross-checking.

- **B. Matching Exercises.** Further reinforcement for key new terms is offered in a matching exercise, which often involves matching the concrete (e.g., an actual research hypothesis) with the abstract (e.g., the term for a specific type of hypothesis). Again, answers are in the Answer Key.

- **C. Study Questions.** Each chapter contains two to five short individual exercises relevant to the materials in the textbook.

- **D. Application Exercises.** These exercises are designed specifically to help you read, comprehend, and critique nursing studies. In each chapter, the application exercises focus on two of the studies in the appendices, and for each study, there are two sets of questions—*Questions of Fact* and *Questions for Discussion*.

  o **Questions of Fact** help you to read the report and find specific types of information related to the content covered in the textbook. For example, a question might ask: How many people participated in this study? For these questions, there are "right" answers, which we provide in the Answer Key.

  o **Questions for Discussion**, by contrast, require an assessment of the merits of various features of the study. For example, a question might ask: Were there *enough* people participating in this study? The second set of questions can be the basis for classroom discussions.

We hope that you will find these activities rewarding, enjoyable, and useful in your effort to develop skills for evidence-based nursing practice.

Denise F. Polit
Cheryl Tatano Beck

EIGHTH EDITION

STUDY GUIDE FOR ESSENTIALS OF NURSING RESEARCH

Appraising Evidence for Nursing Practice

Denise F. Polit, PhD, FAAN

President, Humanalysis, Inc.
Saratoga Springs, New York
Professor
Griffith University School of Nursing
Brisbane, Australia
www.denisepolit.com

Cheryl Tatano Beck, DNSc, CNM, FAAN

Distinguished Professor
School of Nursing
University of Connecticut
Storrs, Connecticut

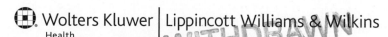 Wolters Kluwer | Lippincott Williams & Wilkins
Health
Philadelphia · Baltimore · New York · London
Buenos Aires · Hong Kong · Sydney · Tokyo

Acquisitions Editor: Christina C. Burns
Product Manager: Helen Kogut
Editorial Assistant: Daniel Reilly
Design Coordinator: Joan Wendt
Illustration Coordinator: Brett MacNaughton
Manufacturing Coordinator: Karin Duffield
Prepress Vendor: SPi Global

Eighth edition

9 8 7 6 5 4 3 2 1

Printed in China

978-1-4511-7683-4

LWW.com

Contents

PART 1

Overview of Nursing Research and Its Role in Evidence-Based Practice

CHAPTER 1

Introduction to Nursing Research in an Evidence-Based Practice Environment

A. FILL IN THE BLANKS

How many terms have you learned in this chapter? Fill in the blanks in the sentences below to find out. Try doing this section with a friend. Which of you is the first one to complete the sentence?

1. A _____ is a world view, a way of looking at natural phenomena.

2. The world view that holds that there are multiple interpretations of reality is _____.

3. _____ is the world view that assumes that there is an orderly reality that can be studied objectively.

4. Research designed to solve a pressing practical problem is _____ (as opposed to basic) research.

5. Nurses have discussions in practice settings to read and evaluate studies in the context of journal _____.

6. Research designed to inform nursing practice is referred to as _____ nursing research.

7. The degree to which research findings can be applied to people who did not participate in a study concerns its _____.

8. Many studies seek to understand determinants of phenomena and are referred to as _____ probing.

9. A principle that is believed to be true without proof or verification is a(n) _____.

10. _____ evidence refers to evidence that is rooted in objective reality and gathered through the senses.

11. The positivist assumption that phenomena are not random but rather have antecedent causes is called _____.

12. _____ is the repeating of a study to determine if findings can be upheld with a new group of people.

13. The techniques used by researchers to structure a study are called research _____.

14. The type of research that analyzes narrative, subjective materials is _____ research.

15. The scientific method involves procedures to enhance objectivity and reduce _____ that could distort the results.

16. _____ research involves the collection and analysis of numeric information and is associated with the traditional scientific method.

B. MATCHING EXERCISES

Match each statement in Set B with one of the paradigms in Set A. Indicate the letter corresponding to the appropriate response next to each entry in Set B.

SET A

a. Positivist/postpositivist paradigm
b. Constructivist paradigm
c. Neither paradigm
d. Both paradigms

SET B   RESPONSES

1. Assumes that reality exists and that it can be objectively studied and known _____

2. Subjectivity in inquiries is considered inevitable and desirable _____

3. Inquiries rely on external (empirical) evidence collected through human senses _____

4. Assumes that reality is a construction and that many constructions are possible _____

5. Method of inquiry relies primarily on collecting and analyzing quantitative information _____

6. Method of inquiry relies primarily on collecting and analyzing narrative, qualitative information _____

7. Provides an overarching framework for inquiries undertaken by nurse researchers _____

8. Inquiries give rise to emerging interpretations that are grounded in people's experiences _____

9. Inquiries are not constrained by ethical issues _____

10. Inquiries focus on discrete, specific concepts while attempting to control others _____

C. STUDY QUESTIONS

1. Why is it important for nurses who will never conduct their own research to understand research methods?

2. What are some potential consequences to the nursing profession if nurses stopped conducting their own research?

3. Below are descriptions of several research problems. Indicate whether you think the problem is best suited to a qualitative or quantitative approach, and explain your rationale.

   a. What is the decision-making process of AIDS patients seeking treatment?

   b. What effect does room temperature have on the colonization rate of bacteria in urinary catheters?

   c. What are sources of daily stress among nursing home residents, and what do these stressors mean to the residents?

   d. Does therapeutic touch affect the vital signs of hospitalized patients?

   e. What is the meaning of *hope* among Stage IV cancer patients?

   f. What are the effects of a formal exercise program on high blood pressure and cholesterol levels of middle-aged men?

   g. What are the health care needs of the homeless, and what barriers do they face in having those needs met?

4. What are some of the limitations of quantitative research? What are some of the limitations of qualitative research? Which approach seems best suited to address problems in which you might be interested? Why is that?

D. APPLICATION EXERCISES

Exercise D.1: Study in Appendix A

Read the abstract and introduction to the report by Weinert and colleagues ("Computer intervention impact") in Appendix A on pages 119–128 and then answer the following questions:

Questions of Fact

a. Does this report describe an example of "disciplined research"?

b. Is this a qualitative or quantitative study?

c. What is the underlying paradigm of the study?

d. Does the study involve the collection of empirical evidence?

e. Is this study applied or basic research?

f. Could this study be described as *cause probing?*

g. Is the specific purpose of this study identification, description, exploration, prediction/control, and (or) explanation?

h. Does this study have an evidence-based practice (EBP)-focused purpose, such as a one related to therapy (treatment), diagnosis, prognosis, etc.?

Questions for Discussion

a. How relevant is this study to the actual practice of nursing?

b. Could this study have been conducted as *either* a quantitative or qualitative study? Why or why not?

Exercise D.2: Study in Appendix B

Read the abstract and introduction of the report by Cricoo-Lizza and colleagues ("Rooting for the breast") in Appendix B on pages 129–138 and then answer the following questions:

Questions of Fact

a. Does this report describe an example of "disciplined research"?

b. Is this a qualitative or quantitative study?

c. What is the underlying paradigm of the research?

d. Does the study involve the collection of empirical evidence?

e. Is this study applied or basic research?

f. Could this study be described as *cause probing?*

g. Is the specific purpose of this study identification, description, exploration, prediction/control, and (or) explanation?

h. Does this study have an EBP-focused purpose, such as one related to therapy (treatment), diagnosis, prognosis, etc.?

Questions for Discussion

a. How relevant is this study to the actual practice of nursing?

b. Could this study have been conducted as *either* a quantitative or qualitative study? Why or why not?

c. Which of the two studies cited in these exercises (the one in Appendix A or Appendix B) is of greater interest and/or relevance to you personally? Why?

CHAPTER 2

Fundamentals of Evidence-Based Nursing Practice

A. FILL IN THE BLANKS

How many terms have you learned in this chapter? Fill in the blanks in the sentences below to find out. Try doing this section with a friend. Which of you is the first one to complete the sentence?

1. A clinical practice _____ based on rigorous systematic evidence is an important tool for evidence-based care.

2. _____ reviews of randomized controlled trails (RCTs) are at the pinnacle of most evidence hierarchies.

3. When a new protocol or guideline is developed in an evidence-based practice (EBP) project, it should be _____ tested to evaluate its utility.

4. The _____ Collaboration is a cornerstone of EBP.

5. When asking clinical questions, the "O" component refers to the _____.

6. When asking clinical questions, the "P" component refers to the _____.

7. A single RCT study would be Level II on an evidence hierarchy for _____ questions.

8. The _____ instrument is an important tool for appraising clinical guidelines.

9. _____ is the acronym for the four-component scheme for asking well-worded clinical questions.

10. _____ is the type of systematic review that involves statistical integration of quantitative research findings.

11. When asking clinical questions, the "C" component refers to the _____.

12. A(n) _____ is a ranked arrangement of the worth of various types of evidence.

13. When asking clinical Therapy questions, the "I" component refers to the _____.

7

14. The integration of multiple qualitative studies can be achieved in a

_____.

15 _____ refers to the conscientious use of the best current evidence when making decisions about patient care.

B. MATCHING EXERCISES

Match each of the statements in Set B with the appropriate phrase in Set A. Indicate the letter(s) corresponding to your response next to each of the statements in Set B.

SET A

a. Research utilization (RU)

b. Evidence-based practice (EBP)

c. Neither RU nor EBP

d. Both RU and EBP

SET B   RESPONSES

1. Has been easily achieved in nursing   _____

2. Evidence hierarchies were developed within this context   _____

3. Is useful only to nurses in academic environments   _____

4. Integrates research findings with clinical expertise and client inputs _____

5. Has given rise to models developed by nurses for guiding the process _____

6. Always begins with a knowledge-focused trigger   _____

7. The CURN project focused on this   _____

8. Sackett and Cochrane were prominent proponents   _____

C. STUDY QUESTIONS

1. For each of the following research questions, identify the component that is underlined as the P, I, C, or O component.

   a. Among community-dwelling elders, does <u>fear of falling</u> affect their quality of life?

   b. Does amount of social support among <u>women with multiple sclerosis</u> affect disability to a greater degree than illness duration?

   c. Among children aged 5 to 10, does participation in the XYZ Youth Fitness Initiative result in better cardiovascular fitness than participation in <u>routine school play activities</u>?

    d. Does <u>chronic stress</u> contribute to fatigue among patients with a traumatic head injury?

    e. Among older adults in a long-term care setting, does a reminiscence program reduce <u>depressive symptoms</u>?

    f. Among <u>methadone maintenance therapy clients,</u> are men more likely than women to be heavy cigarette smokers?

    g. Does <u>family involvement in diabetes management</u> affect glucose control among immigrants with type 2 diabetes?

    h. Among hospitalized adult patients, is greater nurse staffing levels associated with shorter <u>lengths of hospital stay</u>?

    i. Is music more effective treatment than <u>normal hospital sounds</u> in reducing pain in women in labor?

    j. Does self-concept affect <u>dietary intake</u> in moderately obese adults?

2. For each of the following clinical questions, fill in the blank (use your imagination!) for the component that is missing. Do not be concerned with whether the question has been addressed by researchers. The exercise is meant to encourage you to be brave about asking clinical questions, and to help you get in the habit of asking them. There are no right or wrong answers.

    a. Among _____ (P), does intensive exercise (I) affect peak oxygen consumption (O)?

    b. Does _____ (I) reduce cigarette smoking (O) in high school students (P)?

    c. Does fatigue (I) have a bigger effect than _____ (C) on ability to cope (O) in patients undergoing chemotherapy (P)?

    d. Among patients with a chronic health problem (P), does _____ (I) affect their quality of life (O)?

    e. Among caregivers of patients with Alzheimer's disease, do the age and income level of the caregiver (I) affect _____ (O)?

    f. Among adolescent males (P), does/do _____ (I) affect decisions to be sexually abstinent?

    g. Among cognitively impaired elders being relocated to a nursing home (P), does the person's involvement in the decision to relocate (I) affect _____ (O)?

    h. Among _____ (P), does smoking history (I) affect perceptions of acute coronary syndrome (O)?

3. Think about a nursing procedure that you have learned. What is the basis for this procedure? Examine whether the procedure is based on scientific evidence indicating that the procedure is effective. If it is not based on scientific evidence, on what is it based, and why do you think scientific evidence was not used?

4. Identify the factors in your own clinical setting that you think facilitate or inhibit RU and EBP (or, in an educational setting, the factors that promote or inhibit a climate in which EBP is valued).

5. Read one of the following articles and identify the steps of the Iowa model (or an alternative model of EBP) that are represented in the projects described.

   a. Alexander, L., & Allen, D. (2011). Establishing an evidence-based inpatient medical oncology fluid balance measurement policy. *Clinical Journal of Oncology Nursing, 15*, 23–25.

   b. Capasso, V., Collins, J., Griffith, C., Lasala, C., Kilroy, S., Martin, A., et al. (2009). Outcomes of a clinical nurse specialist-initiated wound care education program: using the promoting action on research implementation in health services framework. *Clinical Nurse Specialist, 23*, 252–257.

   c. Long, L., Burkett, K., & McGee, S. (2009). Promotion of safe outcomes: Incorporating evidence into policies and procedures. *Nursing Clinics of North America, 44*, 57–70.

   d. Tschannen, D., Talsma, A., Gombert, J., & Mowry, J. (2011). Using the TRIP Model to disseminate an IT-based pressure ulcer intervention. *Western Journal of Nursing Research, 33*, 427–442.

D. APPLICATION EXERCISES

Exercise D.1: Study in Appendix C

Read the abstract and introduction to the report by Yackel and colleagues ("Nurse-facilitated depression screening program") in Appendix E on pages 157–174 and then answer the following questions:

Questions of Fact

a. What was the purpose of this EBP project?
b. What was the setting for implementing this project?
c. Which EBP model was used as a framework for this project?
d. Did the project have a problem-focused or knowledge-focused trigger?
e. Who were the team members in this study, and what were their affiliations?
f. What, if anything, did the report say about the implementation potential of this project?
g. Was a pilot study undertaken?
h. Did this project involve an evaluation of the project's success?

Questions for Discussion

a. What might be a clinical foreground question that was used in seeking relevant evidence in preparing for this project? Identify the PIO or PICO components of your question.
b. What are some of the praiseworthy aspects of this project? What could the team members have done differently to improve the project?

Exercise D.2: Study in Appendix G

Read the abstract and introduction (from the beginning to the "Methods" section) of the report by Nam and colleagues ("Effect of culturally tailored diabetes education") in Appendix G on pages 183–196 and then answer the following questions:

Questions of Fact

a. Is this report a systematic review? If yes, what type of systematic review was it? Is this an example of preappraised evidence?

b. Where on the evidence hierarchy shown in Figure 2.1 of the textbook would this study belong?

c. What is the stated purpose of this study?

Questions for Discussion

a. What might be a clinical foreground question that was used in seeking relevant evidence in preparing for this project? Identify the PIO or PICO components of your question.

b. What are some of the steps would you need to undertake if you were interested in using this meta-analysis as a basis for an EBP project in your own practice setting?

Key Concepts and Steps in Qualitative and Quantitative Research

A. FILL IN THE BLANKS

How many terms have you learned in this chapter? Fill in the blanks in the sentences below to find out. Try doing this section with a friend. Which of you is the first one to complete the sentence?

1. Another name for outcome variable is _____ variable.
2. To get access to a site and its inhabitants is to _____ entrée into the site.
3. Information gathered in a study is called _____.
4. A(n) _____ is a subset of a population from whom data are gathered.
5. The _____ definition indicates how a variable will be measured or observed.
6. A systematic, abstract explanation of phenomena is a(n) _____.
7. Quantitative researchers perform _____ analyses of their data.
8. Some qualitative researchers do not undertake an upfront _____ review, to avoid having their conceptualization influenced by the work of others.
9. Researchers typically use a(n) _____ design in qualitative studies.
10. The broad class of research that involves an intervention is _____ research.
11. In medical literature, a study that tests the effect of an intervention is a clinical _____.
12. The qualitative research tradition that focuses on lived experiences is _____.
13. A type of qualitative research that focuses on the study of cultures is _____.
14. Data _____ is a principle used to decide when to stop sampling in a qualitative study.

12

15. _____ is the entire aggregate of people in which a researcher is interested (the "P" in PICO).

16. A qualitative tradition that focuses on social psychological processes within a social setting is called _____ theory.

17. A(n) _____ is a somewhat more complex abstraction than a concept.

18. If the independent variable (IV) is the cause, the dependent variable (DV) is the _____.

19. A research _____ is the basic architecture of a study.

20. A relationship in which one variable directly induces changes in another is a _____ relationship.

21. Qualitative analyses usually involve a search for recurrent _____.

22. In quantitative research, a concept is usually referred to as a(n) _____.

23. A person who provides information to researchers in a study is often called a study _____.

24. A(n) _____ is a characteristic or quality that takes on different values—that is, that differs from one person or object to another.

25. The presumed influence on a DV is the _____ variable.

26. A(n) _____ is a bond, connection, or pattern of association between variables.

27. Another name for nonexperimental research, often used in the medical literature, is _____ research.

B. MATCHING EXERCISES

1. Match each statement in Set B with one of the paradigms in Set A. Indicate the letter corresponding to the appropriate response next to each entry in Set B.

SET A

a. Term used in quantitative research
b. Term used in qualitative research
c. Term used in both qualitative and quantitative research

SET B   RESPONSES

1. Subject   _____
2. Study participant   _____
3. Informant   _____
4. Variable   _____
5. Phenomenon   _____
6. Construct   _____
7. Theory   _____
8. Data   _____
9. Emergent design   _____
10. Data analysis   _____

2. Match each term in Set B with one of the terms in Set A. Indicate the letter corresponding to your response next to each item in Set B.

SET A

a. Independent variable

b. Dependent variable

c. Either/both

d. Neither

SET B	**RESPONSES**
1. The variable that is the presumed effect	_____
2. The variable involved in a cause-and-effect relationship	_____
3. The variable that is the presumed cause	_____
4. The variable, "length of stay in hospital"	_____
5. The variable that requires an operational definition	_____
6. The variable that is the main outcome of interest in the study	_____
7. The variable that is constant	_____
8. The variable in a grounded theory study	_____

3. Match each activity in Set B with one of the options in Set A. Indicate the letter corresponding to your response next to each item in Set B.

SET A

a. An activity in quantitative research

b. An activity in qualitative research

c. An activity in both qualitative and quantitative research

d. An activity in neither quantitative nor qualitative research

SET B	**RESPONSES**
1. Choosing between an experimental or nonexperimental design	_____
2. Ending data collection once saturation has been achieved	_____
3. Developing or evaluating measurement instruments	_____
4. Doing a literature review	_____
5. Gaining entrée into a site and negotiating with gatekeepers	_____
6. Taking steps to ensure protection of human rights	_____
7. Developing strategies to avoid collecting new data	_____
8. Disseminating research results	_____
9. Analyzing the data for major themes or categories	_____
10. Formulating hypotheses to be tested statistically	_____

4. Match each activity relating to quantitative studies in Set B with an option in Set A. Indicate the letter corresponding to your response next to each item in Set B.

SET A

a. Conceptual phase
b. Planning phase
c. Empirical phase
d. Analytic phase
e. Dissemination phase

SET B   **RESPONSES**

1. Distributing questionnaires to a group of nursing home residents _____
2. Deciding what type of design to use   _____
3. Conducting a literature review   _____
4. Identifying a suitable theoretical framework   _____
5. Deciding to collect data from 300 alcoholics in treatment   _____
6. Computing what percentage of subjects were clinically depressed   _____
7. Presenting a paper at a meeting of the Eastern Nursing Research Society   _____
8. Designing a training session to be used with data collectors   _____
9. Coding data for entry of information onto a computer file   _____
10. Interpreting findings that were contrary to the hypotheses   _____

C. STUDY QUESTIONS

1. Suggest operational definitions for the following concepts.
   a. Stress:
   b. Prematurity of infants:
   c. Fatigue:
   d. Pain:
   e. Prolonged labor:
   f. Dyspnea:

2. In each of the following research questions, identify the independent variable (IV) and the dependent or outcome variable (DV).
   a. Does assertiveness training improve the effectiveness of psychiatric nurses?
      Independent: _____
      Dependent: _____
   b. Does the postural positioning of patients affect their respiratory function?
      Independent: _____
      Dependent: _____

c. Is the psychological well-being of patients affected by the amount of touch received from nursing staff?

Independent: _____

Dependent: _____

d. Is the incidence of decubitus reduced by more frequent turnings of patients?

Independent: _____

Dependent: _____

e. Are people who were abused as children more likely than others to abuse their own children?

Independent: _____

Dependent: _____

f. Is tolerance for pain related to a patient's age and gender?

Independent: _____

Dependent: _____

g. Are the number of prenatal visits of pregnant women associated with labor and delivery outcomes?

Independent: _____

Dependent: _____

h. Are levels of depression higher among children who experience the death of a sibling than among other children?

Independent: _____

Dependent: _____

i. Is compliance with a medical regimen higher among women than among men?

Independent: _____

Dependent: _____

j. Does participating in a support group enhance coping among family care-givers of AIDS patients?

Independent: _____

Dependent: _____

k. Is hearing acuity of the elderly affected by the time of day?

Independent: _____

Dependent: _____

l. Does home birth affect the parents' satisfaction with the childbirth experience?

Independent: _____

Dependent: _____

m. Does a neutropenic diet in the outpatient setting decrease the positive blood cultures associated with chemotherapy-induced neutropenia?

Independent: _____

Dependent: _____

3. Below is a list of variables. For each, think of a research question for which the variable would be the IV, and a second for which it would be the DV. For example, take the variable "birth weight of infants." We might ask, "Does the age of the mother affect the birth weight of her infant?" (DV). Alternatively, our research question might be, "Does the birth weight of infants (IV) affect their sensorimotor development at 6 months of age?" HINT: For the DV problem, ask yourself, what factors might affect, influence, or cause this variable? For the IV, ask yourself, what factors does this variable influence, cause, or affect—what are the consequences of this variable?

   a. Body temperature

   Independent: _____

   Dependent: _____

   b. Amount of sleep

   Independent: _____

   Dependent: _____

   c. Frequency of practicing breast self-examination

   Independent: _____

   Dependent: _____

   d. Level of hopefulness in cancer patients

   Independent: _____

   Dependent: _____

   e. Stress among victims of domestic violence

   Independent: _____

   Dependent: _____

4. Look at the table of contents of a recent issue of *Nursing Research* (available at www.nursingcenter.com/library) or *Research in Nursing & Health* (available at www.interscience.wiley.com). Pick out a study title (without looking at the abstract or study description at the beginning) that implies that a relationship between variables was studied. Indicate what you think the IV and DV might be, and what the title suggests about the nature of the relationship (i.e., causal or not).

5. Describe what is wrong with the following statements:

   a. Opitz's experimental study was conducted within the ethnographic tradition.

   b. Brusser's experimental study examined the effect of relaxation therapy (the DV) on pain (the IV) in cancer patients.

   c. Ball's grounded theory study of the caregiving process for caretakers of patients with dementia was a clinical trial.

   d. In Lace's phenomenological study of the meaning of futility among AIDS patients, subjects received an intervention designed to sustain hope.

   e. In her experimental study, Gabris developed her data collection plan after she introduced her intervention to a group of patients.

6. Which qualitative research tradition do you think would be most appropriate for the following research questions? Justify your response:

   a. How do the health beliefs and customs of Chinese immigrants influence their health-seeking behavior?

   b. What is the lived experience of being a recovering alcoholic?

   c. What is the process by which husbands adapt to the sudden loss of their wives?

D. APPLICATION EXERCISES

Exercise D.1: Study in Appendix D

Read the abstract, introduction, and first few subsection of the "Methods" section of the report by Jurgens and colleagues ("Why do elders delay responding?") in Appendix D on pages 147–156 and then answer the following questions:

Questions of Fact

a. Who were the researchers and what are their credentials and affiliation?

b. Who were the study participants?

c. What were the site and setting for this study?

d. What is the independent variable (or variables) in this study? Is this variable *inherently* an independent variable?

e. What is the dependent variable (or variables) in this study? Is this variable *inherently* a dependent variable?

f. Did the report actually use the terms "independent variable" or "dependent variable?"

g. How was *depression* operationally defined? Was a conceptual definition provided?

h. Were the data in this study quantitative or qualitative?

i. Were any relationships under investigation? What type of relationship?

j. Is this an experimental or nonexperimental study?

k. Was there any intervention? If so, what is it?

l. Did the study involve statistical analysis of data? Did it involve the qualitative analysis of data?

Questions for Discussion

a. How relevant is this study to the actual practice of nursing?

b. How good a job did the researchers do in summarizing their study in the abstract?

c. How long do you estimate it took for this study to be completed?

Exercise D.2: Study in Appendix F

Read the abstract and introduction of the report by Cummings ("Sharing a traumatic event") in Appendix F on pages 175–182 and then answer the following questions:

Questions of Fact

a. Who was the researcher and what are her credentials and affiliation?

b. Who were the study participants?

c. In what type of setting did the study take place?

d. What was the key concept in this study?

e. Were there any *independent variables* or *dependent variables* in this study?

f. Were the data in this study quantitative or qualitative?

g. Were any relationships under investigation?

h. Could the study be described as an ethnographic, phenomenologic, or grounded theory study?

i. Is this an experimental or nonexperimental study?

j. Does the study involve an intervention? If so, what is it?

k. Did the study involve statistical analysis of data? Did the study involve qualitative analysis of data?

Questions for Discussion

a. How relevant is this study to the actual practice of nursing?

b. How good a job did Cummings do in summarizing her study in the abstract?

c. How long do you estimate it took for this study to be completed?

d. Which of the two studies cited in these exercises (the one in Appendix D or Appendix F) is of greater interest and/or relevance to you personally? Why?

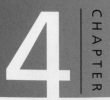

Reading and Critiquing Research Articles

A. FILL IN THE BLANKS

How many terms have you learned in this chapter? Fill in the blanks in the sentences below to find out. Try doing this section with a friend. Which of you is the first one to complete the sentence?

1. _____ is an influence that results in a distortion or error.
2. "The lived experience of caring for a dying spouse" is an example of the section of a research report called the _____.
3. The process of reflecting critically on one's self, used by many qualitative researchers, is _____.
4. One conventional _____ of significance is .05.
5. Qualitative researchers strive to ensure that their findings are _____, which includes enhancing credibility, authenticity, and dependability.
6. If the results of a statistical test indicated a probability of .001, the results would be statistically _____.
7. _____ is the format used to structure most research reports.
8. To address biases stemming from *awareness,* researchers may use a procedure that is usually called _____.
9. A summary of a study, also known as a(n) _____, appears at the beginning of a report.
10. A(n) _____ variable is a variable that is extraneous to the research question but needs to be controlled.
11. Research reports are most likely to be disseminated as _____ articles.
12. Quantitative researchers strive for findings that are reliable and _____.
13. A(n) _____ is a conclusion drawn from the evidence in a study that takes into account the research methods used.
14. _____ is a criterion for evaluating study evidence (mostly in a quantitative study) that concerns the accuracy and consistency of information.

20

15. Research _____ is used by researchers to hold constant outside influences on the dependent variable so that the relationship under study can be better understood.

16. _____ is a strategy used by quantitative researchers to reduce bias and involves having aspects of the study established by chance rather than by personal choices.

17. _____ is to qualitative research what generalizability is to quantitative research.

B. MATCHING EXERCISES

Match each statement in Set B with one of the report sections in Set A. Indicate the letter corresponding to the appropriate response next to each entry in Set B.

SET A

a. Abstract
b. Introduction
c. Method
d. Results
e. Discussion

SET B   RESPONSES

1. Describes the research design   _____

2. In quantitative studies, presents findings from statistical analyses   _____

3. Identifies the research questions or hypotheses   _____

4. Presents a brief summary of the major features of the study   _____

5. Provides information on how study participants were selected   _____

6. Offers an interpretation of the study findings   _____

7. In qualitative studies, describes the themes or categories that emerged from the data   _____

8. Describes the significance of the study   _____

9. Describes how the research data were collected   _____

10. Identifies the study's main limitations   _____

11. This sentence would appear there: "The purpose of this study was to explore the process by which patients cope with a cancer diagnosis."   _____

12. Includes raw data, in the form of excerpts from participants, in qualitative reports   _____

C. STUDY QUESTIONS

1. Why are qualitative research reports typically easier to read than quantitative research reports?

2. Read the following abstract and rewrite it as a "new style" abstract with specific headings: Lee, K., & Gay, C. (2011). Can modifications to the bedroom environment improve the sleep of new parents? Two randomized controlled trials. *Research in Nursing & Health, 34,* 7–19.

   > Postpartum sleep disruption is common among new parents. In this randomized controlled trial, we evaluated a modified sleep hygiene intervention for new parents (infant proximity, noise masking, and dim lighting) in anticipation of night-time infant care. Two samples of new mothers (n = 118 and 122) were randomized to the experimental intervention or attention control, and sleep was assessed in late pregnancy and first 3 months postpartum using actigraphy and the General Sleep Disturbance Scale. The sleep hygiene strategies evaluated did not benefit the more socioeconomically advantaged women or their partners in Sample 1, but did improve postpartum sleep among the less advantaged women of Sample 2. Simple changes to the bedroom environment can improve sleep for new mothers with few resources.

3. Read the titles of the journal articles appearing in the December 2012 issue of *Nursing Research* (or some other issue of this or another nursing journal). Evaluate the titles of the articles in terms of length and adequacy in communicating essential information about the studies.

4. Below is a brief abstract of a fictitious study, followed by a critique. Do you agree with the critique? Can you add other comments relevant to issues discussed in Chapter 4 of the textbook?

FICTITIOUS STUDY
Solomons (2012) prepared the following abstract for her study.

Abstract. Family members often experience considerable anxiety while their loved ones are in surgery. This study examined the effectiveness of a nursing intervention that involved providing oral intraoperative progress reports to family members. Surgical patients undergoing elective procedures were selected to either have family members receive the intervention or not have them receive it. The findings indicated that the family members in the intervention group were less anxious than family members who received the usual care.

Critique. This brief abstract provides a general overview of the nature of Solomons' study. It indicates a rationale for the study (the high anxiety level of surgical patients' family members) and summarizes what the researcher did. However, the abstract could have provided more information while still staying within a 100- or 125-word guideline (the abstract only contains 77 words). For example, the abstract could have better described the nature of the intervention (e.g., at what point during the operation was information given to family members? how much detail was provided? etc.). For a reader to have a preliminary assessment of the worth of the study—and therefore to make a decision about whether to read the entire report—more information about the methods would have been helpful. For example, the abstract should have indicated such methodological features as how the researcher measured anxiety and how many families were in the sample. Also missing is information about how families were allocated to receive the intervention. Some indication of the study's implications might also have enhanced the usefulness of the abstract.

D. APPLICATION EXERCISES

Exercise D.1: Study in Appendix A

Read the abstract and introduction of the report by Weinert and colleagues ("Computer intervention impact") in Appendix A on pages 119–128 and then answer the following questions:

Questions of Fact

a. Does the structure of this article follow the IMRAD format?
b. Is the abstract a traditional narrative or is it a "new style" abstract?
c. Does the abstract summarize information about the study purpose, how the study was done, what the key findings were, and what the findings mean?
d. Skim the Methods section. Is the presentation in the active or passive voice?
e. Is this study experimental or nonexperimental?
f. Was the principle of *randomness* used in this study?

Questions for Discussion

a. What parts of the abstract were most difficult to understand? Identify words that you consider to be research "jargon."
b. Comment on the organization *within* the Methods section of this report.

Exercise D.2: Study in Appendix E

Read the abstract and introduction to the report by Byrne and colleagues ("Care transition experiences") in Appendix E on pages 157–174 and then answer the following questions:

Questions of Fact

a. Does the structure of this article follow the IMRAD format?
b. Is the abstract a traditional narrative or is it a "new style" abstract?
c. Does the abstract include information about the study purpose, how the study was done, what the findings were, and what the findings mean?
d. Skim the Methodology section. Is the presentation in the active or passive voice?
e. Is the study in one of the three main qualitative traditions described in Chapter 3? If so, which tradition?

Questions for Discussion

a. What parts of the abstract were most difficult to understand?

b. Comment on the organization *within* the Results section of this report.

c. Compare the level of difficulty of the abstracts for the two studies used in these exercises—i.e., the studies in Appendix A and E. Why do you think the level of difficulty differs?

d. Which type of abstract do you prefer—the traditional one or the "new" style? Why?

CHAPTER 5

Ethics in Research

A. FILL IN THE BLANKS

How many terms have you learned in this chapter? Fill in the blanks in the sentences below to find out. Try doing this section with a friend. Which of you is the first one to complete the sentence?

1. Most disciplines have developed formal _____ of ethics.
2. _____ is the best method of protecting participants' confidentiality, but is not always possible.
3. Researchers should conduct a(n) _____-benefit assessment to evaluate the ethical aspects of their research plan.
4. _____ is a major ethical principle concerning maximizing benefits of research.
5. _____ is the type of consent procedure that may be required in qualitative research involving multiple points of data collection.
6. A(n) _____ is a payment sometimes offered to participants as an incentive to take part in a study.
7. The _____ report is the basis for ethical regulations for studies funded by the US government.
8. Fraud and misrepresentations are examples of research _____.
9. The return of a questionnaire is often assumed to demonstrate _____ consent.
10. Informal agreement to participate in a study (e.g., by minors) is called _____.
11. Participants' privacy is often protected by _____ procedures, even though the researchers know participants' identities.
12. People can make informed decisions about research participation when there is full _____.
13. A(n) _____ is a committee (in the United States) that reviews the ethical aspects of a study.
14. A conflict between the rights of participants and the demands for rigorous research creates an ethical _____.
15. Prisoners and children involved in research are examples of _____.

25

16. _____ procedures offer prospective participants' information needed to make a reasonable decision about study participation.

17. _____ sessions at the conclusion of a study offer participants an opportunity to learn more about a study, ask questions, and air complaints.

18. A risk no greater than those ordinarily experienced in everyday life is called a(n) _____ risk in research parlance.

B. MATCHING EXERCISES

Match each description in Set B with one of the procedures used to protect study participants listed in Set A. Indicate the letter corresponding to the appropriate response next to each entry in Set B.

SET A

a. Freedom from harm or exploitation

b. Informed consent

c. Anonymity

d. Confidentiality

SET B   RESPONSES

1. A questionnaire distributed by mail bears an identification number in one corner. Respondents are assured that their responses will not be individually divulged.   _____

2. Hospitalized children included in a study, and their parents, are told the study's aims and procedures. Parents are asked to sign an authorization.   _____

3. Participants in a study in which the same people will participate twice by completing questionnaires are asked to place their own four-digit identification number on the questionnaire and to memorize the number for use in the next round. Participants are assured their answers will remain private.   _____

4. Study participants in an in-depth study of family members coping with a natural disaster renegotiate the terms of their participation at successive interviews.   _____

5. Women who recently had a mastectomy are studied in terms of psychological consequences. In the interview, sensitive questions are carefully worded. After the interview, debriefing with the respondent is used to assess the need for psychological support.   _____

6. Women interviewed in the above study (question 5) are told that the information they provide will not be individually divulged.   _____

7. Subjects who volunteered for an experimental treatment for AIDS are warned of potential side effects and are asked to sign an agreement.   _____

8. After determining that a new intervention resulted in discomfort to participants, the researcher discontinued the study.   _____

9. Unmarked questionnaires are distributed to a class of nursing students. The instructions indicate that responses will not be individually divulged. _____

10. The researcher assures participants that they will be interviewed at a single point in time and adheres to this promise. _____

11. A questionnaire distributed to a sample of nursing students includes a statement indicating that completion and submission of the questionnaire will be construed as voluntary participation in a study. _____

12. The names, ages, and occupations of study participants whose interviews are excerpted in the research report are not divulged. _____

C. STUDY QUESTIONS

1. Below are brief descriptions of several studies. Suggest some ethical dilemmas that could emerge for each.
   a. A study of coping behaviors among rape victims
   b. An unobtrusive observational study of fathers' behaviors in the delivery room
   c. An interview study of the determinants of heroin addiction
   d. A study of dependence among mentally retarded children
   e. An investigation of verbal interactions among schizophrenic patients
   f. A study of the effects of a new drug on humans
   g. A study of the relationship between sleeping patterns and acting-out behaviors in hospitalized psychiatric patients

2. Evaluate the ethical aspects of one or more of the following studies using the critiquing guidelines in Box 5.2 on pages 93 in the textbook and available on thePoint. Pay special attention (if relevant) to the manner in which the participants' heightened vulnerability was handled.
   - Champion, J. (2011). Context of sexual risk behaviour among abused ethnic minority adolescent women. *International Nursing Review, 58*, 61–67.
   - Lee, H., & Scherp, K. (2011). Multiple informants in assessing stress and symptoms in adolescents with schizophrenia. *Archives of Psychiatric Nursing, 25*, 120–128.
   - O'Brien, L., Anand, M., Brady, P., & Gillies, D. (2011). Children visiting parents in inpatient psychiatric facilities. *International Journal of Mental Health Nursing, 20*, 137–143.
   - Woods, D., Kim, H., & Yefimova, M. (2011). Morning cortisol in relation to behavioral symptoms of nursing home residents. *Biological Research for Nursing, 13*, 196–203.

3. In the textbook, several actual studies with ethical problems were described (e.g., the study of syphilis among black men and the study in which the mentally retarded children were deliberately infected with the hepatitis virus, p. 81 in the text). Identify which ethical principles were transgressed in these studies.

4. In a study by Byers et al., 2006 (A quasi-experimental trial on individual-ized, developmentally supportive family-centered care. *Journal of Obstetric, Gynecologic, & Neonatal Nursing, 35*, 105–115), the authors indicated that informed consent was not required because there was "no deviation from the standard of care or risk to the subjects" (p. 108).

   Skim the introduction and method section of this paper and comment on the researchers' decision to not obtain informed consent.

5. Below is a brief description of the ethical aspects of a fictitious study, followed by a critique. Do you agree with the critique? Can you add other comments relevant to the ethical dimensions of the study?

FICTITIOUS STUDY

Fortune conducted an in-depth study of nursing home residents to explore whether their perceptions about personal control over decision making differed from the perceptions of the nursing staff. The investigator studied 25 nurse–patient dyads to assess whether there were differing perceptions and experiences regarding control over activities of daily living, such as rising, eating, and dressing. All of the nurses in the study were employed by the nursing home in which the patients resided. Because the nursing home had no Institutional Review Board (IRB), and because Fortune's study was not funded by an organization that required IRB approval, the project was not formally reviewed. Fortune sought permission to conduct the study from the nursing home administrator. She also obtained the consent of the legal guardian or responsible family member of each patient. All study participants were fully informed about the nature of the study. The researcher assured the nurses and the legal guardians and family mem-bers of the patients of the confidentiality of the information and obtained their consent in writing. Data were gathered primarily through in-depth interviews with the patients and the nurses, at separate times. The researcher also observed interactions between the patients and nurses. The findings from the study suggested that patients perceived that they had more control over all aspects of the activities of daily living (except eat-ing) than the nurses perceived that they had. Excerpts from the interviews were used verbatim in the research report, but Fortune did not divulge the location of the nursing home, and she used fictitious names for all participants.

CRITIQUE

Fortune did a reasonably good job of adhering to ethical principles in the conduct of her research. She obtained written permission to conduct the study from the nursing home administrator, and she obtained informed consent from the nurse participants and the legal guardians or family members of the patients. The study participants were not put at risk in any way, and the patients who participated may actually have enjoyed the opportunity to have a conversation with the researcher. Fortune also took appropriate steps to maintain the confidentiality of participants. It is still unclear, however, whether the patients knowingly and willingly participated in the research. Nursing home residents are a vulnerable group. They may not have been aware of their right to refuse to be interviewed without fear of repercussion.

Fortune could have enhanced the ethical aspects of the study by taking more vigorous steps to obtain the informed, voluntary consent of the nursing home residents or to exclude patients who could not reasonably be expected to understand the researcher's request. Given the vulnerability of the group, Fortune probably should have established her own review panel composed of peers and interested lay people to review the ethical dimensions of her project. Debriefing sessions with study participants would also have been appropriate.

D. APPLICATION EXERCISES

Exercise D.1: Study in Appendix D

Read the Method section of the report by Jurgens and colleagues ("Why do elders delay responding") in Appendix D on pages 147–156 and then answer the following questions:

Questions of Fact

a. Does the report indicate that the study procedures were reviewed by an IRB or other similar institutional human subjects group?

b. Would the participants in this study be considered a vulnerable group?

c. Were participants subjected to any physical harm or discomfort or psychological distress as part of the study? What efforts did the researchers make to minimize harm and maximize good?

d. Were participants deceived in any way?

e. Were participants coerced into participating in the study?

f. Were appropriate informed consent procedures used? Was there full disclosure?

g. Does the report discuss steps that were taken to protect the privacy and confidentiality of study participants? Were data collected anonymously?

Questions for Discussion

a. Do you think that the benefits of this research outweighed the costs to participants—what is the overall risk/benefit ratio?

b. Do you consider that the researchers took adequate steps to protect study participants? If not, what else could they have done?

c. The report did not indicate that the participants were paid a stipend. Do you think they should have been?

d. Is there any evidence of discrimination in this study, with regard to people recruited to participate?

e. How comfortable would you feel about having a parent or grandparent participate in this study?

Exercise D.2: Study in Appendix B

Read the Method section of the report by Cricco-Lizza ("Rooting for the breast") in Appendix B on pages 129–138 and then answer the following questions:

Questions of Fact

a. Does the report indicate that the study procedures were reviewed by an IRB or other similar institutional human subjects group?

b. Would the study participants in this study be considered a vulnerable group?

c. Were participants subjected to any physical harm or discomfort or psychological distress as part of this study? What efforts did the researcher make to minimize harm and maximize good?

d. Were participants deceived in any way?

e. Were participants coerced into participating in the study?

f. Were appropriate informed consent procedures used? Was there full disclosure? Was process consent used?

g. Does the report discuss steps that were taken to protect the privacy and confidentiality of study participants?

Questions for Discussion

a. Do you think the benefits of this research outweighed the costs to participants—what is the overall risk/benefit ratio?

b. Do you consider that the researcher took adequate steps to protect the study participants? If not, what else could they have done?

c. Comment on the fact that some of the interviews with the mothers were conducted in the presence of other family members.

PART 2

Preliminary Steps in Research

CHAPTER 6

Research Problems, Research Questions, and Hypotheses

A. FILL IN THE BLANKS

How many terms have you learned in this chapter? Fill in the blanks in the sentences below to find out. Try doing this section with a friend. Which of you is the first one to complete the sentence?

1. A research _____ is an enigmatic or troubling condition.

2. A(n) _____ in a quantitative study states the research aim and indicates the key study variables and the population of interest.

3. A research _____ is what researchers wish to answer through a systematic study.

4. A(n) _____ is the researcher's prediction about variables in the study.

5. Hypotheses predict a(n) _____ between the independent and dependent variables.

6. Hypotheses are typically put to a statistical _____.

7. An hypothesis stipulates the expected relationship between a(n) _____ variable and a dependent variable.

8. A research hypothesis in which the specific nature of the predicted relationship is not stipulated is a(n) _____ hypothesis.

9. The results of hypothesis testing never constitute _____ that a hypothesis is or is not correct.

10. Hypotheses typically involve at least _____ variables.

11. A(n) _____ hypothesis involves a single independent and a single dependent variable.

12. The *actual* hypothesis of an investigator is the _____ hypothesis.

13. The hypothesis that posits the absence of a relationship between variables is called a(n) _____ hypothesis.

Study Guide for Essentials of Nursing Research: Appraising Evidence for Nursing Practice, 8e

B. MATCHING EXERCISES

1. Match each sentence in Set B with one of the phrases listed in Set A. Indicate the letter corresponding to the appropriate response next to each entry in Set B.

SET A

a. Statement of purpose—qualitative study

b. Statement of purpose—quantitative study

c. Not a statement of purpose for a research study

SET B   **RESPONSES**

1. The purpose of this study is to test whether the removal of physical restraints results in behavioral changes in elderly patients.   _____

2. The purpose of this project is to facilitate the transition from hospital to home among women who have just given birth.   _____

3. The goal of this project is to explore the process by which an elderly person adjusts to placement in a nursing home.   _____

4. The investigation was designed to describe the prevalence of smoking, alcohol use, and drug use among urban preadolescents aged 10 to 12.   _____

5. The study's purpose was to describe the nature of touch used by parents in touching their preterm infants.   _____

6. The goal is to develop guidelines for spiritually related nursing interventions.   _____

7. The purpose of this project is to examine the relationship between social support and the use of over-the-counter medications among community-dwelling elders.   _____

8. The purpose is to develop an in-depth understanding of patients' feelings of powerlessness in hospital settings.   _____

2. Match each sentence in Set B with one of the phrases listed in Set A. Indicate the letter corresponding to the appropriate response next to each entry in Set B.

SET A

a. Research hypothesis—directional

b. Research hypothesis—nondirectional

c. Null hypothesis

d. Not a testable hypothesis as stated

SET B   **RESPONSES**

1. First-born infants have higher concentrations of estrogens and progesterone in umbilical cord blood than do later-born infants.   _____

2. There is no relationship between women's participation in prenatal classes and the health outcomes of their infants.   _____

3. Many nursing students are interested in obtaining advanced degrees. _____

4. Functional disability after a cardiac event is higher among patients with comorbidities than among those without comorbidities. _____

5. A person's age is related to his or her difficulty in accessing health care. _____

6. Glaucoma can be effectively screened by means of tonometry. _____

7. Increased noise levels result in increased anxiety among hospitalized patients. _____

8. Media exposure regarding the health hazards of smoking is unrelated to the public's smoking habits. _____

9. Patients' compliance with their medication regimens is related to their perceptions of the consequences of noncompliance. _____

10. Many patients delay seeking health care for symptoms of myocardial infarction because they are afraid. _____

11. Patients from hospitals in the United States and Canada differ with respect to their level of satisfaction with their nursing care. _____

12. A cancer patient's degree of hopefulness regarding the future is unrelated to his or her religiosity. _____

13. The degree of attachment between infants and their mothers is associated with the infant's status as low birthweight or normal birthweight. _____

14. The presence of homonymous hemianopia in stroke patients negatively affects their length of stay in hospital. _____

15. Adjustment to hemodialysis does not vary by the patient's gender. _____

C. STUDY QUESTIONS

1. Below is a list of general topics that could be investigated. Develop at least one research question for each, making sure that some are questions that could be addressed through qualitative research and others are ones that could be addressed through quantitative research. (HINT: For quantitative research questions, think of these concepts as potential independent or dependent variables, and then ask, "What might cause or affect this variable (outcome)?" and "What might be the consequences or effects of this variable on other outcomes?" This should lead to some ideas for research questions.)

   a. Patient comfort _____.
   b. Psychiatric patients' readmission rates _____.
   c. Anxiety in hospitalized children _____.
   d. Elevated blood pressure _____.
   e. Incidence of sexually transmitted infections (STIs) _____.
   f. Patient cooperativeness in the recovery room _____.
   g. Caregiver stress _____.
   h. Mother–infant bonding _____.
   i. Menstrual irregularities _____.

2. Below are five nondirectional hypotheses. Restate each one as a directional hypothesis. Your hypotheses do not need to be "right"—this exercise is designed to encourage familiarity with wording hypotheses.

NONDIRECTIONAL	DIRECTIONAL
a. Tactile stimulation is associated with comparable physiological arousal as verbal stimulation among infants with congenital heart disease.	a.
b. The risk of hypoglycemia in term newborns is related to the infant's birthweight.	b.
c. The use of isotonic sodium chloride solution before endotracheal suctioning is related to oxygen saturation.	c.
d. Fluid balance is related to degree of success in weaning older adults from mechanical ventilation.	d.
e. Nurses administer the same amount of narcotic analgesics to male and female patients.	e.

3. Below are five research hypotheses. Reword them as null hypotheses.

RESEARCH HYPOTHESIS	NULL HYPOTHESIS
a. First-time blood donors experience greater anxiety during the donation than donors who have given blood previously.	a.
b. Nurses who initiate more conversation with patients are rated as more effective in their nursing care by patients than those who initiate less conversation.	b.
c. Surgical patients who give high ratings to the informativeness of nursing communications experience less preoperative stress than do patients who give low ratings.	c.
d. Appendectomy patients who are pregnant are more likely to experience peritoneal infection than female appendectomy patients who are not pregnant.	d.
e. Women who give birth by cesarean delivery are more likely to experience postpartum depression than women who give birth vaginally.	e.

4. In study questions C.2 and C.3 above, 10 research hypotheses were provided. Identify the independent and dependent (outcome) variables in each.

INDEPENDENT VARIABLE(S)	DEPENDENT (OUTCOME) VARIABLE(S)
2a	
2b	
2c	
2d	
2e	
3a	
3b	
3c	
3d	
3e	

5. Below are five statements that are *not* testable research hypotheses as currently stated. Suggest modifications to these statements that would make them testable hypotheses.

ORIGINAL STATEMENT	HYPOTHESIS
a. Relaxation therapy is effective in reducing hypertension.	a.
b. The use of bilingual health care staff produces high utilization rates of health care facilities by ethnic minorities.	b.
c. Nursing students are affected in their choice of clinical specialization by interactions with nursing faculty.	c.
d. Sexually active teenagers have a high rate of using male methods of contraception.	d.
e. In-use intravenous solutions become contaminated within 48 hours.	e.

D. APPLICATION EXERCISES

Exercise D.1: Study in Appendix D

Read the abstract and introduction of the report by Jurgens and colleagues ("Why do elders delay responding") in Appendix D on pages 147–156 and then answer the following questions:

Questions of Fact

a. In which paragraph(s) of this article is the research problem stated? Summarize the problem in a sentence or two.

b. Did the researchers present a statement of purpose? If so, what *verb* did they use in the purpose statement, and is that verb consistent with the type of research that was undertaken?

c. Did the researchers specify a research question? If so, was it well stated? If not, indicate what the question was.

d. Did Jurgens and colleagues specify hypotheses? If there are hypotheses, were they appropriately worded? Are they directional or nondirectional? Simple or complex? Research or null?

e. If no hypotheses were stated, what would one be?

f. Were any hypotheses *tested*?

Questions for Discussion

a. Did the researchers do an adequate job of describing the research problem? Suggest ways in which the problem statement could be improved.

b. Comment on the significance of the study's research problem for nursing.

c. Did the researchers adequately explain the study purpose, research questions, and/or hypotheses?

Exercise D.2: Study in Appendix B

Read the abstract and introduction of the report by Cricco-Lizza ("Rooting for the breast") in Appendix B on pages 129–138 and then answer the following questions:

Questions of Fact

a. In which paragraph(s) of this article is the research problem stated? Summarize the problem in a sentence or two.

b. Did the researcher present a statement of purpose? If so, what *verb* did the researcher use in the purpose statement, and is that verb consistent with the type of research that was undertaken?

c. Did the researcher specify a research question? If so, was it well-stated? If not, indicate what the question was.

d. Did Cricco-Lizza specify hypotheses? If there are hypotheses, were they appropriately worded? Are they directional or nondirectional? Simple or complex? Research or null?

e. Were any hypotheses *tested*?

Questions for Discussion

a. Did the researcher do an adequate job of describing the research problem? Suggest ways in which the problem statement could be improved.

b. Comment on the significance of the study's research problem for nursing.

c. Did the researcher adequately explain the study purpose, research questions, and/or hypotheses?

Finding and Reviewing Research Evidence in the Literature

A. FILL IN THE BLANKS

How many terms have you learned in this chapter? Fill in the blanks in the sentences below to find out. Try doing this section with a friend. Which of you is the first one to complete the sentence?

1. A research journal article written by the researchers who conducted a study is a(n) _____ source for a research review.

2. Descriptions of studies prepared by someone other than the investigators are considered _____ sources.

3. A search strategy sometimes called "footnote chasing" is the _____ approach.

4. A major resource for finding research reports are _____ databases.

5. When doing an electronic database search, one often begins with one or more _____.

6. _____ is the most important bibliographic database for nurses.

7. _____ is a very important bibliographic database for health care professionals around the world.

8. Examples of _____ operators include "AND" and "OR."

9. The controlled vocabulary used to code entries in MEDLINE® is called _____.

10. The MEDLINE® database can be accessed for free through _____.

11. If a researcher has been prominent in an area, it is useful to do a(n) _____ search.

B. MATCHING EXERCISES

Match each statement in Set B with one of the types of literature review listed in Set A. Indicate the letter corresponding to the appropriate response next to each entry in Set B.

SET A

a. CINAHL

b. MEDLINE®

c. Neither CINAHL nor MEDLINE®

d. Both CINAHL and MEDLINE®

SET B   RESPONSES

1. An important bibliographic database for nurses   _____

2. Can be accessed on the Internet through PubMed   _____

3. Does not allow the use of wildcard characters   _____

4. Uses MeSH to index entries   _____

5. Focuses on nursing and allied health   _____

6. Does not provide abstracts, only citations   _____

7. Has over 21 million records   _____

8. The articles in the appendices to this *Study Guide* could
be retrieved in this database   _____

C. STUDY QUESTIONS

1. Below are several research questions. Indicate one or more keywords that you would use to begin a literature search on this topic.

RESEARCH QUESTIONS   KEY WORDS

a. What is the lived experience of being a survivor
of a fatal automobile crash?   _____

b. Does contingency contracting improve patient
compliance with a treatment regimen?   _____

c. What is the decision-making process for a woman
considering having an abortion?   _____

d. Do children raised on vegetarian diets have different
growth patterns than other children?   _____

e. Is a special intervention for spinal cord injury patients
effective in reducing the risk of pressure ulcers?   _____

f. What is the course of appetite loss among cancer
patients undergoing chemotherapy?   _____

g. What is the effect of alcohol skin preparation before insulin
injection on the incidence of local and systemic infection?   _____

h. Are bottle-fed babies introduced to solid foods sooner
than breastfed babies?   _____

2. Below are fictitious excerpts from research literature reviews. Each excerpt has a stylistic problem. Change each sentence to make it acceptable stylistically, inventing citations if necessary.

ORIGINAL	**REVISED**
a. Most elderly people do not eat a balanced diet.	_____
b. Patient characteristics have a significant impact on nursing workload.	_____
c. A child's conception of appropriate sick role behavior changes as the child grows older.	_____
d. Home birth poses many potential dangers.	_____
e. Multiple sclerosis results in considerable anxiety to the family of the patients.	_____
f. Studies have proved that most nurses prefer not to work the night shift.	_____
g. Life changes are the major cause of stress in adults.	_____
h. Stroke rehabilitation programs are most effective when they involve the patients' families.	_____
i. It has been proved that psychiatric outpatients have higher-than-average rates of accidental deaths and suicides.	_____
j. The traditional pelvic examination is sufficiently unpleasant to many women that they avoid having the examination.	_____

3. Read the following research report, McDougall, G., Mackert, M., & Becker, H. (2012). Memory performance, health literacy, and instrument activities of daily living of community residing older adults. *Nursing Research*, *61*(1), 70–75 (or read another article of your choosing).

Use the brief protocol in Figure 7.4 on page 124 in the textbook and note as much information as you can about the report.

4. Read the literature review section from a research article appearing in a nursing journal in the early 2000s (some possibilities are suggested below). Search the literature for more recent research on the topic of the article and update the original researchers' review section. If possible, use the descendancy approach as one of your search strategies. (Don't forget to incorporate in your review the findings from the cited research article itself.) Here are some possible articles:

- Allen Furr, L., Binkley, C., McCurren, C., & Carrico, R. (2004). Factors affecting quality of oral care in intensive care units. *Journal of Advanced Nursing*, *48*, 454–462.
- Lindseth, G., & Bird-Baker, M. (2004). Risk factors for cholelithiasis in pregnancy. *Research in Nursing & Health*, *27*, 382–391.
- Redeker, N., Ruggiero, J., & Hedges, C. (2004). Sleep is related to physical function and emotional well-being after cardiac surgery. *Nursing Research*, *53*, 154–162.
- Winterbottom, A., & Harcourt, D. (2004). Patients' experience of the diagnosis and treatment of skin cancer. *Journal of Advanced Nursing*, *48*, 226–233.

D. APPLICATION EXERCISES

Exercise D.1: Study in Appendix G

Read the abstract, introduction, and the first subsection under "Methods" of the report by Nam and colleagues ("Effect of culturally tailored diabetes education") in Appendix G on pages 183–196 and then answer the following questions:

Questions of Fact

a. What type of research review did the investigators undertake?

b. Did the researchers begin with a problem statement? Summarize the problem in two or three sentences.

c. Did the researchers provide a statement of purpose? If so, what was it?

d. Which bibliographic databases did the researchers search?

e. What keywords were used in the search? Were the keywords related to the independent or dependent variable of interest?

f. Did the researchers restrict their search to English-language reports?

g. Did the researchers restrict their search to published studies?

h. How many studies ultimately were included in the review?

i. Were the studies included in the review qualitative, quantitative, or both?

Questions for Discussion

a. Did the researchers do an adequate job of explaining the problem and their purpose in undertaking the review?

b. Did the researchers appear to do a thorough job in their search for relevant studies?

c. Certain studies that were initially retrieved were eliminated. Do you think the researchers provided a sound rationale for their decisions?

Exercise D.2: Study in Appendix H

Read the following abstract, introduction, and Study Design and Methods sections of the report by Beck ("A metaethnography of traumatic childbirth") in Appendix H on pages 197–208 and then answer the following questions:

Questions of Fact

a. What type of research review did Beck undertake?

b. What was the purpose of this metasynthesis?

c. Did Beck's review involve a systematic search for evidence in bibliographic databases?

d. How many studies were included in the metasynthesis?

e. Which qualitative research traditions were represented in the review?

Questions for Discussion

a. Did Beck do an adequate job of explaining the problem and the study purpose?

b. Should Beck have searched for and included other qualitative studies on birth trauma? If yes, what would have been her keywords?

Theoretical and Conceptual Frameworks

A. FILL IN THE BLANKS

How many terms have you learned in this chapter? Fill in the blanks in the sentences below to find out. Try doing this section with a friend. Which of you is the first one to complete the sentence?

1. The conceptual underpinnings of a study are known as its _____.

2. Abstractions assembled because of their relevance to a core theme form a(n) _____ model.

3. Another term for a schematic model is a conceptual _____.

4. A schematic _____ is a mechanism for representing concepts with a minimal use of words.

5. A(n) _____ theory thoroughly accounts for or describes a phenomenon.

6. A theory that focuses on a specific aspect of human experience is sometimes called _____.

7. The four elements in conceptual models of nursing are _____, _____, _____, and _____.

8. The originator of the Health Promotion Model is Nola _____.

9. _____ is the originator of the Theory of Human Becoming.

10. _____ is the originator of the Science of Unitary Human Beings.

11. Roy conceptualized the _____ Model of nursing.

12. A construct that was fully conceptualized by Bandura, and that is a key mediator in many models of health behavior, is _____.

B. MATCHING EXERCISES

1. Match each statement from Set B with one of the phrases in Set A. Indicate the letter corresponding to your response next to each of the statements in Set B.

SET A

a. Classic theory

b. Conceptual model

c. Schematic model

d. Neither a, b, nor c

e. a, b, *and* c

SET B   RESPONSES

1. Makes minimal use of language   _____

2. Uses concepts as building blocks   _____

3. Is the backbone of evidence-based nursing   _____

4. Can be used as a basis for generating hypotheses   _____

5. Can be proved through empirical testing   _____

6. Incorporates a system of propositions that assert relationships
   among variables   _____

7. Consists of interrelated concepts organized in a rational scheme
   but does not specify formal relationships among the concepts   _____

8. Exists in nature and is awaiting scientific discovery   _____

2. Match each model from Set B with one of the theorists in Set A. Indicate the letter corresponding to your response next to each of the statements in Set B.

SET A

a. Bandura

b. Pender

c. Roy

d. Proshaska

e. Rogers

f. Lazarus-Folkman

g. Mishel

h. Azjen

SET B   RESPONSES

1. Adaptation Model   _____

2. Transtheoretical Model   _____

3. Uncertainty in Illness Theory   _____

4. Social Cognitive Theory _____

5. Theory of Stress and Coping _____

6. Health Promotion Model _____

7. Theory of Planned Behavior _____

8. Science of Unitary Human Beings _____

C. STUDY QUESTIONS

1. Read some recent issues of a nursing research journal. Identify at least three different theories cited by nurse researchers in these research reports.

2. Select one of the research questions/problems listed below. Could the selected problem be developed within one of the models or theories discussed in this chapter? Defend your answer.

   a. How do men cope with a diagnosis of prostate cancer?

   b. What are the factors contributing to perceptions of fatigue among patients with congestive heart failure?

   c. What effect does the presence of the father in the delivery room have on the mother's satisfaction with the childbirth experience?

   d. The purpose of the study is to explore why some women fail to perform breast self-examination regularly.

   e. What are the factors that lead to poorer health among low-income children than higher-income children?

3. Suggest an important health outcome that could be studied using the Health Promotion Model. Identify another theory described in this chapter that could be used to explain or predict the same outcome. Which theory or model do you think would do a better job? Why?

4. Read the following article, Su, S. F., et al. (2011). Nurses' perceptions of leadership style in hospitals: A grounded theory study. *Journal of Clinical Nursing*, *21*, 272–280, and then assess the following:

   a. What evidence do the researchers offer to substantiate that their grounded theory is a good fit with her data?

   b. To what extent is it clear or unclear in the article that symbolic interaction-ism (or some other theoretical perspective) was the theoretical underpin-ning of the study?

D. APPLICATION EXERCISES

Exercise D.1: Study in Appendix D

Read the introduction and methods section of the report by Jurgens and colleagues ("Why do elders delay responding") in Appendix D on pages 147–156 and then answer the following questions:

Questions of Fact

a. Does the study by Jurgens and colleagues involve a conceptual or theoretical framework? What is it called?

b. Is this framework one of the models of nursing cited in the textbook? Is it related to one of those models?

c. Does the report include a schematic model?

d. What are the key concepts in the model?

e. According to the framework, what factors *directly* affect the decision to seek care?

f. According to the framework, what factors *indirectly* affect the decision to seek care?

g. Did the report present conceptual definitions of key concepts?

h. Did the report explicitly present hypotheses deduced from the framework?

Questions for Discussion

a. Does the link between the problem and the framework seem contrived? Do the hypotheses (if any) naturally flow from the framework?

b. Do you think any aspects of the research would have been different without the framework?

c. Could the study have been undertaken using Pender's Health Promotion Model as its framework (see Figure 8.1 on page 134 in the textbook)? Why or why not?

d. Would you describe this study as a model-testing inquiry or do you think the model was used more as an organizing framework?

Exercise D.2: Study in Appendix E

Read the report by Byrne and colleagues ("Care transition experiences") in Appendix E on pages 157–174 and then answer the following questions:

Questions of Fact

a. Did this article describe a conceptual or theoretical framework for the study? What is it called?

b. Did the study result in the generation of a theory? What was it called?

c. Did the report include a schematic model? If so, what are the key concepts in the framework?

d. Did the report explicitly present hypotheses deduced from the framework? Did they undertake hypothesis-testing statistical analyses?

Questions for Discussion

a. What framework might be appropriate for this study?

b. Do you think any aspects of the research would have been different with an explicit theoretical framework?

Quantitative Research

Quantitative Research Design

A. FILL IN THE BLANKS

How many terms have you learned in this chapter? Fill in the blanks in the sentences below to find out. Try doing this section with a friend. Which of you is the first one to complete the sentence?

1. Good research design in quantitative studies involves achieving four types of _____.

2. A(n) _____ design refers to a study design in which the same participants are exposed to two or more conditions, in random order.

3. The loss of subjects from a study over time is called _____.

4. A key threat to internal validity stemming from preexisting group differences is the _____ threat.

5. The allocation of participants to groups by chance is called _____ assignment.

6. Researchers use the strategy of _____ to guard against expectation biases.

7. Techniques of research _____ include randomization, homogeneity, and matching.

8. _____ is a threat to internal validity stemming from differential loss of participants from groups.

9. In a(n) _____ design, data about causes are collected before data about effects.

10. Demonstrating the existence of a relationship between an independent variable and an outcome contributes to _____ conclusion validity.

11. The degree to which it can be inferred that the independent variable caused the outcome variable is _____ validity.

12. The type of validity referring to the generalizability of results is _____ validity.

13. Data are collected at a single point in time in a _____ study.

14. A(n) _____ represents what would have happened to the same people simultaneously exposed and not exposed to a hypothesized causal factor.

49

15. A(n) _____ study is a nonexperimental study involving the comparison of *cases* and matched counterparts.

16. A(n) _____ study is designed to collect data over an extended period of time.

17. _____ involves the deliberate pairing of participants in different groups as a method of controlling confounding variables.

18. Statistical _____ refers to the ability of the design to detect true relationships among variables.

19. A(n) _____ is an internal validity problem that concerns the effect of other things co-occurring with the independent variable.

20. In a delayed treatment design, control group members are _____ for the intervention.

21. In an intervention study, data collected before implementing the intervention are often called _____ data.

22. Intervention studies in which there is no randomization to treatment conditions are called _____.

23. Correlational studies examine _____ between variables but involve no intervention.

24. In _____ studies, researchers search for antecedent causes of an effect occurring in the present.

B. MATCHING EXERCISES

Match each research question from Set B with one (or more) of the phrases from Set A that indicates a potential reason for using a nonexperimental design. Indicate the letter(s) corresponding to your response next to each statement in Set B.

SET A

a. Independent variable cannot be manipulated

b. Possible ethical constraints on manipulation

c. Practical constraints on manipulation

d. No constraints on manipulation

SET B   RESPONSES

1. Does the use of certain tampons cause toxic shock syndrome? _____

2. Does heroin addiction among mothers affect Apgar scores of infants? _____

3. Is the age of a hemodialysis patient related to the incidence of the disequilibrium syndrome? _____

4. What body positions aid respiratory function? _____

5. Does the ingestion of saccharin cause cancer in humans? _____

6. Does a nurse's attitude toward the elderly affect his or her choice of a clinical specialty? _____

7. Does the use of touch by nursing staff affect patient morale?   _____

8. Does a nurse's gender affect his or her salary and rate of promotion?   _____

9. Does extreme athletic exertion in young women cause amenorrhea?   _____

10. Does assertiveness training affect a psychiatric nurse's job performance?   _____

C. STUDY QUESTIONS

1. Suppose you wanted to study self-efficacy among successful dieters who lost 20 or more pounds and maintained their weight loss for at least 6 months. Specify at least two different types of comparison strategies that might provide a useful comparative context for this study. Do your strategies lend themselves to experimental manipulation? If not, why not?

2. Refer to the 10 hypotheses in Chapter 6 Exercises C.2 and C.3 on page 36. Indicate below whether these hypotheses could be tested using an experimental/quasi-experimental approach, a nonexperimental approach, or both.

Question No	Experimental/ Quasi-Experimental	Nonexperimental	Both
2a			
2b			
2c			
2d			
2e			
3a			
3b			
3c			
3d			
3e			

3. In the following study, Yeh, M., Chung, Y., Chen, K., & Chen, H. (2011). Pain reduction of acupoint electrical stimulation for patients with spinal surgery. *International Journal of Nursing Studies, 48,* 703–709, the researchers used two comparison groups.

   a. Review the design for this study, and comment on the appropriateness of having three groups.

   b. What biases were the researchers trying to avoid? Do you think they were successful?

4. Suppose that you were studying the effects of range-of-motion exercises on radical mastectomy patients. You start your experiment with 50 experimental subjects and 50 control subjects. Your intervention requires the experimental subjects to come for daily sessions over a 2-week period, while control subjects

come only once at the end of 2 weeks. Your final group sizes are 40 for the experimental group and 49 for the control group. The results of your study indicate that women in the experimental group did better in raising the arm of the affected side above head level. What effects, if any, do you think the attrition might have on the internal validity of your study?

5. Suppose that you were interested in testing the hypothesis that regular ingestion of aspirin reduced the risk of colon cancer. Describe how such a hypothesis could be tested using a retrospective case–control design. Now describe a prospective cohort design for the same study. Compare the strengths and weaknesses of the two approaches.

D. APPLICATION EXERCISES

Exercise D.1: Study in Appendix A

Read the Methods section of the report by Weinert and colleagues ("Computer intervention impact") in Appendix A on pages 119–128 and then answer the following questions:

Questions of Fact

a. Was there an intervention in this study?

b. Is the design for this study experimental, quasi-experimental, or nonexperimental?

c. What were the independent and dependent variables?

d. Was randomization used? If yes, what method was used to assign participants to groups?

e. In terms of the control group strategies described in the textbook, what approach did the researchers use?

f. What is the specific name of the research design used in this study?

g. Was any blinding used in this study?

h. Would this study be described as longitudinal?

i. Which of the methods of research control described in this chapter were used to control confounding variables?

j. Which confounding variables were controlled?

k. Was there any attrition in this study?

l. Is there evidence that constancy of conditions was achieved?

m. Were group treatments as distinct as possible to maximize power? If not, why not?

Questions for Discussion

a. What was the intervention? Comment on how well the intervention was described, including a description of how it was developed and refined.

b. Comment on the researchers' control group strategy. Could a more powerful or effective strategy have been used?

c. Discuss ways in which this study achieved or failed to achieve the criteria for making causal inferences.

d. Comment on the researchers' use or nonuse of blinding.

e. Comment on the timing of postintervention data collection

f. Is this study *cause-probing?* Is this study strong in internal validity? What, if any, are the threats to the internal validity of this study?

g. Is this study strong on external validity? What, if any, are the threats to the external validity of this study?

Exercise D.2: Study in Appendix D

Read the Methods section of the report by Jurgens and colleagues ("Why do elders delay responding") in Appendix D on pages 147–156 and then answer the following questions:

Questions of Fact

a. Was there an intervention in this study?

b. Is the design for this study experimental, quasi-experimental or nonexperimental?

c. What were the independent and dependent variables in this study?

d. Was the independent variable amenable to manipulation?

e. What is the name of the research design used in this study?

f. Was randomization used to control confounding variables in this study? Was matching used? Was homogeneity used?

g. Was any blinding used in this study?

h. Would this study be described as longitudinal or cross-sectional?

i. In terms of the EBP-type questions described in Chapters 1 and 2, what type of question did these researchers ask?

Questions for Discussion

a. Could this study be described as cause-probing? Discuss ways in which this study achieved or failed to achieve the criteria for making causal inferences.

b. Comment on the timing of data collection.

c. Is this study strong in internal validity? What, if any, are the threats to the internal validity of this study?

d. Is this study strong on external validity? What, if any, are the threats to the external validity of this study?

Sampling and Data Collection in Quantitative Studies

A. FILL IN THE BLANKS

How many terms have you learned in this chapter? Fill in the blanks in the sentences below to find out. Try doing this section with a friend. Which of you is the first one to complete the sentence?

1. _____ sampling involves recruiting *every* eligible person over a specified period of time.
2. Specifications for a population are identified in the _____ criteria.
3. The total number of participants in a study is known as the study's sample _____.
4. An aggregate set of people/objects with specified characteristics is a(n) _____.
5. Subdivisions of a population are called _____.
6. _____ sampling involves sampling by convenience within specified subgroups of the population, to enhance representativeness.
7. The _____ population is the group to which the researcher wants to generalize.
8. The broad class of sampling in which every element of a population has an equal chance of being selected is _____ sampling.
9. In quantitative studies, the key criterion for evaluating a sample is its _____ of the population.
10. _____ sampling is the most widely used type of sampling in quantitative research.
11. Probability sampling involves the selection of sample members at _____.
12. Sampling _____ is the systematic overrepresentation or underrepresentation of some segment of the population.
13. In _____ sampling, the researcher samples every k^{th} case, with the interval established by dividing the population size by the desired sample size.
14. In quantitative studies, researchers use _____ _____ to estimate how large a sample they need.

54

15. The most widely used method of data collection by nurse researchers is _____.

16. The type of questions prevalent in mailed questionnaires are _____ questions.

17. The question, "What is it like to be a cancer survivor?" is a(n) _____ question.

18. A composite _____ yields a score that places people on a continuum with regard to an attribute.

19. The type of self-report strategy that typically yields better quality data than self-administered questionnaires is called a(n) _____.

20. A(n) _____ scale is a summated rating scale used to measure agreement or disagreement with statements.

21. A scaling procedure to measure clinical symptoms is a(n) _____ analog scale.

22. The tendency to distort self-report information in characteristic ways is called a response _____ bias.

23. A bias stemming from people wanting to "look good" is called a(n) _____ desirability bias.

24. Methods of collecting data by watching behaviors and events are referred to as _____ methods.

25. In a structured observation, a(n) _____ is used with a category system to record frequencies of observed events or behaviors.

26. _____ sampling in observational studies is used to select periods when observations are made, either systematically or randomly.

B. MATCHING EXERCISES

1. Match each statement relating to sampling for quantitative studies from Set B with one of the phrases from Set A. Indicate the letter corresponding to your response next to each of the statements in Set B.

SET A

a. Probability sampling

b. Nonprobability sampling

c. Both probability and nonprobability sampling

d. Neither probability nor nonprobability sampling

SET B   RESPONSES

1. Includes systematic sampling   _____

2. Allows an estimation of the magnitude of sampling error   _____

3. Guarantees a representative sample   _____

4. Includes quota sampling   _____

5. Requires a sample size of at least 100 subjects _____
6. Elements are selected by nonrandom methods _____
7. Can be used with entire populations or with selected strata from the populations _____
8. Used to select populations _____
9. Elements have an equal chance of being selected _____
10. Is most widely used by nurse researchers _____

2. Match each descriptive statement regarding data collection methods from Set B with one (or more) of the statements from Set A. Indicate the letter(s) corresponding to your response next to each item in Set B.

SET A

a. Self-reports
b. Observations
c. Biophysiologic measures
d. None of the above

SET B   RESPONSES

1. Cannot easily be gathered unobtrusively _____
2. Can be biased by the participants' desire to "look good" _____
3. Can be used to gather data from infants _____
4. Is a good way to obtain information about human <u>behavior</u> _____
5. Can be biased by the researcher's values and beliefs _____
6. Can be combined with other data collection methods in a single study _____
7. Can yield quantitative information _____
8. Benefits from pretesting _____

3. Match each descriptive statement regarding self-report methods from Set B with one of the statements from Set A. Indicate the letter corresponding to your response next to each item in Set B.

SET A

a. Interviews
b. Questionnaires
c. Both interviews and questionnaires
d. Neither interviews nor questionnaires

SET B   RESPONSES

1. Can provide participants the protection of anonymity _____
2. Can be used with illiterate participants _____

3. Can contain both open- and closed-ended questions   _____

4. Is the best way to measure human behavior   _____

5. Generally yields high response rates   _____

6. Is generally an inexpensive method of data collection   _____

7. Can be used in descriptive studies   _____

8. Can be distributed by mail   _____

C. STUDY QUESTIONS

1. Identify the type of quantitative sampling design used in the following examples:

   a. A sample of 250 members randomly selected from a roster of American Nurses Association members

   b. All the oncology nurses participating in a continuing education seminar

   c. Every 20th patient admitted to the emergency room between January and June

   d. Twenty male and twenty female patients admitted to the hospital with hypothermia

   e. Twenty-five internationally renowned experts in critical care nursing

   f. All patients receiving hospice services from Capital District Hospice in 2013.

2. Suppose you have decided to use systematic sampling for a study. The known population size is 5,000, and the sample size desired is 250. What is the sampling interval? If the first element selected is 23, what would be the second, third, and fourth elements selected?

3. Suppose you were interested in studying the attitude of nurse practitioners toward autonomy in work situations. Suggest a possible target and accessible population. What strata might be useful if quota sampling were used?

4. Below are several research questions. Indicate what methods of data collection (self-report, observation, biophysiologic measures, records) you might recommend using for each. Defend your response.

   a. What are the predictors of intravenous site symptoms?

   b. What are the health and mental health consequences of a sedentary lifestyle among community-dwelling elders?

   c. To what extent and in what manner do nurses interact differently with male and female patients?

   d. What are the effects of a HIV-prevention intervention on the risk-taking behavior of urban adolescents?

5. Identify five constructs of clinical relevance that would be appropriate for measurement using a visual analog scale (VAS).

6. Below are several research questions in which the dependent variable is amenable to observation. For each question, specify whether you think a time sampling or event sampling approach would be preferable. Justify your response.

   a. What is the effect of touch on the crying behavior of hospitalized children?

   b. What is the effect of increased patient/staff ratios in psychiatric hospitals on interpersonal conflict among patients?

   c. Are the self-grooming activities of nursing home patients related to the frequency of visits from friends and relatives?

   d. What types of patient behavior are most likely to elicit empathic behaviors in nurses?

   e. Do nurses reinforce passive behaviors among female patients more than among male patients?

D. APPLICATION EXERCISES

Exercise D.1: Quantitative Appendix Studies

Which of the studies in Appendices A (by Weinert et al.) on pages 119–128, C (by Yackel et al.) on pages 139–146, and D (by Jurgens et al.) on pages 147–156 used the following sampling methods?

a. Probability sampling

b. Convenience sampling

c. Consecutive sampling

Exercise D.2: Quantitative Appendix Studies

Which of the studies in Appendices A (by Weinert et al.) on pages 119–128, C (by Yackel et al.) on pages 139–146, and D (by Jurgens et al.) on pages 147–156 used the following data collection methods?

a. Self-reports

b. Observational methods

c. Biophysiologic measures

d. Records

Exercise D.3: Study in Appendix D

Read the Methods and first part of the Results sections of the report by Jurgens and colleagues ("Why do elders delay responding") in Appendix D on pages 147–156 and then answer the following questions:

Questions of Fact

a. What was the target population of this study? How would you describe the accessible population?

b. What were the eligibility criteria for the study?

c. Was the sampling method probability or nonprobability? What specific sampling method was used?

d. How were study participants recruited?

e. What was the response rate in this study?

f. What was the sample size that Jurgens and colleagues achieved? How long did it take them to enroll their sample?

g. Was a power analysis used to determine sample size needs? If yes, what number of subjects did the power analysis estimate as the minimum needed number?

h. Were sample characteristics described? If yes, what were those characteristics?

i. Did the researchers develop their own measures, or did they use instruments or scales that had been developed by others?

j. Who gathered the data in this study? How were the data collectors trained?

Questions for Discussion

a. Comment on the adequacy of the researchers' sampling plan and recruitment strategy. What types of sampling biases might be of special concern?

b. Comment on efforts the researchers made (or did not make) to ensure a diverse sample of study participants.

c. Could the researchers have used quota sampling in this study? If so, what stratifying variables do you think they should have used?

d. Assume that you had no resource constraints to conduct this study. What sampling plan would you recommend?

e. Do you think the sample size in this study was adequate? Why or why not?

f. How representative do you think the sample in this study was of the target population? Comment on issues relating to the generalizability of the results.

g. Comment on the adequacy of the data collection approaches used in this study. Did Jurgens and her colleagues operationalize their outcome measures in the best possible manner?

h. Comment on factors that could have biased the data in this study.

Measurement and Data Quality

A. FILL IN THE BLANKS

How many terms have you learned in this chapter? Fill in the blanks in the sentences below to find out. Try doing this section with a friend. Which of you is the first one to complete the sentence?

1. The _____ level of measurement rank orders phenomena but provides no information about distance between values.

2. A(n) _____ -level measurement has a rational zero point.

3. The lowest level of measurement is _____ measurement, which places objects into mutually exclusive categories.

4. Psychological scales yield _____ -level measures

5. Measurement involves assigning numbers according to established _____.

6. The most widely evaluated aspect of reliability is an instrument's _____ consistency.

7. A thorough evaluation of an instrument's quality is called a(n) _____ assessment.

8. The difference between an obtained score and the true score is the _____ of measurement.

9. A(n) _____ score is the score on a measure that would be obtained if the measure were infallible.

10. _____ is the degree of consistency or accuracy of a measure.

11. The method used to assess an instrument's stability is _____ reliability.

12. Inter _____ reliability assesses degree of equivalence of codings or ratings.

13. A scale's internal consistency is usually measured through an index called coefficient _____.

14. _____ is the extent to which an instrument actually is measuring what it purports to measure.

15. _____ validity is the type of validity concerned with adequate representation of all aspects of a concept.

60

16. Predictive validity and concurrent validity are aspects of _____ -related validity.

17. One means of assessing construct validity is through the known- _____ technique.

18. An instrument's ability to identify a case correctly is its _____.

19. The _____ of a screening or diagnostic instrument is the extent to which it is able to identify noncases accurately.

20. In evaluating screening instruments, "cases" are separated from "noncases" at a _____ point on a continuous scale.

B. MATCHING EXERCISES

1. Match each variable in Set B with the level of measurement from Set A that captures the highest possible level for that variable. Indicate the letter corresponding to your response next to each variable in Set B.

SET A

a. Nominal scale

b. Ordinal scale

c. Interval scale

d. Ratio scale

SET B   RESPONSES

1. Hours spent in labor before childbirth   _____

2. Religious affiliation   _____

3. Time for first postoperative voiding   _____

4. Responses to a single Likert scale item   _____

5. Temperature on the centigrade scale   _____

6. Nursing specialty area   _____

7. Status on the following scale: in poor health; in fair health; in good health; in excellent health   _____

8. Pulse rate   _____

9. Score on a 25-item Likert scale   _____

10. Highest college degree attained (bachelor's, master's, doctorate)   _____

11. Apgar scores   _____

12. Membership in the American Nurses Association   _____

2. Match each statement from Set B with one of the phrases from Set A. Indicate the letter corresponding to your response next to each of the statements in Set B.

SET A

a. Reliability

b. Validity

c. Both reliability and validity

d. Neither reliability nor validity

SET B   **RESPONSES**

1. Is concerned with the accuracy of measures   _____

2. The measures must be high on this for the results of a study
   to be valid   _____

3. If a measure possesses this, then study findings are necessarily
   sound   _____

4. Can often be estimated by procedures that yield a quantified
   coefficient   _____

5. An aspect can be assessed by evaluating the relevance of each
   component (the items) of the measure   _____

6. Is concerned with whether the researcher has adequately
   conceptualized the variables under investigation   _____

7. Coefficient alpha is one index for this   _____

8. Psychometric assessments evaluate this   _____

C. STUDY QUESTIONS

1. The reliability of measures of which of the following attributes would *not* be appropriately assessed using a test–retest procedure with 1 month between administrations. Why?

   a. Attitudes toward abortion

   b. Stress

   c. Achievement motivation

   d. Nursing effectiveness

   e. Depression

2. In the following situation, what might be some of the sources of measurement error?

> One hundred nurses who worked in a large metropolitan hospital were asked to complete a 10-item Likert scale designed to measure job satisfaction. The questionnaires were distributed by nursing supervisors at the end of shifts. The staff nurses were asked to complete the forms and return them immediately to their supervisors.

3. Identify what is incorrect about the following statements:

   a. "My scale is highly reliable, so it must be valid."

   b. "My instrument yielded an internal consistency coefficient of .80, so it must be stable."

   c. "The validity coefficient between my scale and a criterion measure was .40; therefore, my scale must be of low validity."

   d. "My scale had a reliability coefficient of .80. Therefore, an obtained score of 20 is indicative of a true score of 16."

   e. "The validation study proved that my scale has construct validity."

   f. "My advisor examined my new scale of dependence in nursing home residents and, based on its content, assured me it was valid."

4. In the following situations, for which instrument or situation would reliability be expected to be higher, all else equal? Why?

   a. An 8-item scale measuring self-efficacy or a 15-item scale of self-efficacy?

   b. A stress scale administered to patients just diagnosed with cancer, or the same stress scale administered to patients just diagnosed with hyperthyroidism?

   c. A test of nursing knowledge administered to freshmen nursing students or senior nursing students?

D. APPLICATION EXERCISES

Exercise D.1: Studies in Appendices A and D

In the studies in Appendices A (Weinert et al.) on pages 119–128 and D (Jurgens et al.) on pages 147–156, identify which variables (sample description variables, independent variables, or outcome variables) were measured on the nominal scale, ordinal scale, interval scale, or ratio scale.

Exercise D.2: Study in Appendix A

Read the Method section of the report by Weinert and colleagues ("Chronically ill rural women") in Appendix A on pages 119–128. Pay special attention to the subsections labeled "Measures" and then answer the following questions:

Questions of Fact

a. For the following instruments (which measured the key outcome variables), did the researchers select measures with previously documented good reliability? Also, describe what methods (if any) were reported as having been used by the researchers themselves to assess the reliability of the following instruments, and indicate what the reliability coefficients were in each case:

   • The Personal Resource Questionnaire (PRQ2000)
   • Rosenberg Self-Esteem Scale
   • Acceptance of Illness Scale

- Perceived Stress Scale
- CES-D Depression Scale
- UCLA Loneliness Scale

b. What type of validity assessment (if any) were reported as having been made to assess the validity of the same six instruments?

c. Did Weinert and colleagues rely on assessments of quality from other researchers, or did they perform any data quality assessments themselves?

d. Was information about the specificity or sensitivity of any of the instruments provided in the report?

Questions for Discussion

a. Describe what some of the sources of measurement error might have been in this study. Did the researchers take adequate steps to minimize measurement error?

b. Comment on the adequacy of information in the report about efforts to select or develop high quality instruments.

c. Comment on the quality of the measures that Weinert and colleagues used in their study. Do you feel confident that instruments yielded adequately reliable and valid indicators of the key constructs?

CHAPTER 12

Statistical Analysis of Quantitative Data

A. FILL IN THE BLANKS

How many terms have you learned in this chapter? Fill in the blanks in the sentences below to find out. Try doing this section with a friend. Which of you is the first one to complete the sentence?

1. _____ statistics is the broad class of statistics used to draw conclusions about a population.

2. Distributions with a tail pointing to the left have a(n) _____ skew; those with a tail pointing to the right have a(n) _____ skew.

3. Distributions with a single high point are _____; those with two high points are _____.

4. A bell-shaped curve is a popular name for a(n) _____ distribution.

5. A distribution without a skew is a(n) _____ distribution.

6. The most stable, and most frequently used, index of central tendency is known as the _____.

7. An index of central tendency that indicates the most "popular" value in a distribution is called _____.

8. The range and SD are two indexes for describing a distribution's _____.

9. The most common index of variability is the _____ deviation.

10. An index indicating the highest score value minus the lowest score value in a distribution is called the_____.

11. The distributions for two nominal-level variables can be displayed in a _____ table.

12. _____ is a widely used risk index that summarizes the ratio of two probabilities—the likelihood of occurrence versus nonoccurrence.

13. The standard deviation in a sampling distribution of means is called the _____.

14. _____ is the criterion used to establish the risk of a Type I error.

15. The class of inferential statistics without rigorous assumptions about distributional properties of variables are _____.

65

16. A _____ error involves the incorrect rejection of a true null hypothesis.

17. _____ error is the error committed when a false null hypothesis is accepted.

18. The risk of making a Type II error is called _____; one minus this risk value is the _____ of the statistical test.

19. The statistic r = .85 indicates a strong, _____ relationship between two variables.

20. The symbol used to designate total sample size is _____.

21. The _____ of significance is the researcher's risk of making a Type I error.

22. The statistical test used to compare two group means is the _____.

23. Researchers establish a(n) _____ interval around a statistic to indicate the range within which a population parameter probably lies (indicates the precision of the estimate).

24. The statistical test used to compare means of three or more group means is _____.

25. A(n) _____ size index summarizes the magnitude of an impact of the independent variable on the outcome variable.

26. The direction and magnitude of relationships between two variables are summarized in _____ coefficients.

27. A Type II error can occur when the analysis has insufficient _____, usually reflecting too small a sample.

28. The index designating a correlation coefficient is called _____.

29. The _____ test is used to test hypotheses about differences in proportions.

30. Multiple _____ analysis could be used to predict body weight based on data about height, gender, and caloric intake of people.

31. ANCOVA is an acronym for _____.

32. An effect size indicator that captures the magnitude of difference between two group means is known as _____.

33. _____ regression is a type of regression used to predict a nominal-level dependent variable from multiple predictors.

B. MATCHING EXERCISES

Match each statement or phrase from Set B with one of the phrases from Set A. Indicate the letter corresponding to your response next to each of the statements in Set B.

SET A

a. Index(es) of central tendency

b. Index(es) of variability

c. Index(es) of neither central tendency nor variability

d. Index(es) of both central tendency and variability

SET B   **RESPONSES**

1. The range   _____
2. In lay terms, an average   _____
3. A percentage   _____
4. Descriptor(s) of a distribution of scores   _____
5. Descriptor(s) of how heterogeneous a set of values is _____
6. The standard deviation   _____
7. The mode   _____
8. The median   _____
9. A normal distribution   _____
10. The mean   _____

C. STUDY QUESTIONS

1. Prepare a frequency distribution and frequency polygon for the set of scores below, which represent the ages of 30 women receiving a mammogram:

   47 50 51 50 48 51 50 51 49 51

   54 49 49 53 51 52 51 52 50 53

   49 51 52 51 50 55 48 54 53 52

Describe the resulting distribution in terms of its symmetry and modality (i.e., whether it is unimodal or multimodal).

2. Calculate the mean, median, and mode for the following pulse rates:

   78 84 69 98 102 72 87 75 79 84 88 84 83 71 73

   Mean:_____   Median:_____   Mode:_____

3. Suppose a researcher has conducted a study concerning lactose intolerance in children. The data reveal that 12 boys and 16 girls have lactose intolerance, out of a sample of 60 children of each gender. Construct a contingency table and calculate the column percentages for each cell in the table, with gender listed in the columns (similar to Table 12.10 on page 235 in the textbook). Discuss the meaning of these statistics.

4. Suppose that 400 subjects (200 per group) were in the intervention study described in connection with Table 12.7 on page 224 in the textbook, and that 60% of those in the experimental group and 90% of those in the control group continued smoking. Compute the absolute risk reduction (ARR) and the odds ratio in this scenario.

5. A group of nurse researchers measured the amount of time (in minutes per week) spent in recreational activities by a sample of 200 hospitalized paraplegic patients. They compared male and female patients as well as those aged 50 and younger versus those over 50 years old. The four group means (50 subjects per group) were as follows:

Age	Male	Female
≤50 years	98.2	70.1
>50	50.8	68.3

A two-way ANOVA yielded the following results

	F	*df*	*p*
Gender	3.61	1, 196	*ns*
Age group	5.87	1, 196	<.05
Gender × Age group	6.96	1, 196	<.01

Interpret the meaning of these results.

6. The correlation between the number of days absent per year and annual salary in a sample of 100 nurses was found to be –.23, $p < .05$. What does this result mean?

7. Indicate which statistical tests you would use to analyze data for the following variables:

   a. Variable 1 is psychiatric patients' gender; variable 2 is whether or not the patient has attempted suicide in the past 6 months.

   b. Variable 1 is the participation versus nonparticipation of patients with a pulmonary embolus in a special treatment group; variable 2 is the pH of the patients' arterial blood gases.

   c. Variable 1 is serum creatinine concentration levels; variable 2 is daily urine output.

   d. Variable 1 is patients' marital status (married vs. divorced/separated/widowed vs. never married); variable 2 is the patients' degree of self-reported depression (measured on a 20-item depression scale).

8. In the following examples, which multivariate procedure is most appropriate for analyzing the data?

   a. A researcher is testing the effect of verbal expressiveness, self-esteem, age, and the availability of family supports among a group of recently discharged psychiatric patients on recidivism (i.e., whether they will be readmitted within 12 months after discharge).

   b. A researcher is comparing daily hours of sleep of recently widowed and divorced individuals, controlling for their age.

   c. A researcher wants to test the effects of two drug treatments and two dosages of each drug on blood pressure, and the pH and PO_2 levels of arterial blood gases.

   d. A researcher wants to predict hospital staff absentee rates (number of days absent per year) based on staff rank, shift, number of years with the hospital, and marital status.

9. Below is a list of variables. Assume that you have data from 500 nurses on these variables. Develop two or three hypotheses regarding the relationships among these variables, and indicate which statistical tests you would use to test your hypotheses.

- Number of years of nursing experience
- Type of employment setting (hospital, nursing home, public school system, other)
- Annual salary
- Marital status (single, married, other)
- Job satisfaction (as measured on a 10-item Likert-type scale)
- Number of children under 18 years of age
- Gender
- Type of nursing preparation (diploma, Associate's, Bachelor's)

D. APPLICATION EXERCISES

Exercise D.1: Quantitative Appendix Studies

Which of the studies in Appendices A (by Weinert et al.) on pages 119–128, C (by Yackel et al.) on pages 139–146, and D (by Jurgens et al.) on pages 147–156 used the following descriptive statistical methods:

a. Percentages
b. Means and standard deviations
c. Medians
d. Mode

Exercise D.2: Study in Appendix A

Read the Results section of the report by Weinert and colleagues ("Computer intervention impact") in Appendix A on pages 119–128, and then answer the following questions:

Questions of Fact

a. Did Weinert and colleagues analyze the comparability of the intervention and control group subjects to assess potential selection biases? If yes, what statistical tests did they perform? If not, what statistical tests could they have used?

b. Was there any attrition in this study (i.e., did some participants drop out of the study?) Did Weinert and colleagues analyze the comparability of participants who remained and those who dropped out to assess potential attrition biases?

c. What statistical test discussed in Chapter 12 was used to assess attrition bias?

d. Which statistical tests discussed in Chapter 12 did Weinert and colleagues use to assess the effects of the intervention on study participants?

e. Did Weinert and colleagues present information about confidence intervals (estimation of parameters) for the means of the six outcomes over time?

f. Referring to Table 3, answer the following questions:
- For which outcomes (if any) were the mean group scores at 24 weeks significantly different?
- For which outcome was the level of significance greatest (i.e., strongest evidence that the group differences were not spurious)?
- What does the value of −1.8 represent in the fourth column for the outcome Loneliness?
- For the self-esteem scale, what is the 95% confidence interval around the mean difference? Do these values communicate whether or not the difference was significant?

g. Did the report indicate that a power analysis was done while planning the study to estimate sample size needs?

Questions for Discussion

a. Discuss the effectiveness of the presentation of information in the tables. What, if anything, could be done to make the tables more informative, more comprehensible, or more efficient? Should there have been additional tables? Create one such table, using information summarized in the text of the article.

b. Did Weinert and colleagues use the appropriate statistical tests to analyze their data? If not, what tests should have been performed?

c. Did the researchers present a sufficient amount of information about their statistical tests? What additional information would have been helpful?

d. Discuss the possibility of selection and attrition biases in this study.

e. Discuss the possibility of Type I and/or Type II errors.

Rigor and Interpretation in Quantitative Research

A. FILL IN THE BLANKS

How many terms have you learned in this chapter? Fill in the blanks in the sentences below to find out. Try doing this section with a friend. Which of you is the first one to complete the sentence?

1. Both researchers and consumers of quantitative research must develop a(n) _____ of the accuracy, meaning, and importance of the study results.

2. A famous research precept is that _____ does not prove that one variable caused another.

3. _____ size estimates such as d help to better understand the importance of the results.

4. The _____ guidelines for preparing research reports include a flow chart documenting participant flow in a study.

5. When some hypotheses are supported and others are not, the results are _____.

6. Researchers should take both the strengths and the _____ of their study into account when interpreting their findings.

7. A research _____ that is actually null is difficult to evaluate through standard statistical methods.

8. An important aspect of interpretation for clinical decision-making is the degree of _____ of effects, usually communicated through confident intervals (CIs).

9. Researchers' interpretations are presented in the _____ section of a report.

10. Results that are non _____ are especially difficult to interpret because of the possibility of a Type II error.

B. MATCHING EXERCISES

Match each statement or phrase from Set B with one or more of the phrases from Set A. Indicate the letter(s) corresponding to your response next to each of the statements in Set B.

SET A

a. Credibility of results
b. Precision of results
c. Magnitude of effects and importance
d. Generalizability of results
e. Implications of results

SET B   RESPONSES

1. Confidence intervals provide information about this   _____
2. An analysis of threats to study validity is a way to
   address this   _____
3. A consideration of how study limitations could be corrected
   in subsequent research is part of this   _____
4. In addressing this, consideration is given to the characteristics
   of the study sample and the research setting   _____
5. Effect size information can be especially useful for
   considering this   _____
6. An analysis of the success of the researcher's "proxies" is an
   approach to this   _____
7. Biases can reduce this   _____
8. Statements about the utility of findings for clinical practice
   are part of this   _____

C. STUDY QUESTIONS

1. Read one of the following studies and evaluate the extent to which the researchers assessed and considered possible biases and commented on them in their discussions.
   • Nyamathi, A., Sinha, K., Greengold, B., Cohen, A., & Marfisee, M. (2010). Predictors of HAV/HBV vaccination completion among methadone maintenance clients. *Research in Nursing & Health, 33*, 120–132.
   • Oh, P. J., & Kim, S. H. (2010). Effects of a brief psychosocial intervention in patients with cancer receiving adjuvant therapy. *Oncology Nursing Forum, 37*, E98–E104.
2. In a research article by D. McDonald and colleagues, 2010 (Motivating people to learn cardiopulmonary resuscitation and use of automated external defibrillators. *Journal of Cardiovascular Nursing, 25*, 69–74) the researchers reported that they obtained some nonsignificant results that were not consistent with expectations.

Review and critique the researchers' interpretation of the findings and suggest some possible alternatives.

3. In a report by Osterman and Dyehouse, 2012 (Effects of a motivational interviewing intervention to decrease prenatal alcohol use. *Western Journal of Nursing Research, 34*(4), 434–454), the researchers did not present a flow chart to track participant flow, as recommended in the CONSORT guidelines. Use information in the report (see the section "Description of sample") to create one, to the extent possible.

4. Skim one of the following articles, the titles for which imply a causal connection between phenomena. Do you think a causal inference is warranted—why or why not?

   • Emmanuel, E., Creedy, D., St. John, W., & Brown, C. (2011). Maternal role development: the impact of maternal distress and social support following childbirth. *Midwifery, 27*, 265–272.

   • Sullivan, M. C., et al. (2012). 17-year outcome of preterm infants with diverse neonatal mobidities:Impact on physical, neurological, and psychological health status. Journal for Specialists in Pediatric Nursing, 17, 226–241.

5. Below are a fictitious research report and a critique of various aspects of it. This example is designed to highlight features about the form and content of both a written report and a written evaluation of the study's worth. To economize on space, the report is brief, but it incorporates essential elements for a meaningful appraisal. Read the report and critique, and then determine whether you agree with the critique. Can you add other comments relevant to a critical appraisal of the study?

THE REPORT
The Role of Health Care Providers in Teenage Pregnancy by Phyllis Clinton

Background. Of the 20 million teenagers living in the United States, about one in four is sexually active by age 14; more than half have had sexual intercourse by age 17 (Kelman and Saner, 2001).[1] Despite increased availability of contraceptives, the number of teenage pregnancies has remained fairly stable over the past two decades. About 1 million girls under age 20 become pregnant each year and, of these, about 500,000 become teenaged mothers (U.S. Bureau of the Census, 2002).

Public concern regarding teenage pregnancy stems not only from the high rates but also from the extensive research that has documented the adverse consequences of early parenthood in the health arena. Pregnant teenagers have been found to receive less prenatal care (Tremain, 2000), to be more likely to develop toxemia (Schendley, 1999; Waters, 2004), to be more likely to experience prolonged labor (Curran, 1999), to be more likely to have low-birth-weight babies (Tremain, 2003; Beach, 2004), and to be more likely to have babies with low Apgar scores (Beach, 2004) than older mothers. The long-term consequences to the teenaged mothers themselves are also extremely bleak: teenaged mothers get less schooling, are more likely to be on public assistance, are likely to earn lower wages, and are more likely to get divorced if they marry than their peers who postpone parenthood (Jamail, 1999; North, 2002; Smithfield, 2001).

---

[1]All references in this example are fictitious.

The 1 million teenagers who become pregnant each year are caught up in a tough emotional decision—to carry the pregnancy to term and keep the baby, to have an abortion, or to deliver the infant and surrender it for adoption. Despite the widely reported adverse consequences of young parenthood cited above, most young women today are opting for delivery and child-rearing, often out of wedlock (Jaffrey, 2007; Henderson, 2001). Relatively few young mothers in recent years have been relinquishing their babies for adoption, forcing many couples with fertility problems to seek adoption options overseas (Smith, 2002).

The purpose of this study was to test the effect of a special intervention based in an outpatient clinic of a Chicago hospital on improving the health outcomes of a group of pregnant teenagers. Specifically, it was hypothesized that pregnant teenagers who were in the special program would receive more prenatal care, be less likely to develop toxemia, be less likely to have a low-birth-weight baby, spend fewer hours in labor, have babies with higher Apgar scores, and be more likely to use a contraceptive at 6 months postpartum than pregnant teenagers not enrolled in the program.

The theoretical model on which this research was based is an ecologic model of personal behavior (Brandenburg, 1984). A schematic diagram of the ecologic model is presented in Figure A. In this framework, the actions of the person are the focus of attention, but those actions are believed to be a function not only of the person's own characteristics, attitudes, and abilities but also of other influences in their environment. Environmental influences can be differentiated according to their proximal relationship with the target person. Health care workers and institutions are, according to the model, more distant influences than family, peers, and boyfriends. Yet it is assumed that these less immediate forces are real and can intervene to change the behaviors of the target person. Thus, it is hypothesized that pregnant teenagers can be influenced

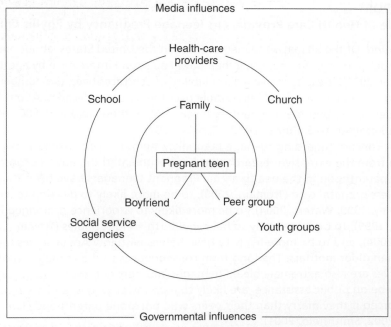

FIGURE A   Model of ecologic contexts

by increased exposure to a health care team providing a structured program of services designed to promote improved health outcomes.

Method. A special program of services for pregnant teenagers was implemented in the outpatient clinic of an inner-city public hospital in Chicago. The intervention involved 8 weeks of nutrition education and counseling, parenting education, instruction on prenatal health care, preparation for childbirth, and contraceptive counseling.

All teenagers with a confirmed pregnancy attending the clinic were asked if they wanted to participate in the special program. The goal was to enroll 150 pregnant teenagers during the program's first year of operation. A total of 276 teenagers attending the clinic were invited to participate; of these, 59 had an abortion or miscarriage and 108 declined to participate, yielding an experimental group sample of 109 girls.

To test the effectiveness of the special program, a comparison group of pregnant teenagers was needed. Another inner-city hospital agreed to cooperate in the study. Staff obtained information on the labor and delivery outcomes of the 120 teenagers who delivered at the comparison hospital, where no special teen-parent program was available. For both experimental group and comparison group subjects, a follow-up telephone interview was conducted 6 months postpartum to determine if the teenagers were using birth control.

The outcome variables in this study were the teenagers' labor, delivery, and post-partum outcomes, and their contraceptive behavior. Operational definitions of these variables were as follows:

Prenatal care: Number of visits made to a physician or nurse during the pregnancy, exclusive of the visit for the pregnancy test

Toxemia: Presence versus absence of preeclamptic toxemia as diagnosed by a physician or nurse midwife

Labor time: Number of hours elapsed from the first contractions until delivery of the baby, to the nearest half hour

Low infant birth weight: Infant birth weights of <2,500 g versus those of 2,500 g or greater

Apgar score: The summary rating (from 0 to 10) of the health of the infant, taken at 3 minutes after birth

Contraceptive use postpartum: Self-reported use of any form of birth control 6 months postpartum versus self-reported nonuse

The two groups were compared on these six outcome measures using t-tests and chi-squared tests.

Results. The teenagers in the sample were, on average, 17.6 years old at the time of delivery. The mean age was 17.0 in the experimental group and 18.1 in the comparison group ($p < .05$).

By definition, all the teenagers in the experimental group had received prenatal care. Two of the teenagers in the comparison group had no health care treatment before delivery. The distribution of visits for the two groups is presented in Figure B. The experimental group had a higher mean number of prenatal visits than the comparison group, as shown in Table A, but the difference was not statistically significant at the .05 level, using a *t*-test for independent groups.

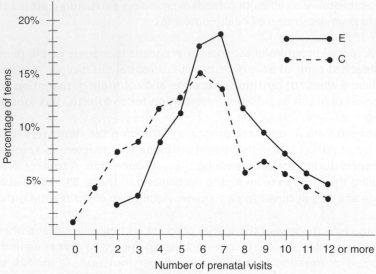

FIGURE B Frequency distribution of prenatal visits, by expirimental versus comparison group. (E, experimental group; c, comparision group)

In the sample as a whole, about 1 girl in 10 was diagnosed as having preeclamptic toxemia. The difference between the two groups was in the hypothesized direction, with 1.6% more of the comparison group teenagers developing this complication, but the difference was not significant using a chi-squared test.

The hours spent in labor ranged from 3.5 to 29.0 in the experimental group and from 4.5 to 33.5 in the comparison group. On average, teenagers in the experimental group spent 14.3 hours in labor, compared with 15.2 for the comparison group teenagers. The difference was not statistically significant.

TABLE A Summary of Experimental and Comparison Group Differences

	Group			
Outcome Variable	Experimental (n = 109)	Comparison (n = 120)	Difference	Test Statistic
Mean number of prenatal visits	7.1	5.9	1.2	$t = 1.83$, $df = 227$, NS
Percentage with toxemia	10.1%	11.7%	−1.6%	$\chi^2 = 0.15$, $df = 1$, NS
Mean hours spent in labor	14.3	15.2	−.09	$t = 1.01$, $df = 227$, NS
Percentage with low-birth-weight baby	16.5%	20.9%	−4.4%	$\chi^2 = 0.71$, $df = 1$, NS
Mean Apgar score	7.3	6.7	.6	$t = 0.98$, $df = 227$, NS
Percentage adopting contraception postpartum	81.7%	62.5%	19.2%	$\chi^2 = 10.22$, $df = 1$, $p < .01$

With regard to low-birth-weight babies, a total of 43 girls out of 229 in the sample gave birth to babies who weighed <2,500 g (5.5 lb).[2] More of the comparison group teenagers (20.9%) than experimental group teenagers (16.5%) had low-birth-weight babies, but, once again, the group difference was not significant.

The 3-minute Apgar scores in the two groups were quite similar—7.3 for the experimental group and 6.7 for the comparison group. This difference was nonsignificant.

Finally, the teenagers were compared with respect to their use of birth control 6 months after delivering their babies. For this variable, teenagers were coded as users of contraception if they were either using some method of birth control at the time of the follow-up interview or if they were nonusers but were sexually inactive (i.e., were using abstinence to prevent a repeat pregnancy). The results of the chi-squared test revealed that a significantly higher percentage of experimental group teenagers (81.7%) than comparison group teenagers (62.5%) reported using birth control after delivery. This difference was significant beyond the .01 level.

Discussion. The results of this evaluation were disappointing but not discouraging. There was only one outcome for which a significant difference was observed. The experimental program significantly increased the percentage of teenagers who used birth control after delivering their babies. Thus, one highly important result of participating in the program is that an early repeat pregnancy will be postponed. There is abundant research that has shown that repeat pregnancy among teenagers is especially damaging to their educational and occupational attainment and leads to particularly adverse labor and delivery outcomes in the higher-order births (Klugman, 1995; Jackson, 2007).

The experimental group had more prenatal care, but not significantly more. Part of the difficulty may be that the program can only begin to deliver services once pregnancy has been diagnosed. If a teenager does not come in for a pregnancy test until her fourth or fifth month, this obviously puts an upper limit on the number of visits she will have; it also gives less time for her to eat properly, avoid smoking and drinking, and take other steps to enhance her health during pregnancy. Thus, one implication of this finding is that the program needs to do more to encourage early pregnancy screening. Perhaps a joint effort between the clinic personnel and school nurses in neighboring middle schools and high schools could be launched to publicize the need for a timely pregnancy test and to inform teenagers where such a test could be obtained. The two groups performed similarly with respect to the various labor and delivery outcomes chosen to evaluate the effectiveness of the new program. The issue of timeliness is again relevant here. The program may have been delivering services too late in the pregnancy for the instruction to have made much of an impact on the health of the mother and her child. This interpretation is supported, in part, by the fact that the one variable for which timeliness was *not* an issue (postpartum contraception) was, indeed, positively affected by program participation. Another possible implication is that the program itself should be made more powerful, for example, by lengthening or adding to instructional sessions.

Given that the experimental and comparison group differences were all in the hypothesized direction, it is also tempting to criticize the study's sample size. A larger sample (which was originally planned) might have yielded some significant differences.

---

[2] All mothers gave birth to live infants; however, there were two neonatal deaths within 24 hours of birth in the comparison group.

In summary, the experimental intervention is not without promise. A particularly exciting finding is that participation in the program resulted in better contraceptive use, which will presumably lower the incidence of repeat pregnancy. It would be interesting to follow these teenagers 2 years after delivery to see if the groups differ in the rates of repeat pregnancy. It appears that more needs to be done to get these teenagers into the program early in their pregnancies. Perhaps then the true effectiveness of the program would be demonstrated.

CRITIQUE OF THE RESEARCH REPORT

In the following critique, we present some comments on various aspects of this research report. You are urged to read the report and form your own opinion about its strengths and weaknesses before reading our critique. An evaluation of a study is necessarily partly subjective. Therefore, you might disagree with some of the points made below, and you might have additional criticisms and comments. We believe, however, that most of the serious methodologic flaws of the study are highlighted in our critique.

Title. The title for the study is misleading. The research does *not* investigate the role of health care professionals in serving the needs of pregnant teenagers. A more appropriate title would be "Effects of an Intervention to Improve Pregnant Teenagers' Health-Related Outcomes."

Background. The background section of this report consists of three distinct elements that can be analyzed separately: a literature review, statement of the problem, and a theoretical framework.

The literature review is relatively clearly written and well organized. It serves the important function of establishing a need for an intervention by documenting the prevalence of teenage pregnancy and some of its adverse consequences. However, the literature review could be improved. First, an inspection of the citations suggests that the author is not as up-to-date on research relating to teenage pregnancy as she might have been. Most of the references date before 2005, and so the review might be different if more recent studies were cited. Second, there is material in the literature review section that is not relevant and should be removed. For example, the paragraph on the options with which a pregnant teenager is faced (paragraph 3) is not germane to the research problem. A third and more critical flaw is what the review does *not* cover. Given the research problem, there are probably four main points that should be addressed in the review:

1. How widespread is teenage pregnancy and parenthood?
2. What are the social and health consequences of early child-bearing?
3. What has been done by healthcare researchers to address the problems associated with teenage parenthood?
4. How successful have other interventions been?

The review adequately handles the first question: the need for concern is established. The second question is covered in the review, but perhaps more depth and more recent research is needed here. The new study is based on an assumption of negative health outcomes in teenaged mothers. The author has strung together a series of references without giving the reader any clues about the reliability of the information. The author would have made her point more convincingly if she had added a sentence such as "For example, in a carefully executed prospective study involving nearly 8,000 pregnant women, Beach (2004) found that young maternal age was significantly associated with higher rates of prematurity and other negative neonatal outcomes." The third and fourth points that should have been covered are totally absent from the review. Surely the author's intervention does not represent the first attempt to address the needs of pregnant teenagers. How is Clinton's intervention different from or better than other interventions? What reason does she have to believe that such an intervention might be successful? Clinton has provided a rationale for addressing the problem but no rationale for the manner in which she has addressed it. If, in fact, there is little information about other interventions and their effectiveness in improving health outcomes, then the review should say so.

The problem statement and hypothesis were stated succinctly and clearly. The hypothesis is complex (there are multiple dependent variables) and directional (it predicts better outcomes among teenagers participating in the special program).

The third component of the Background section of the report is the theoretical framework. In our opinion, the theoretical framework chosen does little to enhance the research. The hypothesis is not generated on the basis of the model, nor does the intervention itself grow out of the model. One gets the feeling that the model might have been tacked on as an afterthought to try to make the study seem more theoretical. Actually, if more thought had been given to this conceptual framework, it might have proved useful. According to this model, the most immediate and direct influences on a pregnant teenager are her family, friends, and sexual partner. One programmatic implication of this is that the intervention should involve one or more of these influences. For example, a workshop for the teenagers' parents could have been developed to reinforce the teenagers' need for adequate nutrition and prenatal care. A research hypothesis that could have been tested in the context of the model is that teenagers who are missing one of the direct influences would be especially susceptible to the influence of less proximal health care providers (i.e., the program). For example, it might be hypothesized that pregnant teenagers who do not live with both parents have to depend on alternative sources of social support (such as health care personnel) during the pregnancy. Thus, it is not that the theoretical context selected is far-fetched but rather that it was not convincingly linked to the actual research problem.

Method. The design used to test the research hypothesis was a widely used quasi-experimental design. Two groups, whose equivalence is assumed but not established, were compared on several outcome measures. The design is one that has serious problems because the preintervention comparability of the groups is unknown.

The most serious threat to the internal validity of the study is selection bias. Selection bias can work both ways—either to mask true treatment effects or to create the illusion of a program effect when none exists. This is because selection bias can be either positive (i.e., the experimental group can be initially advantaged in relation to the comparison group) or negative (i.e., the experimental group can have pretreatment disadvantages). In the present study, it is possible that the two hospitals served clients of different economic circumstances, for example. If the average income of the families of the experimental group teenagers was higher, then these teenagers would probably have a better opportunity for adequate prenatal nutrition than the comparison group teenagers. Or the comparison hospital might serve older teens, or a higher percentage of married teens, or a higher percentage of teens attending a special school-based program for pregnant students. None of these confounding variables, which could affect the mother's health, has been controlled.

Another way in which the design was vulnerable to selection bias is the high refusal rate in the experimental group. Of the 217 eligible teenagers, half declined to partici- pate in the special program. We cannot assume that the 109 girls who participated were a random sample of the eligible girls. Again, biases could be either positive or negative. A positive selection bias would be created if, for example, the teenagers who were the most motivated to have a healthy pregnancy selected themselves into the experimental group. A negative selection bias would result if the teenagers from the most disadvan- taged households or from families offering little support elected to participate in the program.

The researcher could have taken a number of steps to either control selection biases or, at the least, estimate their direction and magnitude. The following are among the most critical confounding variables: social class and family income, age, race and ethnic- ity, parity, participation in another pregnant teenager program, marital status, and prepregnancy experience with contraception (for the postpartum contraception out- come). The researcher should have attempted to gather information on these variables from experimental group and comparison group teenagers *and* from eligible teenagers in the experimental hospital who declined to participate in the program. To the extent that these groups were similar on these variables, the internal validity of the study, and thus the credibility of the results, would be enhanced. If sizable differences were observed, the researcher would at least know or suspect the direction of the biases and could factor that information into her interpretation and conclusions.

Had the researcher gathered information on the confounding variables, another pos- sibility would have been to match experimental and comparison group subjects on one or two variables, such as family income and age. Matching is not an ideal method of controlling confounding variables; for one thing, matching on two variables would not equate the two groups in terms of the other confounding variables. However, matching is preferable to doing nothing to control extraneous variation.

So far we have focused our attention on the research design, but other aspects of the study are also problematic. Let us consider the decision the researcher made about the population. The target population is not explicitly defined by the researcher, but we can perhaps infer that the target population is pregnant young women under age 20 who carry their infants to delivery. The accessible population is pregnant teenagers from one area in Chicago. It cannot reasonably be assumed that the accessible population is representative of the target population. It is likely that the accessible population is quite different with regard to health care, family intactness, and many other characteristics. The researcher should have more clearly discussed who the target population of this research was.

Clinton would have done well, in fact, to delimit the target population; had she done so, it might have been possible to control some of the confounding variables discussed previously. For example, Clinton could have established eligibility criteria that excluded multigravidas, very young teenagers (e.g., under age 15), or married teenagers. Such a specification would have limited the generalizability of the findings, but it would have enhanced the internal validity of the study because it probably would have increased the comparability of the experimental and comparison groups.

The sample was a sample of convenience, the least effective sampling design for a quantitative study. There is no way of knowing whether the sample represents the accessible and target populations. Although probability sampling likely was not feasible, the researcher might have improved her sampling design by using a quota sampling plan. For example, if the researcher knew that in the accessible population, half of the families received public assistance, then it might have been possible to enhance the representativeness of the samples by using a quota system to ensure that half of the research participants came from welfare-dependent families.

Sample size is a difficult issue. Many of the reported results were in the hypothesized direction but were nonsignificant. When this is the case, the adequacy of the sample size is always suspect, as Clinton pointed out. Each group had about 100 subjects. In many cases, this sample size would be considered adequate, but in the present case, it is not. One of the difficulties in testing the effectiveness of new interventions is that, generally, the experimental group is not being compared with a no-treatment group. Although the comparison group in this example was not getting the special program services, it cannot be assumed that this group was getting no services at all. Some comparison group members may have had ample prenatal care during which the health care staff may have provided much of the same information as was taught in the special program. The point is not that the new program was not needed but rather that unless an intervention is extremely powerful and innovative, the incremental improvement will typically be small. When relatively small effects are anticipated, the sample must be very large for differences to be statistically significant. Indeed, power analysis can be performed using the study findings. For example, a power analysis indicates that to detect a significant difference between the two groups with respect to one outcome— the incidence of toxemia—a sample of over 5,000 pregnant teenagers would have been needed. Had the researcher done a power analysis before conducting the study, she might have realized the insufficiency of her sample for some of the outcomes and might have developed a different sampling plan or identified different outcome variables.

The third major methodologic decision concerns the measurement of the research variables. For the most part, the researcher did a good job in selecting objective, reliable, and valid outcome measures. Also, her operational definitions were clearly worded and unambiguous. Two comments are in order, however. First, it might have been better to operationalize two of the variables differently. Infant birth weight might have been more sensitively measured as actual weight (a ratio-level measurement) or as a three-level ordinal variable (<1,500 g; ≥1,500 but <2,500 g; and ≥2,500 g) instead of as a dichotomous variable. The contraceptive variable could also have been operationalized to yield a more sensitive (i.e., more discriminating) measure. For example, rather than measuring contraceptive use as a dichotomy, Clinton could have measured frequency of using contraception (e.g., never, sometimes, usually, or always), effectiveness of the *type* of birth control used, or a combination of these two.

A second consideration is whether the outcome variables adequately captured the effects of program activities. It would have been more directly relevant to the intervention to capture group differences in, say, dietary practices during pregnancy than in infant birth weight. Also, none of the outcome variables was a measure of the effects of parenting education. In other words, Clinton could have added additional and more directly relevant measures of the effectiveness of the intervention.

One other point about the methods should be made, and that relates to ethical considerations. The article does not specifically say that the teenagers were asked for their informed consent, but that does not necessarily mean that no written consent was obtained. It is quite likely that the experimental group members, when asked to volunteer for the special program, were advised about their participation in the study and asked to sign a consent form. But what about teenagers in the control group? The article implies that comparison group members were given no opportunity to decline participation and were not aware of having their birth outcomes used as data in the research. In some cases, this procedure is acceptable. For example, a hospital or clinic might agree to release patient information without the patients' consent if the release of such information is done anonymously—that is, if it can be provided in such a way that even the researcher does not know the identity of the patients. In the present study, however, it is clear that the names of the comparison group teenagers *were* given to the researcher because she had to contact the comparison group at 6 months post-partum to determine their contraceptive practices. Thus, this study does not appear to have adequately safeguarded the rights of the comparison group participants.

In summary, the researcher appears not to have given the new program, a particularly fair test. Clinton should have taken a number of steps to control confounding variables and should have attempted to get a larger sample (even if this meant waiting for additional subjects to enroll in the program). In addition to concerns about the internal validity of the study, its generalizability is also questionable.

Results. Clinton did an adequate job of presenting the results of the study. The presentation was straightforward and succinct and was enhanced by the inclusion of a good table and figure. The style of this section was also appropriate: it was written objectively and was well organized.

The statistical analyses were also reasonably well done. The descriptive statistics (means and percentages) were appropriate for the level of measurement of the variables. The two types of inferential statistics used (the *t*-test and chi-squared test) were also appropriate, given the levels of measurement of the outcome variables. The results of these tests were efficiently presented in a single table. Of course, more powerful statistics could have been used to control confounding variables (e.g., analysis of covariance). It appears, however, that the only confounding variable that could have been controlled statistically was the participants' ages; no data were apparently collected on other confounding variables (social class, ethnicity, parity, and so on).

Discussion. Clinton's discussion section fails almost entirely to take the study's limitations into account in interpreting the data. The one exception is her acknowledgment that the sample size was too small. She seems unconcerned about the many threats to the internal or external validity of her research.

Clinton lays almost all the blame for the nonsignificant findings on the program rather than on the research methods. She feels that two aspects of the program should be changed: (1) recruitment of teenagers into the program earlier in their pregnancies and (2) strengthening program services. Both recommendations might be worth pursuing, but there is little in the data to suggest these modifications. With nonsignificant results such as those that predominated in this study, there are two possibilities to consider: (1) the results are accurate—that is, the program was not effective for those outcomes examined (though it might be effective for other measures), and (2) the results are false—that is, the existing program was effective for the outcomes examined, but the tests failed to demonstrate it. Clinton concluded that the first possibility was correct and therefore recommended that the program be changed. Equally plausible is the possibility that the study methods were too weak to demonstrate the program's true effects.

We do not have enough information about the characteristics of the sample to conclude with certainty that there were substantial selection biases. We do, however, have a clue that selection biases were operative in a direction that would make the program look less effective than it actually was. Clinton noted in the beginning of the results section that the average age of the teenagers in the experimental group was 17.0, compared with 18.1 in the comparison group—a difference that was significant. Age is inversely related to positive labor and delivery outcomes, indeed, that is the basis for having a special program for teenaged mothers. Therefore, the experimental group's performance on the outcome measures was possibly depressed by the youth of that group. Had the two groups been equivalent in terms of age, group differences on the outcomes might have been larger and could have reached levels of statistical significance. Other uncontrolled pretreatment differences could also have masked true treatment effects.

For the one significant outcome, we cannot rule out the possibility that a Type I error was made—that is, that the null hypothesis was in fact true. Again, selection biases could have been operative. The experimental group might have contained many more girls who had preprogram experience with contraception; it might have been comprised of more highly motivated teenagers, or more teenagers who had already had multiple pregnancies than the comparison group. There simply is no way of knowing whether the significant outcome reflects true program effects or initial group differences.

Aside from Clinton's disregard for the problems of internal validity, she overstepped the bounds of scholarly speculation. She assumed that the program *caused* contraceptive improvements: "the experimental program significantly increased the percentage of teenagers who used birth control…" Worse yet, she went on to conclude that repeat pregnancies will be postponed in the experimental group, although she does not know whether the teenagers used an effective contraception, whether they used it all the time, or whether they used it correctly.

As another example of going beyond the data, Clinton became overly invested in the notion that teenagers need greater and earlier exposure to the program. It is not that her hypothesis has no merit—the problem is that she builds an elaborate rationale for program changes with no apparent empirical support. She probably had information on when in the pregnancy the teenagers entered the program, but that information was not shared with readers. Her argument about the need for more publicity on early screening would have had more clout if she had reported that most teenagers entered the program during the fourth month of their pregnancies or later. Additionally, she could have marshaled more evidence in support of her proposal if she had been able to show that earlier entry into the program was associated with better health outcomes. For example, she could have compared the outcomes of teenagers entering the program in the first, second, and third trimesters of their pregnancies.

In conclusion, the study has several positive features. As Clinton noted, there is some reason to be cautiously optimistic that the program *could* have some beneficial effects. However, the existing study is too seriously flawed to reach any conclusions, even tentatively. A replication with improved research methods is needed to solve the research problem.

D. APPLICATION EXERCISES

Exercise D.1: Study in Appendix A

Read the "Results," and "Discussion" sections of the report by Weinert and colleagues ("Computer intervention impact") in Appendix A on pages 119–128 and then answer the following questions:

Questions of Fact

a. Was a CONSORT-type flow chart included in this report? If yes, what did it show?

b. Did the researchers provide evidence about the success of randomization—i.e., whether experimentals and controls were equivalent at the outset and, thus, whether selection biases were absent?

c. Did the researchers report an analysis of attrition biases? Was attrition taken into account in the analysis of group differences on the outcomes?

d. With regard to the primary aim of the study, to compare intervention and control group outcomes on psychosocial variables following the computer intervention, were hypotheses supported, nonsupported, or mixed?

e. Did the report provide information about the precision of results via confidence intervals?

f. Did the report provide information about magnitude of effects via calculation of effect sizes?

g. In the Discussion section, was there any explicit discussion about the study's internal validity?

h. In the Discussion section, was there any explicit discussion about the study's external validity?

i. In the Discussion section, was there any explicit discussion about the study's statistical conclusion validity?

j. Did the Discussion section link study findings to findings from prior research— i.e., did the authors place their findings into a broader context?

k. Did the Discussion section explicitly mention any study limitations?

Questions for Discussion

a. Critique the analysis of biases in this report and possible resulting effects on the interpretation of the findings.

b. Do you agree with the researchers' interpretations of their results? Why or why not?

c. Discuss the extent to which the Discussion addressed all major findings.

d. What is your assessment of the internal and external validity of the study?

e. To what extent do you think the researchers adequately described the study's limitations and strengths?

Exercise D.2: Study in Appendix D

Read the "Results" and "Discussion" sections of the report by Jurgens and colleagues ("Why do elders delay responding") in Appendix D on pages 147–156 and then answer the following questions:

Questions of Fact

a. Did any study participants withdraw from the study? Did the researchers report an analysis of attrition biases?

b. Were any other biases analyzed in this study? If yes, what was the analysis and what type of bias was addressed?

c. Did the researchers state or imply any hypotheses? With regard to any hypotheses, were they supported, nonsupported, or mixed?

d. Did the report provide information about the precision of results via confidence intervals?

e. Did the report provide information about magnitude of effects via calculation of effect sizes?

f. In the Discussion section, was there any explicit discussion about the study's internal validity?

g. In the Discussion section, was there any explicit discussion about the study's external validity?

h. In the Discussion section, was there any explicit discussion about the study's statistical conclusion validity?

i. Did the Discussion section link study findings to findings from prior research—i.e., did the authors place their findings into a broader context?

j. Did the Discussion section explicitly mention any study limitations?

Questions for Discussion

a. Do you agree with the researchers' interpretations of their results? Why or why not?

b. Discuss the extent to which the Discussion addressed all major findings.

c. To what extent do you think the researchers' adequately described the study's limitations and strengths?

Qualitative Research

Qualitative Designs and Approaches

A. FILL IN THE BLANKS

How many terms have you learned in this chapter? Fill in the blanks in the sentences below to find out. Try doing this section with a friend. Which of you is the first one to complete the sentence?

1. Participatory _____ research is designed to be empowering for the group under study.

2. _____ was Leininger's phrase for research at the interface between culture and nursing.

3. In _____ analysis, the focus is on a *story*.

4. _____ research focuses on gender domination.

5. The two originators of grounded theory were _____ and _____.

6. Ethnographers typically undertake _____ observation as a data collection strategy during their fieldwork.

7. Grounded theory researchers often identify the _____ social process (BSP) that explains how people resolve a problem.

8. Phenomenologists study _____ experiences.

9. The systematic collection and analysis of materials relating to the past is known as _____ research.

10. _____ phenomenology focuses on the *meaning* of experiences; another term used for this type of phenomenology is _____.

11. A phenomenological question is: What is the _____ of this phenomenon?

12. Grounded theorists use an analytic strategy called _____ comparison.

13. Ethnographers rely on one or more key _____ to help them understand and interpret a culture.

14. Research that seeks to be transformative is based on _____ theory.

15. In a(n) _____ study, a single person or group is at center stage.

16. Descriptive phenomenologists use the strategy called _____ to hold in abeyance their presuppositions about a phenomenon.

89

B. MATCHING EXERCISES

Match each descriptive statement from Set B with one of the research traditions from Set A. Indicate the letter corresponding to your response next to each item in Set B.

SET A

a. Ethnography

b. Phenomenology

c. Grounded theory

d. Ethnography, phenomenology, and grounded theory

SET B   RESPONSES

1. Is rooted in a philosophical tradition developed by Husserl and Heidegger   _____

2. Involves the study of both broadly defined cultures and more narrowly defined ones   _____

3. Uses qualitative data to address questions of interest   _____

4. Is an approach to the study of social processes and social structures   _____

5. Is concerned with the lived experiences of humans   _____

6. Strives to achieve an emic perspective on the members of a group   _____

7. Is closely related to a research tradition called hermeneutics   _____

8. Uses a procedure referred to as constant comparison   _____

9. Stems from a discipline other than nursing   _____

10. Developed by the sociologists Glaser and Strauss   _____

11. Is a tradition that is particularly well suited to a critical theory perspective   _____

12. Typically involves interviews with study participants.   _____

C. STUDY QUESTIONS

1. For each of the research questions below, indicate what type of qualitative research tradition would likely guide the inquiry and why you think that would be the case.

   a. What is the social psychological process through which couples deal with the abrupt loss of an infant through Sudden Infant Death Syndrome (SIDS)?

   b. How does the culture of a suicide survivors' self-help group adapt to a successful suicide attempt by a former member?

   c. What is the lived experience of the spousal caretaker of an Alzheimer patient?

   d. What is the meaning of loneliness to childless widows with chronic health problems?

2. Skim the following two studies, which are examples of ethnographic and phenomenological studies that focused on alcohol and drinking. What were the central phenomena under investigation? Compare and contrast the methods used in these two studies (e.g., how were data collected? How many study participants were there? To what extent did the design unfold while the researchers were in the field?)

   • *Ethnographic Study*: Chang, L., Lo, S., & Hayter, M. (2011). Drinking behaviors: the life narratives of indigenous Bunun women in Taiwan. *Journal of Nursing Research, 19*, 83–93.

   • *Phenomenological Study*: Thurang, A., Rydstrom, J., & Bentsson-Tops, A. (2011). Being in a safe haven and struggling against alcohol dependency. *Issues in Mental Health Nursing, 32*, 401–407.

3. Skim one of the following participatory action research studies and comment on the roles of participants and researchers. In what ways would the study have been different if a participatory approach had not been used?

   • Findholt, N., Michael, Y., & Davis, M. (2011). Photovoice engages rural youth in childhood obesity prevention. *Public Health Nursing, 28*, 186–192.

   • Pierre-Lousi, B., Akoh, V., White, P., & Pharris, M. (2011). Patterns in the lives of African American women with diabetes. *Nursing Science Quarterly, 24*, 227–236.

4. Read one of the case studies suggested below, and evaluate the extent to which a case study approach was appropriate. What were the drawbacks and benefits of using this approach?

   • Mawn, B., Siquiera, E., Koren, A., Slatin, C., Devereux-Melillo, K., Pearce, C., & Hoff, L. (2010). Health disparities among health care workers. *Qualitative Health Research, 20*, 68–80.

   • Zuñiga, J. (2012). A woman's lived experience with directly observed therapy for tuberculosis—a case study. *Health Care for Women International, 33*, 19–28.

   • Wilkinson, J., Nutley, S., & Davies, H. (2011). An exploration of the roles of nurse managers in evidence-based practice implementation. *Worldviews on Evidence-Based Nursing, 8*, 236–246.

5. Read one of the studies below, and evaluate the extent to which the problem was amenable to the grounded theory research tradition. Which school of grounded theory thought was followed in this study? Does the report explicitly discuss how the constant comparative method was used?

   • Pieters, H., Heilemann, M., Maliski, S., Dornig, K.,& Mentes, J. (2012). Instrumental relating and treatment decision-making among older women with early-stage breast cancer. *Oncology Nursing Forum, 39*, E10–E19.

   • Chen, P., & Chang, H. (2012). The coping process of patients with cancer. *European Journal of Oncology Nursing, 16*, 10–16.

   • Stewart, J., Pyke-Grimm, K., & Kelly, K. (2012). Making the right decision for my child with cancer: The parental imperative. *Cancer Nursing , 21*, 89–97.

6. Read one of the studies below and think about how the researcher could have adopted a critical theory or feminist perspective. In what ways might the methods for such a modification differ from the methods used?

   • Annan, S. L. (2011). "It's not just a job. This is where we live. This is our backyard": The experiences of expert legal and advocate providers with sexually assaulted women in rural areas. *Journal of the American Psychiatric Nurses Association, 17*, 138–147.

- Gurnah, K., Khoshnood, K., Bradley, E., & Yuan, C. (2011). Lost in translation: Reproductive health care experiences of Somali Bantu women in Hartford, Connecticut. *Journal of Midwifery & Women's Health, 56,* 340–346.
- Lowe, J., & Gibson, S. (2011). Reflections of a homeless population's lived experience with substance abuse. *Journal of Community Health Nursing, 28,* 92–104.
- Sawin, E., & Parker, B. (2011). "If looks could kill then I would be dead": Intimate partner abuse and breast cancer in older women. *Journal of Gerontological Nursing, 37,* e26–35.

D. APPLICATION EXERCISES

Exercise D.1: Study in Appendix E

Read the Methodology section of the report by Byrne and colleagues ("Care transition experiences") in Appendix E on pages 157–174 and then answer the following questions:

Questions of Fact

a. In which tradition was this study based?

b. Which specific approach was used—that of Glaser and Strauss, Strauss and Corbin, or Charmaz?

c. What is the central phenomenon under study?

d. Was the study longitudinal or cross-sectional?

e. What was the setting for this research?

f. Did the report indicate or suggest that constant comparison was used?

g. Was a core variable or basic social process identified? If yes, what was it?

h. Did the researchers use methods that were congruent with the qualitative research tradition?

i. Did this study have an ideological perspective? If so, which one?

Questions for Discussion

a. How well is the research design described in the report? Were design decisions explained and justified?

b. Does it appear that the researchers made all design decisions up-front, or did the design emerge during data collection, allowing them to capitalize on early information?

c. Were there any elements of the design or methods that appear to be more appropriate for a qualitative tradition other than the one the researchers identified as the underlying tradition?

d. Could this study have been undertaken within an ideological framework? If so, what changes to the research methods would be necessary?

Exercise D.2: Study in Appendix F

Read the Methods section of the report by Cummings ("Sharing a traumatic event") in Appendix F on pages 175–182 and then answer the following questions:

Questions of Fact

a. In which tradition was this study based? Within which specific school of inquiry was the study based?

b. What is the central phenomenon under study?

c. Was the study longitudinal or cross-sectional?

d. What was the setting for this research?

e. Did the researcher make explicit comparisons?

f. Did the researchers use methods that were congruent with the qualitative research tradition?

g. Did this study have an ideological perspective?

Questions for Discussion

a. How well is the research design described? Were design decisions explained and justified?

b. Does it appear that the researcher made all design decisions up-front, or did the design emerge during data collection, allowing researchers to capitalize on early information?

c. Could this study have been undertaken within an ideological perspective? Why or why not?

Sampling and Data Collection in Qualitative Studies

A. FILL IN THE BLANKS

How many terms have you learned in this chapter? Fill in the blanks in the sentences below to find out. Try doing this section with a friend. Which of you is the first one to complete the sentence?

1. _____ sampling is a type of sampling based on referrals from early participants.

2. _____ sampling is preferred by grounded theory researchers.

3. A sampling approach in which participants are intentionally selected by the researchers to fulfill the needs of the study is known as _____ sampling.

4. A type of purposive sampling that involves deliberate attempts to draw from diverse groups is _____ variation sampling.

5. The principle used by qualitative researchers to determine when to stop sampling is called data _____.

6. The _____ incidents technique involves in-depth exploration of specific events or episodes.

7. _____ involves the use of photographs as a stimulus for conversations in qualitative studies.

8. A(n) _____ guide is used in some qualitative studies to ensure that important question areas are covered in an interview.

9. A(n) _____ interview is guided by an established list of topics or broad questions _____.

10. A completely _____ interview typically begins with a grand tour question to begin an undirected conversation.

11. _____ is a technique wherein participants take pictures of their own environments and then explain the pictures to the researcher.

12. Participant observers record their observations, thoughts, and interpretations in _____ notes; they also maintain a daily _____ to record activities and events.

13. A technique for gathering in-depth information from 5 to 10 people simultaneously is called a(n) _____ interview.

B. MATCHING EXERCISES

1. Match each type of sampling approach from Set B with one of the phrases from Set A. Indicate the letter corresponding to your response next to each of the statements in Set B.

SET A

a. Sampling approach for quantitative studies
b. Sampling approach for qualitative studies
c. Sampling approach for either quantitative or qualitative studies
d. Sampling approach for neither quantitative nor qualitative studies

SET B   RESPONSES

1. Typical case sampling   _____
2. Purposive sampling   _____
3. Systematic sampling   _____
4. Weighted sampling   _____
5. Consecutive sampling   _____
6. Snowball sampling   _____
7. Stratified random sampling   _____
8. Quota sampling   _____
9. Power sampling   _____
10. Theoretical sampling   _____

2. Match each descriptive statement regarding data collection methods from Set B with one of the statements from Set A. Indicate the letter corresponding to your response next to each item in Set B.

SET A

a. Self-reports
b. Observations
c. Both self-reports and observations
d. Neither self-reports nor observations

SET B   RESPONSES

1. Is the primary source of data in phenomenological research   _____
2. The critical incidents technique is one approach   _____
3. Data are recorded in logs and field notes   _____
4. Ethnographies rely on this as a data source   _____
5. Photovoice is one approach   _____
6. Mobile positioning is a strategy for collecting such data   _____
7. Artifact scrutiny is one approach   _____

8. Can be either structured for quantitative inquiries or unstructured for qualitative inquiries _____

9. Can be audio- or video-recorded _____

10. Can rely on a topic guide _____

C. STUDY QUESTIONS

1. Below are several research questions. Indicate which methods of sampling you might recommend using for each, and what you think the sample size might be. Defend your response.

   a. How does an elderly person manage the transition from a nursing home to a hospital and then back again?

   b. What is it like to be an in vitro fertilization patient and not get pregnant after many months of treatment?

   c. What is the process by which patients adjust to postdischarge life following a spinal cord injury?

   d. What are the health beliefs and risk-taking behaviors of adolescent members of a vampire cult?

2. Suppose a qualitative researcher wanted to study the life quality of cancer survivors. Suggest what the researcher might do to obtain a maximum variation sample and an extreme case sample.

3. Each of the following studies relied primarily on a sample of convenience. Suggest ways in which the researcher might have improved the study by using a different sampling approach:

   • Mendias, E., Clark, M., Guevera, E., & Svrcek, C. (2011). Low-income Euro-American mothers' perceptions of health and self-care practices. *Public Health Nursing, 28*, 233–242.

   • Sawin, B., & Parker, B. (2011). If looks would kill then I would be dead: Intimate partner abuse and breast cancer in older women. *Journal of Gerontological Nursing, 37*, e26–e35.

   • Steeves, R., Parker, B., Laughon, K., Knopp, A., & Thompson, M. (2011). Adolescents' experiences with uxoricide, *Journal of the American Psychiatric Nurses Association, 17*, 115–123.

4. Below are several research problems. Indicate which type of unstructured self-report approach you might recommend using for each. Defend your response.

   a. How do parents of autistic children manage their frustration and fears?

   b. What are the barriers to preventive health care practices among the urban poor?

   c. What stresses does the spouse of a terminally ill patient experience?

   d. What are the coping mechanisms and perceived barriers to coping among severely disfigured burn patients?

5. Suppose you were interested in studying the patients' impatience and anxiety waiting for treatment in the waiting area of an emergency department. Develop a topic guide for a semi-structured interview on this topic.

6. Suggest how you might collect data to address the following research question: *To what extent and in what manner do male and female nurses interact differently with male and female patients?* Would *participant* observation be appropriate? What are the possible advantages and drawbacks of such an approach?

7. Read one of the following articles, and indicate how, if at all, you would augment the self-report data collected in the study with participant observation:

   • Ames, K., Rennick, J., & Baillargeon, S. (2011). A qualitative interpretive study exploring parents' perception of the parental role in the paediatric intensive care unit. *Intensive Critical Care Nursing, 27*, 143–150.

   • Lin, Y. P., & Tsai, Y. F. (2011). Maintaining patients' dignity during clinical care. *Journal of Advanced Nursing, 67*, 340–348.

   • McDowell, L., Hilfinger-Messias, D., & Estrada, R. (2011). The work of language interpretation in health care. *Journal of Transcultural Nursing, 22*, 137–147.

   • Fisher, C., & O'Connor, M. (2012). "Motherhood" in the context of living with breast cancer. *Cancer Nursing, 35*, 157–163.

D. APPLICATION EXERCISES

Exercise D.1: Study in Appendix B

Read the Methods sections of the report by Cricco-Lizza ("Rooting for the Breast") in Appendix B on pages 129–138 and then answer the following questions:

Questions of Fact

a. What were the eligibility criteria for this study?

b. How were study participants recruited?

c. What type of sampling approach was used?

d. How many participants constituted the sample?

e. Was data saturation achieved?

f. Were sample characteristics described? If yes, what were those characteristics?

g. Did the researcher collect any self-report data? If yes, what concepts were captured by self-report?

h. What specific types of qualitative self-report methods were used?

i. Were examples of the interview questions included in the report?

j. Does the report provide information about how long interviews took, on average?

k. How were the self-report data recorded?

l. Did this study collect any data through observation? If no, could observation have been used? If yes, what concepts were captured through observation?

m. If there were observations, how were observational data recorded?

n. Were any other types of data collected in this study?

o. Who collected the data in this study?

Questions for Discussion

a. Comment on the adequacy of the researcher's sampling plan and recruitment strategy for achieving the goals of an ethnographic study.

b. Do you think Cricco-Lizza's sample size was adequate? Why or why not?

c. Cricco-Lizza used nurse experience as her key dimension of variability in selecting key informants. What other dimensions might have been used productively?

d. Comment on the adequacy of the researcher's description of her data collection methods.

e. Comment on the data collection approaches Cricco-Lizza used. Did she fully capture the concepts of interest in the best possible manner?

f. Comment on the procedures used to record data in this study. Were adequate steps taken to ensure the highest possible quality data?

Exercise D.2: Study in Appendix E

Read the Methodology section of the article by Byrne and colleagues ("Care transition experiences") in Appendix E on pages 157–174 and then answer the following questions:

Questions of Fact

a. What were the eligibility criteria for this study?

b. How were study participants recruited?

c. What type of sampling approach was used?

d. How many study participants constituted the sample?

e. Was data saturation achieved?

f. Did the sampling strategy include confirming and disconfirming cases?

g. Were sample characteristics described? If yes, what were those characteristics?

h. Did the researcher collect any self-report data? If no, could self-reports have been used? If yes, what concepts were captured by self-report?

i. What specific types of qualitative self-report methods were used?

j. Were examples of questions included in the report?

k. Does the report provide information about how long interviews took, on average?

l. How were the self-report data recorded?

m. Did this study collect any data through observation? If no, could observation have been used? If yes, what concepts were captured through observation?

Questions for Discussion

a. Comment on the adequacy of the researchers' sampling plan and recruitment strategy for achieving the goals of an in-depth study.

b. Assume that you had no resource constraints to address the research questions in this study. What sampling plan would you recommend?

c. Do you think the sample size in this study was adequate? Why or why not?

d. Comment on issues relating to the transferability of findings from this study.

CHAPTER 16

Analysis of Qualitative Data

A. FILL IN THE BLANKS

How many terms have you learned in this chapter? Fill in the blanks in the sentences below to find out. Try doing this section with a friend. Which of you is the first one to complete the sentence?

1. Qualitative descriptive studies typically rely on _____ analysis to discover key themes and patterns.

2. Sometimes themes are validated through the use of quasi-_____.

3. In ethnographies, a broad unit of cultural knowledge is called a(n) _____.

4. The hermeneutic _____ involves movement between parts and whole of a text being analyzed.

5. In Diekelmann's analytic approach, the discovery of a(n) _____ pattern forms the highest level of analysis.

6. Van Manen's _____ approach involves analyzing every sentence.

7. Grounded theorists document an idea in an analytic _____.

8. After a category system is developed, the next task involves _____ the data.

9. A recent approach to grounded theory analysis is called _____ grounded theory.

10. In Glaserian grounded theory, the type of coding focused on the core variable is _____ coding.

11. A(n) _____ is a literary device sometimes used as part of an analytic strategy, especially by interpretive phenomenologists.

12. The concept of _____ fit in grounded theory involves comparing identified concepts with similar concepts from previous studies.

13. In grounded theory, the _____ category is a central pattern that is relevant to participants.

14. In Benner's hermeneutic approach, the presentation of _____ in reports allows readers to draw conclusions about the validity of the results.

15. The second level of analysis in Spradley's ethnographic method, yielding an organizational structure for the data, is called _____.

16. The first stage of grounded theory analysis involves _____ coding.

17. _____ cases, in one approach to hermeneutic analysis, are strong examples of ways of being in the world.

B. MATCHING EXERCISE

Match each descriptive statement from Set B with one or more types of qualitative analyses from Set A. Indicate the letter(s) corresponding to your response next to each item in Set B.

SET A

   a. Grounded theory analysis
   b. Phenomenologic/hermeneutic analysis
   c. Ethnographic analysis
   d. None of the above

SET B   RESPONSES

1. Involves the development of coding categories   _____
2. Begins with "open coding"   _____
3. One method of analysis was developed by Colaizzi   _____
4. Data can be organized using computer software   _____
5. One method of analysis was developed by Glaser and Strauss   _____
6. May involve the development of a taxonomy   _____
7. One analytic approach involves identifying paradigm cases   _____
8. Requires the use of quasi-statistics   _____

C. STUDY QUESTIONS

1. What is wrong with the following statements?

   a. Perez conducted a grounded theory study about coping with a miscarriage and she was able to identify four major themes.

   b. Schwartz's ethnographic analysis of Haitian clinics involved gleaning related thematic material from French poetry.

   c. Titterton's phenomenological study of the lived experience of Parkinson's disease focused on the domain of fatigue.

   d. Levine's grounded theory study of widowhood yielded a taxonomy of coping strategies.

   e. In her ethnographic study of the culture of a nursing home, Stimpfle used a rural nursing home as a paradigm case.

2. Use the category scheme presented in Box 16.1 on page 303 in the textbook (also available on thePoint) to code the following segments from actual interviews:

> My first birth was horrendous. As soon as I became pregnant with my second child I read absolutely everything I could possibly get my hands on about childbirth from midwifery textbooks to independent research papers. I was determined that this next time was going to be very different. I would be very aware of the facts and I would have a better understanding of my own needs for privacy, control, and emotional support.
>
> I then went about choosing an independent midwife. I interviewed 2 lovely women, and asked them identical questions. I told them both that I had not dilated beyond 3 cm in my first birth and asked what they would do if I got to 3 cm and then progress slowed. Midwife #1 said she would probably transfer me to the hospital. Midwife #2 said she would just wait until things changed. She talked about how much faith she had in the female body. I went with midwife #2.
>
> During my pregnancy I bought a copy of *Birthing from Within* and spent a lot of time painting my previous birth experience and how I envisioned birth #2. I truly nurtured myself. I swam, did yoga, walked, and spent lots of time outdoors and enjoyed being with my 2-year-old.
>
> Over my pregnancy I felt very supported by my midwife and I became able to trust her. My husband and I also hired a doula to make sure both he and I would be supported during this labor and delivery.

3. Suppose a researcher was studying people with hypertension who were struggling unsuccessfully for months to manage their weight. The researcher plans to interview 10 to 20 people for this study. Answer the following questions:

    a. What might be the research question that a phenomenologist would ask relating to this situation? And what might the research question be for a grounded theory researcher?

    b. Which do you think would take longer to do—the analysis of data for the phenomenological or the grounded theory? Why?

    c. What would the final "product" of the analyses be for the two different studies?

    d. Which study would have more appeal to you? Why?

 4. Read the following study, Marcuccilli, L., Casida, J., Peters, R., & Wright, S. (2011). Sex and intimacy among patients with implantable left-ventricular assist devices. *Journal of Cardiovascular Nursing, 26*, 504–511. Critique how well the researchers described the analytic process for this phenomenological study.

D. APPLICATION EXERCISES

Exercise D.1: Study in Appendix E

Read the "Design and Methods" and "Findings" sections of the report by Byrne and colleagues ("Care transition experiences") in Appendix E on pages 157–174 and then answer the following questions. (Note: The following questions supplement the critical thinking questions for Example 1 in the textbook on page 317):

Questions of Fact

a. Did the researchers audiotape and transcribe the interviews? If yes, who did the transcription? Did the report state how many pages of data comprised the data set?

b. Did data collection and data analysis occur concurrently?

c. Was a computer used to analyze the data? If yes, what software was used?

d. Did the researchers calculate any quasi-statistics?

e. Were there any metaphors used to highlight key findings?

f. Did the researchers prepare any analytic memos?

g. Did the authors describe the coding process? If so, what did they say?

Questions for Discussion

a. Discuss the effectiveness of the researchers' presentation of results. Does the analysis seem sensible, thoughtful, and thorough?

b. Were data presented in a manner that allows you to be confident about the researchers' conclusions? Comment on the inclusion or noninclusion of figures that graphically represent the grounded theory.

c. Comment on the amount of verbatim quotes from study participants that were included in this report.

Exercise D.2: Study in Appendix F

Read the "Data Analysis" and "Results" sections of the article by Cummings ("Sharing a traumatic event") in Appendix F on pages 175–182 and then answer the following questions:

Questions of Fact

a. Did Cummings audiotape and transcribe the interviews?

b. Did Cummings organize her data manually or with the assistance of computer software? If the latter, what software was used?

c. Did Cummings calculate any quasi-statistics?

d. Which phenomenologic analytic approach was adopted in this study?

e. Did Cummings prepare any reflective memos or keep a reflective journal?

f. Did Cummings describe the coding process? If so, what did she say?

g. How many themes emerged in Cummings' analysis? What were they?

h. Did Cummings provide supporting evidence for her themes, in the form of excerpts from the data?

Questions for Discussion

a. Discuss the thoroughness of Cummings' description of her data analysis efforts. Did the report present adequate information about the steps taken to analyze the data?

b. Was there any evidence of "method slurring"—that is, did Cummings apply any analytic procedures that are inappropriate for a phenomenological approach?

c. Discuss the effectiveness of Cummings' presentation of results. Does the analysis seem sensible, thoughtful, and thorough? Was sufficient evidence provided to support the findings? Were data presented in a manner that allows you to be confident about Cummings' conclusions?

CHAPTER 17

Trustworthiness and Integrity in Qualitative Research

A. FILL IN THE BLANKS

How many terms have you learned in this chapter? Fill in the blanks in the sentences below to find out. Try doing this section with a friend. Which of you is the first one to complete the sentence?

1. _____ is a key criterion for assessing quality in qualitative studies, concerning confidence in the truth value of the findings.

2. Use of multiple means of converging on the truth is called _____.

3. The stability of data over time and conditions, analogous to reliability, is called _____.

4. The quality criterion concerning the extent to which qualitative findings can be applied to other settings is called _____.

5. The dependability of an inquiry can be enhanced by a(n) _____ trail that documents judgments and choices.

6. Transferability is enhanced through the researcher's use of _____ in a research report.

7. The criterion of _____ refers to the potential for congruence between independent coders, analysts, or interpreters of qualitative data—its analog in quantitative studies is objectivity.

8. Credibility in qualitative inquiry has been described as analogous to _____ validity in quantitative inquiry.

9. Persistent _____ refers to a focus on the aspects of a situation that are relevant to the phenomena being studied.

10. A process by which researchers revise their interpretations by including cases that appear to disconfirm earlier hypotheses is a(n) _____ case analysis.

11. One method of addressing credibility is to do _____ checks, which involve going back to participants to have them review preliminary findings.

12. _____ triangulation is achieved by having two or more researchers make key decisions and interpretations.

13. _____ is a quality criterion indicating the extent to which the researchers fairly and faithfully portray a range of different realities.

103

14. The strategy of _____ debriefing involves seeking the input from other researchers regarding the analysis of interpretation of qualitative data.

15. The strategy of _____ engagement involves a researcher's investment of sufficient time collecting and analyzing qualitative data.

B. MATCHING EXERCISES

Match each statement from Set B with one of the phrases from Set A. Indicate the letter corresponding to your response next to each of the statements in Set B.

SET A

a. Data source triangulation

b. Investigator triangulation

c. Theory triangulation

d. Method triangulation

SET B   RESPONSES

1. A researcher studying health beliefs of the rural elderly
interviews old people and health care providers in the area   _____

2. A researcher tests narrative data, collected in interviews with
people who attempted suicide, against two alternative
explanations of stress and coping   _____

3. Two researchers independently interview 10 informants in a
study of adjustment to a cancer diagnosis and debrief with
each other to review what they have learned   _____

4. A researcher studying embarrassment in school-based clinics
observes interactions in the clinics and also conducts in-depth
interviews with students   _____

5. A researcher studying the process of resolving an infertility
problem interviews husbands and wives separately   _____

6. Themes emerging in the field notes of an observer on a
psychiatric ward are categorized and labeled independently
by the researcher and an assistant   _____

C. STUDY QUESTIONS

1. Suppose you were conducting a grounded theory study of couples' coming to terms with infertility. What might you do to incorporate various types of triangulation into your study?

2. What is your opinion about the value of member checking as a strategy to enhance credibility? Defend your position.

3. Read a research report in a recent issue of the journal *Qualitative Health Research*. Identify several examples of "thick description." Also, identify areas of the report in which you feel additional thick description would have enhanced the transferability of the evidence.

4. Read the abstract, and then the Method section, of one of the following studies. Comment on the amount of information the researchers provided regarding the integrity and trustworthiness of the study:

   • Hadders, H. (2011). Negotiating leave-taking events in the palliative medicine unit. *Qualitative Health Research, 21*, 223–232.

   • McNiesh, S., Benner, P., & Chesla, C. (2011). Learning formative skills of nursing practice in an accelerated program. *Qualitative Health Research, 21*, 51–61.

   • Wang, Y., Chen, S., Jou, H., Tsao, L. (2011). Doing the best to control: The experiences of Taiwanese women with lower urinary tract symptoms. *Nursing Research, 60*, 66–72.

D. APPLICATION EXERCISES

Exercise D.1: Study in Appendix E

Read the report by Byrne and colleagues ("Care transition experiences") in Appendix E on pages 157–174 and then answer the following questions:

Questions of Fact

a. Did the researchers devote a section of their report to describing their quality-enhancement strategies? If so, what was it labeled? If not, where was information about such strategies located?

b. What types of triangulation, if any, were used in this study?

c. Were any of the following methods used to enhance the credibility of the study and its data:

   • Prolonged engagement and/or persistent observation
   • Member checks
   • Search for disconfirming evidence
   • Reflexivity
   • Audit trail

Questions for Discussion

a. Discuss the thoroughness with which Byrne and colleagues described their efforts to enhance and evaluate the quality and integrity of their study.

b. How would you characterize the integrity and trustworthiness of this study, based on the researchers' documentation? How would you describe the credibility, dependability, confirmability, authenticity, and transferability of this study?

Exercise D.2: Study in Appendix F

Read the report by Cummings and colleagues ("Sharing a traumatic event") in Appendix F on pages 175–182 and then answer the following questions:

Questions of Fact

a. Did the researchers devote a section of their report to describing their quality-enhancement strategies? If so, what was it labeled? If not, where was information about such strategies located?

b. What types of triangulation, if any, were used in this study?

c. Were any of the following methods used to enhance the credibility of the study and its data:

- Prolonged engagement and/or persistent observation
- Peer review and debriefing
- Member checks
- Search for disconfirming evidence
- Reflexivity
- Audit trail
- Researcher credibility

Questions for Discussion

a. Discuss the thoroughness with which Cummings described her efforts to enhance and evaluate the quality and integrity of her study.

b. How would you characterize the integrity and trustworthiness of this study, based on the researchers' documentation? How would you describe the credibility, dependability, confirmability, authenticity, and transferability of this study?

Special Topics
in Research

CHAPTER 18

Mixed Methods and Other Special Types of Research

A. FILL IN THE BLANKS

How many terms have you learned in this chapter? Fill in the blanks in the sentences below to find out. Try doing this section with a friend. Which of you is the first one to complete the sentence?

1. The type of research that integrates qualitative and quantitative data is mixed _____ research.

2. Mixed methods designs can be characterized by decisions on _____ and _____.

3. In the notation QUAL + quan, the dominant strand is the _____ component.

4. The notation QUAN(qual) signifies a(n) _____ design.

5. In mixed methods research, the design notation of an arrow (→) designates a design that is _____.

6. In mixed methods research, the design notation of a plus sign ("+") designates a design that is _____.

7. The paradigm most often associated with mixed methods research is called _____.

8. A(n) _____, which involves collecting self-report data about people's opinions, characteristics, and intentions, can be administered by telephone, by mail, over the Internet, or in person.

9. A(n) _____ is a multiphase effort to refine and test the effectiveness of a clinical treatment.

10. A Phase II trial often involves a pilot _____ of a new treatment.

11. Phase IV clinical trials are sometimes called _____ studies.

12. In nursing intervention research, the construct validity of a new intervention is enhanced by the construction of a(n) _____.

13. A(n) _____ analysis in evaluation research provides information about the net effects of a program over and above what is standard or usual, usually using an experimental design.

109

14. An evaluation of how a new intervention gets implemented is a(n) _____ analysis.

15. _____ research involves efforts to understand the end results of health care practices.

16. In the Donabedian framework, the three key factors are process, outcomes, and _____.

17. A(n) _____ analysis involves undertaking a study using an existing dataset to answer new questions.

18. The type of research that focuses on improving research strategies is called _____ research.

19. Phase III of a clinical trial is a(n) _____ controlled trial.

B. MATCHING EXERCISES

Match each feature from Set B with one (or more) of the phrases from Set A that indicates a type of quantitative research. Indicate the letter(s) corresponding to your response next to each statement in Set B.

SET A

a. Clinical trial

b. Evaluation research

c. Methodological research

d. Survey research

e. Outcomes research

f. Secondary analysis

SET B   RESPONSES

1. Can involve an experimental design   _____

2. Examines the global effectiveness of nursing services   _____

3. Data are always from self-reports   _____

4. The aim is to develop better instruments and procedures for doing substantive research   _____

5. Often designed in a series of phases (typically four)   _____

6. Includes process analyses   _____

7. Donabedian's framework is often used in this research   _____

8. Avoids time-consuming and costly research steps   _____

C. STUDY QUESTIONS

1. Read one of the following studies, in which quantitative data were gathered and analyzed to address a research question. Suggest ways in which the collection of qualitative data might have enriched the study, strengthened its validity, or enhanced its interpretability:

- Coyle, S. B. (2011). Maternal concern, social support, and health-related quality of life across childhood. *Research in Nursing & Health, 34*, 297–309.
- Ham, O. K. (2011). Predictors of quality of life among low-income women. *Western Journal of Nursing Research, 33*, 63–78.
- Suh, E. E. (2012). The effects of P6 acupressure and nurse-provided counseling on chemotherapy-induced nausea and vomiting in patients with breast cancer. *Oncology Nursing Forum, 39*, E1–E9.

2. Read one of the following qualitative studies. Suggest ways that the findings could be validated or the emergent hypotheses could be tested in a quantitative study:

- DeSantis, J., & Barroso, S. (2011). Living in silence: A grounded theory study of vulnerability in the context of HIV infection. *Issues in Mental Health Nursing, 32*, 345–354.
- Foulkes, M. (2011). Enablers and barriers to seeking help for a postpartum mood disorder. *Journal of Obstetric, Gynecologic, & Neonatal Nursing, 40*, 450–457.
- Myers, J. S. (2012). Chemotherapy-related cognitive impairment: The breast cancer experience. *Oncology Nursing Forum, 39*, E31–E40.

3. Below is a brief description of a mixed methods study, followed by a critique. Do you agree with this critique? Can you add other comments regarding the study design?

FICTITIOUS STUDY

Garvey conducted a study to examine the emotional well-being of women who had a mastectomy. Garvey wanted to develop an in-depth understanding of the emotional experiences of women as they recovered from their surgery, including the process by which they handled their fears, their concerns about their sexuality, their levels of anxiety and depression, their methods of coping, and their social supports.

Garvey's basic study design was a descriptive qualitative study. She gathered information from a sample of 26 women, primarily by means of in-depth interviews with the women on two occasions. The first interviews were scheduled within 1 month after the surgery. Follow-up interviews were conducted about 12 months later. Several women in the sample participated in a support group, and Garvey attended and made observations at several meetings. Additionally, Garvey decided to interview the "significant other" (usually the husbands) of most of the women, when it became clear that the women's emotional well-being was linked to the manner in which the significant other was reacting to the surgery.

In addition to the rich, in-depth information she gathered, Garvey wanted to be able to better interpret the emotional status of the women. Therefore, at both the original and follow-up interviews with the women, she administered a psychological scale known as the Center for Epidemiological Studies Depression Scale (CES-D), a quantitative measure that has scores that can range from 0 to 60. This scale has been widely used in community populations and has cut-off scores designating when a person is at risk of clinical depression (i.e., a score of 16 and above).

Garvey's qualitative analysis showed that the basic process underlying psychological recovery from the mastectomy was something she labeled "Gaining by Losing," a process that involved heightened self-awareness and self-respect after an initial period of despair and self-pity. The process also involved, for some, a strengthening of personal relationships with significant others, whereas for others, it resulted in the birth of awareness of fundamental deficiencies in their relationships. The quantitative findings confirmed that a very high percentage of women were at risk of being depressed at 1 month after the mastectomy, but at 12 months, the average level of depression was modestly lower than in the general population of women.

CRITIQUE

In her study, Garvey embedded a quantitative measure into her field work in an interesting manner. The bulk of data were qualitative—in-depth interviews and in-depth observations. However, she also opted to include a well-known measure of depression, which provided her with an important context for interpreting her data. A major advantage of using the CES-D is that this scale has known characteristics in the general population, and therefore provided a built-in "comparison group."

Garvey used a flexible design that allowed her to use her initial data to guide her inquiry. For example, she decided to conduct in-depth interviews with significant others when she learned their importance to the women's process of emotional recovery. Garvey did do some advance planning, however, that provided general guidance. For example, although her questioning likely evolved while in the field, she had the foresight to realize that to capture a process as it evolved, she would need to collect data longitudinally. She also made the up-front decision to use the CES-D to supplement the in-depth interviews.

In this study, the findings from the qualitative and quantitative portions of the study were complementary. Both portions of the study confirmed that the women initially had emotional "losses," but eventually they recovered and "gained" in terms of their emotional well-being and their self-awareness. This example illustrates how the validity of study findings can be enhanced by the blending of qualitative and quantitative data. If the qualitative data alone had been gathered, Garvey might not have gotten a good handle on the degree to which the women had actually "recovered" (vis-à-vis women who had never had a mastectomy). Conversely, if she had collected only the CES-D data, she would have had no insights into the process by which the recovery occurred.

 4. Read the following mixed methods study, Dickson, V., McCarthy, M., Howe, A., Schipper, J., & Katz, S. (2012). Sociocultural influences on heart failure self-care among an ethnic minority black population. *Journal of Cardiovascular Nursing, 26*, E1-E10.

Describe how the study would have yielded less complete information if only qualitative or only quantitative data had been gathered.

D. APPLICATION EXERCISES

Exercise D.1: All Studies in Appendices

Which of the studies in the appendices of this *Study Guide* (if any) could be considered:

a. a clinical trial?

b. an economic analysis?

c. outcomes research?

d. survey research?

e. a secondary analysis?

f. methodological research?

Exercise D.2: Study in Appendix B

Read the article by Cricco-Lizza ("Rooting for the breast") in Appendix B on pages 129–138.

    Was this a mixed methods study? If yes, describe its design. If no, redesign the study in such a fashion that it would involve mixed methods. In your design, specify the following: (a) the new question(s) that would be addressed; (b) the specific design, using symbols to designate priority and sequence; (c) the sampling design that would be used; and (d) the additional data that would be collected.

Exercise D.3: Study in Appendix D

Read the article by Jurgens and colleagues ("Responding to heart failure symptoms") in Appendix D on pages 147–156 and then answer the following questions:

Questions of Fact

a. Was this a mixed methods study? If yes, what was the purpose of the quantitative strand, and what was the purpose of the qualitative strand?
b. Which strand had priority in the study design?
c. Was the design sequential or concurrent?
d. Using the design names used in the textbook, what would the design be called?
e. How would the design be portrayed using the notation system described in the textbook? Did the researchers themselves use this notation?
f. What sampling design was used in this study?
g. What did the report say about integrating the two strands?

Questions for Discussion

a. Evaluate the use of a mixed methods approach in this study. Did the approach yield richer or more useful information than would have been achieved with a single-strand study?
b. Discuss the researchers' choice of a specific research design and the sampling design. Would an alternative mixed methods design have been preferable? If so, why?

Systematic Reviews: Meta-Analysis and Metasynthesis

A. FILL IN THE BLANKS

How many terms have you learned in this chapter? Fill in the blanks in the sentences below to find out. Try doing this section with a friend. Which of you is the first one to complete the sentence?

1. A systematic review that integrates study findings statistically is called a(n) _____.

2. Statistical _____ concerns dissimilarity among the effect size estimates of different primary studies in a meta-analysis.

3. Another name for the effect index d for comparing two group means is *standardized mean* _____.

4. One way to address primary study quality is to do a(n) _____ analysis that includes and then excludes studies of low quality.

5. A(n) _____ analysis involves examining the extent to which effects differ for different types of studies or types of people—i.e., whether effects are *moderated* by other factors.

6. The type of meta-analytic model that is preferred when heterogeneity is high is called a(n) _____ effects model.

7. There tends to be a bias against the _____ hypothesis in studies that get published.

8. For some outcomes, the effect size index is the odds _____.

9. The body of unpublished studies is sometimes referred to as _____ literature.

10. To use a(n) _____ effects model to analyze aggregate effects, heterogeneity should be low.

11. A(n) _____ plot is a graphic display of the effect size (including CIs around it for each primary study in a meta-analysis.

12. In a synthesis of qualitative studies, a(n) _____ effect size is the ratio of the number of themes represented in one report, divided by all relevant themes relating to a phenomenon across all reports.

13. A concern in a systematic review is the _____ bias that stems from identifying only studies in journals and books.

114

14. A(n) _____ effect size in a synthesis of qualitative studies is the ratio of reports with a particular thematic finding, divided by all reports describing study results on a phenomenon.

15. A(n) _____, which involves calculating manifest effect sizes, can lay the foundation for a metasynthesis.

B. MATCHING EXERCISE

Match each of the statements in Set B with the appropriate phrase in Set A. Indicate the letter(s) corresponding to your response next to each of the statements in Set B.

SET A

a. Meta-analysis

b. Metasynthesis

c. Neither meta-analysis nor metasynthesis

d. Both meta-analysis and metasynthesis

SET B   RESPONSES

1. Involves gathering data from human participants   _____

2. Focuses on synthesizing information from prior studies   _____

3. Relies on findings from qualitative studies   _____

4. May involve an assessment of publication bias   _____

5. Sandelowski developed important approaches for this   _____

6. Often involves calculating *d* or OR statistics   _____

7. CINAHL likely would be used for this in searching for primary studies   _____

8. Can involve the calculation of a frequency effect size   _____

C. STUDY QUESTIONS

1. Read one of the following meta-analysis reports:
   - Beck, C. T., (2001). Predictors of postpartum depression: An update. *Nursing Research, 50*, 275–285.
   - Conn, V., Valentine, J., & Cooper, H. (2002). Interventions to increase physical activity among aging adults: A meta-analysis. *Annals of Behavioral Medicine, 24*, 190–200.
   - Fetzer, S. J. (2002). Reducing venipuncture and intravenous insertion pain with eutectic mixture of local anesthetic. *Nursing Research, 51*, 119–124.

Then, search the literature for related quantitative primary studies published *after* this meta-analysis. Are new study results consistent with the conclusions drawn in the meta-analytic report? Are there enough new primary studies to warrant a new meta-analysis?

2. Read one of the following metasynthesis reports:

- Beck, C. T. (2002). Postpartum depression: A metasynthesis. *Qualitative Health Research*, *12*, 453–472.
- Lefler, L., & Bondy, L. (2004). Women's delay in seeking treatment with myocardial infarction: A meta-synthesis. *Journal of Cardiovascular Nursing, 19*, 251–268.
- Nelson, A. M. (2002). A metasynthesis: Mothering other-than-normal children. *Qualitative Health Research, 12*, 515–530.

Then, search the literature for related qualitative primary studies published *after* this metasynthesis. Are new study results consistent with the conclusions drawn in the metasynthesis report? Are there enough new primary studies to warrant a new metasynthesis?

3. Skim the following report, which involved a systematic review without a meta-analysis. Did the authors adequately justify their decision not to conduct a meta-analysis?

- Shepherd, C., & While, A. (2012). Cardiac rehabilitation and quality of life: A systematic review. *International Journal of Nursing Studies, 49*, 755–771.

D. APPLICATION EXERCISES

Exercise D.1: Study in Appendix G

Read the report on the meta-analysis by Nam and colleagues ("Effect of culturally tailored diabetes education") in Appendix G on pages 183–196 and then answer the following questions:

Questions of Fact

a. What was the stated purpose of this review? What were the independent and dependent variables in this review?

b. What inclusion criteria were stipulated? How many studies met all inclusion criteria?

c. How many of the studies included in this meta-analysis used an experimental (randomized) design? How many were nonexperimental or quasi-experimental?

d. Did the researchers rate each study in the dataset for its quality? If yes, what aspects of the study were appraised? What was the highest possible quality score? How many people scored the studies for quality? Was interrater agreement assessed?

e. What was the cutoff score for high versus low quality? How many studies were rated low quality and how many were high quality? Did the researchers set a threshold for study quality as part of their inclusion criteria? If yes, what was it? Were any studies excluded because of a low quality rating?

f. What effect size measure was used in the analysis?

g. Did the researchers perform any tests for statistical heterogeneity? Was a fixed effects or random effects model used?

h. How many participants were there in total, in all studies combined?

i. Overall, what was the value of the average effect size for the tailored interventions? Was this effect size significant?

j. Considering the information in Figure 2, answer the following questions:
   - In which study was the effect size the largest? Was this effect size statistically significant?
   - Were effect sizes nonsignificant in any studies? If yes, which one(s)?
   - Were there any studies where the effect size was in the opposite direction from what was anticipated?

k. Were subgroup analyses undertaken? If yes, what subgroups were examined? What were the key findings?

Questions for Discussion

a. Was the size of the sample (studies and subjects) sufficiently large to draw conclusions about the overall intervention effects and about subgroup effects?

b. What other subgroups might have been interesting to examine (assume there was sufficient information in the original studies)?

c. How would you assess the overall rigor of this meta-analysis?

d. Based on this review, what is the evidence regarding interventions for ethnic minorities with type 2 diabetes? What are the implications for nursing practice?

Exercise D.2: Study in Appendix H

Read the report on the metasynthesis by Beck ("A metaethnography of traumatic childbirth") in Appendix H on pages 197–208 and then answer the following questions:

Questions of Fact

a. In what way was this metasynthesis different from a typical metasynthesis?

b. What was Beck's position in the controversy regarding integration across different research traditions?

c. Were the data in the primary studies derived from interviews, observations, or both?

d. How many mothers participated in the six primary studies?

e. What approach was used to conduct this metasynthesis? Was the analytic process described?

f. Was a meta-summary performed?

g. How many shared themes were identified in this metasynthesis? What were those themes?

h. Was Beck's analysis supported through the inclusion of raw data from the primary studies?

Questions for Discussion

a. Was the size of the sample (studies and subjects) sufficiently large to conduct a meaningful metasynthesis? Comment on the extent to which the diversity of the sample enhanced or weakened the metasynthesis.

b. Did the analysis and integration appear reasonable and thorough?

c. Were primary studies adequately described?

d. How would you assess the overall rigor of this metasynthesis? What would you recommend doing to improve its quality?

e. Based on this metasynthesis, what is the evidence regarding the experiences of birth trauma for mothers?

Nursing Research • March/April 2011 • Vol 60, No 2, 82–91

Computer Intervention Impact on Psychosocial Adaptation of Rural Women With Chronic Conditions

Clarann Weinert ▾ Shirley Cudney ▾ Bryan Comstock ▾ Aasthaa Bansal

▶ **Background:** Adapting to living with chronic conditions is a life-long psychosocial challenge.

▶ **Objective:** The purpose of this study was to report the effect of a computer intervention on the psychosocial adaptation of rural women with chronic conditions.

▶ **Methods:** A two-group study design was used with 309 middle-aged, rural women who had chronic conditions, randomized into either a computer-based intervention or a control group. Data were collected at baseline, at the end of the intervention, and 6 months later on the psychosocial indicators of social support, self-esteem, acceptance of illness, stress, depression, and loneliness.

▶ **Results:** The impact of the computer-based intervention was statistically significant for five of six of the psychosocial outcomes measured, with a modest impact on social support. The largest benefits were seen in depression, stress, and acceptance.

▶ **Discussion:** The women-to-women intervention resulted in positive psychosocial responses that have the potential to contribute to successful management of illness and adaptation. Other components of adaptation to be examined are the impact of the intervention on illness management and quality of life and the interrelationships among environmental stimuli, psychosocial response, and illness management.

▶ **Key Words:** computer-based intervention · psychosocial health · rural · women

C hronic illness has been described as a *constant shadow* (Massie, 1984) that pervades the lives of 133 million Americans (Centers for Disease Control and Prevention, 2010) who have chronic conditions. Adapting to living under this shadow is a life-long psychosocial challenge for persons with long-term health problems as they struggle to find a balance between the demands of their illness and their capacity to respond to these demands (Pollock, Christian, & Sands, 1990). Individuals contending with an enduring illness must deal with countless psychological issues because they are frightened by persistent symptoms, given fleeting hope by remissions, frustrated by the unpredictability of the course of the illness, and exhausted by its progression. The onset of chronic illness may challenge individuals' assump-

tions about their sense of self-worth, sense of invulnerability, and optimism about the future (Helgeson & Reynolds, 2002). The chronic illness experience can engender a *loss of self*—a fundamental form of suffering in those with chronic conditions (Charmaz, 1983) or, as one affected individual expressed it, "I feel like I have been robbed of my person-hood sometimes" (Weinert, 2009).

Persons with chronic health conditions also must deal with people who fail to understand the condition. One woman who lived the experience offered her explanation of this phenomenon:

> You have to remember that no matter how supportive our spouses, family or regular friends might be, they really don't understand everything there is to know about our diseases. They can hear us telling them things, they can read up on the disease, they can even ask our doctors, but unless they have the same disease, they just can't fully understand it. It's like trying to explain to a man, what it's like to give birth. They will never know (Weinert, 2009).

Such psychological and social challenges can result in an imbalance or disorganization of body, mind, and spirit (Royer, 1998).

The way individuals respond to these psychosocial assaults determines how well they adjust to living with the chronic illness. Adaptation to a chronic condition is relentless and requires making day-to-day adjustments to achieve an acceptable quality of life. The journey for rural dwellers is made more difficult by isolation as well as limited access to support systems and health services. Often, these individuals work alone to meet the psychosocial challenges of adapting to their chronic illnesses. Technology-based interventions have shown promise of being viable resources for providing social support and health information that rural dwellers need to help them adapt more successfully to living with their

Clarann Weinert, SC, PhD, RN, FAAN, is Professor, College of Nursing, Montana State University, Bozeman.

Shirley Cudney, MA, RN, is Associate Professor (Retired), College of Nursing, Montana State University, Bozeman.

Bryan Comstock, MS, is Biostatistician, Department of Biostatistics, University of Washington, Seattle.

Aasthaa Bansal, MS, is Biostatistics Research Assistant, Department of Biostatistics, University of Washington, Seattle.

DOI: 10.1097/NNR.0b013e3181ffbcf2

119

chronic conditions (Griffiths, Lindenmeyer, Powell, Lowe, & Thorogood, 2006; Weinert, Cudney, & Hill, 2008).

Background

Helping individuals adapt successfully to living with their chronic conditions has become a daunting task for America's healthcare system, especially providing appropriate care for those 20% who live in rural locations and experience higher rates of chronic illness than their urban counterparts (Rural Assistance Center, 2010). Fortunately, in recent years, the Internet has increased the potential for healthcare providers to reach out to geographically isolated people with chronic conditions. Bandura (2004) commented that by designing interventions that link the interactive aspects of chronic illness self-management education to the Internet, its availability could be expanded "to people wherever they may live at whatever time they may choose to use it" (p. 624). The proportion of use of the Internet by rural dwellers grew from 39.2% in March 2000 to 63.1% in May 2008 (Hale, Cotten, Brentea, & Goldner, 2010). Thus, they had access to a huge fund of health information at a distance and without having to consult a health professional (Norman, 2009). Of rural people with chronic conditions who used the Internet, 86% reported seeking health information, and the information gained was used by 75% to influence a health-related decision (Fox, 2007).

Concurrent with the growth and utilization of the Internet, research about the potential effects of Web-based interventions on the psychosocial well-being of affected adults and, ultimately, their ability to *adapt* to living with chronic illness proliferated (Bond, Burr, Wolf, & Feldt, 2010). However, studies targeting rural populations with chronic conditions were few. In a global study of 37 health interventions using the Internet (Griffiths et al., 2006), only five stated *geographical isolation* as their reason for using the technology. Thus, the need for the provision of Internet-based interventions for rural dwellers that could support them in their quest to adapt to and lift the shadow of living with a chronic condition was evident.

Adaptation is a dynamic, complex process that has been evaluated from many perspectives by different sets of criteria. From the myriad of possible empirical indicators of psychosocial adaptation reported, those selected for examination in this study were social support, self-esteem, acceptance of illness, stress, depression, and loneliness.

Social support can help persons with chronic conditions to adopt positive health behaviors, minimize risky behaviors, diminish physiologic reactivity to stress, and decrease depression (Helgeson & Reynolds, 2002). The level of perceived support has been linked also to positive adaptive outcomes including physical health, mental well-being, and successful social functioning (White, Richter, & Fry, 1992).

Self-esteem is related to self-concept and how others respond, and the character of these responses can impact the psychological well-being of the individual significantly (Falvo, 2005). Maintaining self-esteem in the chronically ill is essential because people with a sense of high self-esteem adjust more successfully to chronic illness (Helgeson & Reynolds, 2002).

The process of adaptation also includes a search for meaning in the illness experience, culminating in the acceptance of the condition and associated limitations (Falvo, 2005).

Acceptance of illness is defined as the recognition by individuals that they are ill, prepared to relinquish the old definition of self and life before becoming ill, and ready to deal with the restrictions and changes in everyday life imposed by the illness (Juczynski, 2001).

Psychological threats, those that tax or exceed resources and endanger well-being, are the most important stressors with which humans have to cope. Stress can precipitate illness and has a disruptive impact on chronic health conditions (Carnegie Mellon University, 2007). Effectively managing disease-related stressors is key to finding meaning and purpose in life and moving toward acceptance (White et al., 1992).

Depression, one of the most common complications of chronic illness, has been identified as a negative indicator of psychological adaptation to chronic illness (Buchanan & Abram, 1975). Because of the negative impact on lifestyle, mobility, independence, recreational activities, and physical comfort, chronic illness can result in feelings of despair and sadness (Chakraburtty, 2007). Depression is closely linked with loneliness (Shaver & Brennan, 1991), a complex set of feelings arising from the absence of intimate and social resources (Ernst & Cacioppo, 1999).

Social isolation can be a major detrimental consequence of chronic illness and puts all persons with long-term health problems at high risk for a negative sense of aloneness or reduced participation in social relationships (Royer, 1998). Thus, loneliness can be thought of as a negative indicator of adaptation.

Purpose

To provide persons with long-term illnesses the support, the skills, and the resources needed to adapt successfully to living with their illnesses and to maintain quality of life, chronic care interventions are emerging (Lorig & Holman, 2003). However, such programs may be inaccessible to underserved populations such as chronically ill rural women who live in health service-deficient areas. In an attempt to bridge the accessibility gap to enhance the potential for rural women to adapt more successfully to their chronic illnesses, the women-to-women (WTW) computer-based research project was launched in 1995 and has evolved continuously. Historically, the design of the study was influenced by the pioneering efforts of Brennan, Ripich, and Moore's (1991) use of computers to provide support to persons living with AIDS and later the Stanford Chronic Disease Self-Management Program (Lorig, Ritter, Laurent, & Plant, 2006). The latest phase of the WTW project, consistent with the evolving adaptation to chronic illness conceptual base, was designed to test the effectiveness of a computer-based intervention on psychosocial adaptation, illness management, and quality of life. The specific purpose of this article is to report the effect of the latest phase of the WTW intervention on psychosocial adaptation as measured by selected positive and negative empirical indicators.

Methods

The WTW study was approved and monitored by the University Institutional Review Board for the Protection of Human Subjects. Participants were required to be between the ages of 35 and 65 years and live at least 25 miles outside a town or a city of 12,500 or more on a ranch, on a farm, or in a small town in Idaho, Montana, Nebraska, Iowa, North Dakota, Oregon, South Dakota, Washington, or Wyoming. They were recruited through mass media, agency and service organization newsletters, and word of mouth. Those who contacted the research office were screened via a telephone interview and then randomized into an intervention or control group (Figure 1). The project has been described in detail in previous publications (Weinert, Cudney, & Hill, 2008); therefore, only a limited description will be provided here.

Design

A randomized controlled study design was used with participants assigned to either a computer-based intervention or a control group. For practical convenience, study participants were enrolled into one of eight cohorts, with each cohort consisting of approximately 20 participants in each of the two groups. Data were collected via mailed questionnaires from both groups at baseline, at the end of the intervention, and 6 months later. The research staff was not blinded to the participant groups.

The computer group participated in an 11-week intervention that gave the women 24-hour access to (a) a peer-led virtual support group and (b) a series of self-study health teaching units focused on Web skills and the five skills of self-management (problem solving, decision making, resource utilization, forming partnerships with healthcare providers, and taking action; Lorig & Holman, 2003). The virtual support group consisted of an asynchronous forum, Sharing Circle, in which the women exchanged feelings and life experiences, gave and received support, discussed issues related to the self-study health teaching units, and shared discoveries of pertinent Internet-based health information (Weinert, Cudney, & Spring, 2008). The control group had no access to the intervention, and their sole responsibility was to complete the questionnaires. To help maintain the sample, after the return of the last questionnaire, a monetary incentive of $75 was provided to all participants (intervention and control) along with *Living a Healthy Life With Chronic Conditions* (Lorig et al., 2000). Data were collected between 2007 and 2009.

Measures

This latest phase of the WTW project was guided by *The Women to Women Conceptual Model for Adaptation to Chronic Illness* (Figure 2). The basic tenets of the model are that people are bombarded with environmental stimuli (such as chronic illnesses) that evoke psychosocial responses that, in turn, can be a positive or a negative influence on their ability to self-manage their condition and on their overall

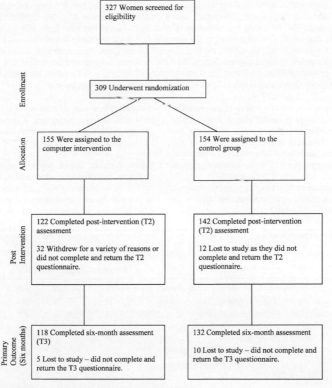

FIGURE 1. Randomization and follow-up of women-to-women study participants.

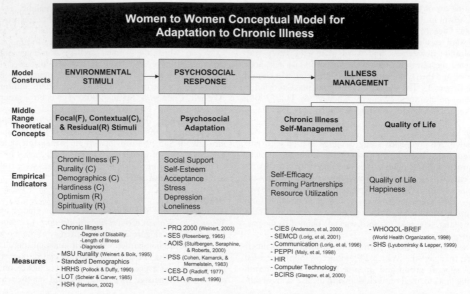

FIGURE 2. The *Women to Women Conceptual Model for Adaptation to Chronic Illness*. Adapted from "Evolution of a conceptual model for adaptation to chronic illness," by C. Weinert, S. Cudney, & A. Spring, 2008, *Journal of Nursing Scholarship, 40*, p. 366. Copyright 2008 by John Wiley & Sons. Reprinted with permission. MSU = Montana State University; HRHS = Health-Related Hardiness Scale; LOT = Life Orientation Test; HSH = Harrison Spirituality Scale; PRQ = Personal Resource Questionnaire; BCIRS = Brief Chronic Illness Resources Survey; SES = Self-esteem Scale; AOIS = Acceptance of Illness Scale; PSS = Perceived Stress Scale; CES-D = Center for Epidemiologic Studies–Depression Scale; UCLA = University of California, Los Angeles Loneliness Scale; CIES = Chronic Illness Empowerment Scale; SEMCD = Self-Efficacy for Managing Chronic Disease; PEPPI = Perceived Efficacy in Patient–Physician Interactions Questionnaire; HIR = Health Information Resources; WHOQOL-BREF = World Health Organization Quality of Life–BREF; SHS = Subjective Happiness Scale.

quality of life. The task was to select a representative number of pertinent indicators to be targeted for change from among the many that make up the complex concept of adaptation. On the basis of the literature and the experience of the investigators, the selected psychosocial indicators were social support, self-esteem, acceptance of illness, stress, depression, and loneliness.

The selected measurement instruments were not designed specifically for use in rural environments but had wide application in a variety of populations and in chronic illness research. They were chosen on the basis of the strength of their psychometric properties, conceptual fit, amenability to change by an appropriate intervention, and experiential use by the research team (Table 1).

Social Support Social support was described by Weiss (1969) as the provision of intimacy, facilitation of social integration, opportunity for nurturant behavior, reassurance of self-worth, and availability of assistance. Social support can influence management of chronic illness positively

TABLE I. Psychosocial Factors

Empirical Indicators	Measures	No. Items	Reported α	Study α	Validity
Social support	Personal Resource Questionnaire 2000 (Weinert, 2003)	15	.87–.92	.933	Construct divergent
Self-esteem	Self-esteem Scale (Rosenberg, 1965)	10	.77–.88	.901	Convergent discriminant
Acceptance of illness	Acceptance of Illness Scale (Stuifbergen et al., 2000)	14	.81–.84	.824	Content
Depression	Center for Epidemiologic Studies–Depression Scale (Devine & Orme, 1985)	20	.84–.90	.922	Convergent discriminant
Stress	Perceived Stress Scale (Cohen et al., 1983)	14	.84–.86	.899	Convergent discriminant
Loneliness	University of California, Los Angeles Loneliness Scale (Russell, 1996)	20	.94	.921	Convergent discriminant

(Symister & Friend, 2003) and contribute to the desired outcome of successful adaptation. The Personal Resource Questionnaire 2000 has undergone psychometric evaluation systematically over the past 20 years and was considered the instrument of choice to measure social support. The Personal Resource Questionnaire 2000 has 15 items, each with a 7-point Likert item response set, with higher scores indicating a higher level of perceived support (Weinert, 2003).

Self-esteem Self-esteem is considered an indicator of psychological well-being and is thought by some to be a dimension of the potential to manage chronic illness. The Rosenberg Self-esteem Scale was selected as an easily administered, 10-item tool designed to measure global feelings of self-worth or self-acceptance (Rosenberg, 1965). It has been used widely in clinical practice and has been shown to be a reliable, internally consistent measure of global self-esteem (Gray-Little, Williams, & Hancock, 1997). Higher scores are indicative of higher levels of self-esteem.

Acceptance Acceptance of illness is defined not as resignation but as an integration of the disease into one's overall lifestyle. It is the notion that the illness must be accepted to *get on with living*. The Acceptance of Illness Scale (Stuifbergen, Seraphine, & Roberts, 2000) was included in the battery of indicators because it has been shown to influence health promotion and quality of life for persons with chronic illnesses. Potential scores range from 14 to 70, and higher scores indicate greater acceptance.

Depression Depression can be characterized by all-encompassing feelings of sadness, feelings of guilt or worthlessness, trouble concentrating or making decisions, and decreased interest or pleasure in what were normally enjoyable activities (Chakraburtty, 2007). Recognizing depression is important because it can undermine confidence, concentration, energy, and motivation—essential ingredients in adapting effectively to chronic illness (Simon, Von Korff, & Lin, 2005). The widely used Center for Epidemiologic Studies–Depression Scale (Devine & Orme, 1985) was selected as the appropriate measure for depressive symptomatology. Potential scores range from 0 to 60, with higher scores indicating higher levels of distress. A score of 16 or greater is considered to suggest a clinically significant level of psychological distress.

Stress Health- or illness-related stressors are events, situations, conditions, or cues that are generally unpredictable, result in dire consequences, and require adjustment or adaptation (Lyon, 2000). Developing the capacity to manage stress is often helpful in managing and adapting to the additional problems of a chronic illness (Cagle, 2004). The Perceived Stress Scale (Cohen, Kamarck, & Mermelstein, 1983) was used to assess the level of stress being experienced by the study participants. Scores on this 14-item scale can range from 0 to 56.

Loneliness Loneliness can be defined as a deficit in human intimacy and negative feelings about being alone (Hall & Havens, 1999). Rural women with chronic conditions may be at particular risk for loneliness because they are often geographically isolated. The University of California, Los Angeles Loneliness Scale (Russell, 1996), a well-recognized measure of loneliness, consisted of 20 Likert items rated on a 4-point scale, with potential scores ranging from 20 to 80; the higher the score, the higher degree of self-reported loneliness. The positive factors of social support, self-esteem, and acceptance and negative factors of depression, stress, and loneliness can be conceptualized as psychosocial health indicators of an individual's potential to manage and adapt to chronic illness.

Analysis

For the primary analysis, an analysis of covariance model was fit for each psychosocial outcome measured at 24 weeks, with treatment group as the independent variable of interest and adjusted for the baseline value of the outcome measure and cohort as a fixed effect covariate. An intention-to-treat approach was taken; the women were analyzed in accordance with the randomized group to which they were assigned, regardless of how closely they adhered to the assigned intervention. As a secondary analysis, the same models were fit as above, including an interaction between the treatment group and the cohort to test whether there were significant differences in treatment among the eight cohorts.

Because of a differential proportion of dropout by group (intervention vs. control), a sensitivity analysis was conducted to assess whether individuals with missing outcome data influenced the results of the primary analysis; that is, if study participants who failed to follow through with the computer-based intervention also tended to be sicker or have worse psychosocial health, there may be a potential for bias toward better psychosocial improvement with the computer-based intervention. In separate logistic regression models with dropout status indicator as the outcome, all available demographic or psychosocial variables were assessed as predictors of missing data at 24 weeks. These analyses were then repeated for each treatment group by including an interaction term between the treatment group assignment and the baseline variable. Finally, missing 24-week outcome measures were imputed using the last-value-carried-forward method (e.g., baseline or 12 week outcome measures), and the six primary regression models were recalculated with the imputed data to assess the impact on intervention effectiveness (van Belle, Fisher, Heagerty, & Lumley, 2004).

Statistical analyses were performed using Stata (Version 10; StataCorp, College Station, TX) and R statistical software (Version 2.10.1; R Development Core Team, Vienna, Austria). All reported p values were two-sided, with statistical significance taken to be $p < .05$. There was no adjustment for multiple testing.

Results

A total of 309 women in rural communities were enrolled, 155 in the computer intervention and 154 in the control group. By the end of data collection, 37 women (23.8%) had dropped out of the intervention group and 22 women (14.3%) had dropped out of the control group. Of those who began the study, 250 completed and provided data at all three time points, resulting in an overall retention rate of 80.9%. There were a variety of reasons that 59 women did not complete the study: failure to return a questionnaire ($n = 29$), increased family responsibilities ($n = 9$), exacerbation of their illness ($n = 8$), lack of participation in the intervention ($n = 6$), did not relate well to using the computer ($n = 4$), computer or Internet irresolvable problems ($n = 2$), and deceased ($n = 1$).

Participants

Participants were 35 to 65 years old (mean = 55.5 years, median = 56 years, mode = 60 years), primarily Caucasian (91.0%) rural women who had been dealing with one or more chronic illnesses for an average length of illness of 16.5 years (median = 13 years, mode = 12 years). More than three quarters (76.9%) were married, with a similar percentage (77.7%) having no children in the home. Fifty-three percent were employed outside the home, and the mean years of education for the group was 14.7 (Table 2).

Outcomes

In Figure 3, the mean scores and the 95% confidence intervals (CIs) of each outcome measure are shown for each treatment group across the three data collection time points (T1—baseline, T2—12 weeks, and T3—24 weeks). By the end of the 11-week intervention, women in the intervention group improved across all psychosocial outcome measures, whereas women in the control group experienced little or no improvement. Differences in psychosocial outcomes observed between groups at T2 persisted to the end of the study at 24 weeks (T3).

In Table 3, the psychosocial outcome measures at T3 (24 weeks) were assessed with separate analysis of covariance models. The impact of the intervention was statistically significant for five of six of the psychosocial outcomes measured, with the intervention having only a modest impact on social support (effect = 2.5 points, 95% CI = -0.05 to 5.5, $p = .097$). In terms of the size of the effect relative to the scale of the outcome measure, the largest benefits of the intervention were observed on the acceptance, depression, and stress measures. The computer-based group was estimated to have an acceptance of illness score of 2.0 points higher (95% CI = 0.8–3.3, $p = .001$) on a scale of 14 to 70, a depression score of 3.1 points lower (95% CI = 0.8–5.4, $p = .010$) on a scale of 0 to 60, and a stress score of 2.4 points lower (95% CI = 0.7–4.1, $p = .005$) on a scale of 0 to 56.

Relative to the width of each scale, the intervention had a small- to medium-sized impact on women's self-esteem and loneliness outcomes than those in the control group. Compared with controls, women in the intervention scored 1.2 points higher on the self-esteem scale (95% CI = 0.2–2.1, $p = .018$) and 1.8 points lower (95% CI = 0.1–3.6, $p = .040$) on the loneliness scale.

Sensitivity Analysis

Compared with the control group, more women dropped out of the intervention group ($p = .024$), potentially impacting the reliability of the intervention effects observed and reported at 24 weeks. The reasons given for dropping out included deteriorating health, family problems, competing demands on time, computer technical difficulties, or moving away from a rural area.

All baseline characteristics were assessed and are displayed in Table 2 in separate univariate models as predictors of missing data at 24 weeks, both overall and separately, for each group. Divorcees were almost twice as likely to drop out as married women (odds ratio = 1.95, $p = .090$).

TABLE 2. Baseline Characteristics of Study Participants

Characteristic	Computer Intervention ($n = 155$)	Control Group ($n = 154$)
Age (years)	56.1 ± 7.7	55.0 ± 9.1
Caucasian	144 (93)	137 (89)
Marital status		
Married, common law, or living together	126 (81)	118 (77)
Divorced or separated	19 (12)	24 (16)
Other	9 (6)	12 (8)
Education (years)	14.8 ± 2.4	14.5 ± 2.6
Income		
Less than $15,000	18 (12)	25 (16)
$15,000–$34,999	45 (29)	54 (35)
$35,000–$64,999	59 (38)	50 (32)
More than $65,000	28 (18)	23 (15)
Homemaker	74 (48)	69 (45)
Hours/week worked outside home	29.5 ± 14.6	28.0 ± 16.0
Years since onset of symptoms	13 (8–23)	13.50 (7–23.75)
Years since diagnosis[a]	10 (5–16)	9 (4–16)
Primary health condition		
Arthritis	31	25
Diabetes	24	19
Multiple sclerosis	24	26
Fibromyalgia	22	22
Lupus	11	1
Cancer	6	8
Other	37	53
Degree of difficulty with vision, hearing, mobility, pain, fatigue, and coordination	10.7 ± 5	10.3 ± 5.1
Psychosocial outcome measures		
Social support (Personal Resource Questionnaire)	79.2 ± 16.4	77.7 ± 19.7
Self-esteem (Rosenberg Self-esteem Scale)	30.8 ± 5.6	29.9 ± 5.8
Acceptance of illness (Acceptance of Illness Scale)	51.0 ± 7.9	49.6 ± 7.9
Depression (Center for Epidemiologic Studies–Depression Scale)	15.5 ± 11.0	17.0 ± 12.1
Stress (Perceived Stress Scale)	38.8 ± 8.3	39.4 ± 8.7
Loneliness (University of California, Los Angeles Loneliness Scale)	44.8 ± 10.7	45.3 ± 11.3

Note. Values are presented as mean ± *SD*, frequency (%), and median (IQR). IQR = interquartile range.
[a]IQR is presented as the 25th and 75th percentiles.

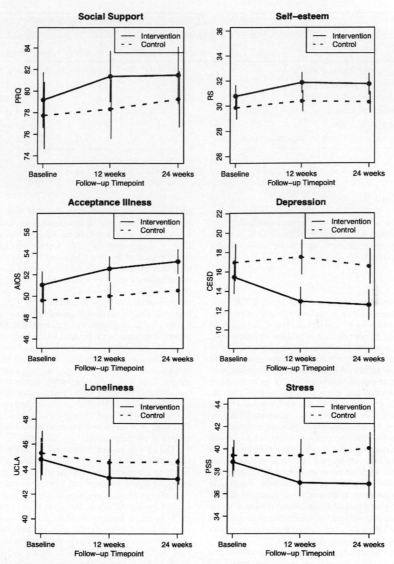

FIGURE 3. Mean values (95% confidence intervals) of six psychosocial outcome measures over the three study time points.

Similarly, women in either group who self-identified as homemakers were almost twice as likely to drop out (odds ratio = 1.82, p = .053). The factors found to have an association with dropout by treatment group were social support and loneliness. Women with higher levels of social support before the study tended to drop out of the intervention group more than those from the control group (p = .092); women scoring higher on the loneliness scale tended to stay with intervention more than women assigned to the control group (p = .077).

To adjust for women with missing data at 24 weeks, each of the models were reassessed for the six psychosocial outcome measures by imputing missing data using the last known value. For 33 women in the intervention and 12 in the control groups, the outcomes measured at baseline were imputed. Outcome measures collected at 12 weeks were used for 5 and 10 additional women in the intervention and control groups, respectively. Using last-value-carried-forward imputation for women who dropped out of the study, the five psychosocial outcome measures remained statistically

TABLE 3. Intervention Impact on Psychosocial Variables at 24 Weeks

Variable	Intervention, M (SD)	Control, M (SD)	Intervention Effect[a]	p
Social support (Personal Resource Questionnaire)	81.4 (17.0)	79.2 (16.5)	2.5 (−0.5 to 5.5)	.097
Self-esteem (Rosenberg Self-esteem Scale)	31.8 (5.5)	30.3 (5.5)	1.2 (0.2 to 2.1)	.018
Acceptance (Acceptance of Illness Scale)	53.2 (7.2)	50.5 (8.2)	2.0 (0.8 to 3.3)	.001
Depression (Center for Epidemiologic Studies–Depression Scale)	12.6 (10.0)	16.6 (11.6)	−3.1 (−5.4 to −0.8)	.010
Stress (Perceived Stress Scale)	36.9 (8.0)	40.1 (9.0)	−2.4 (−4.1 to −0.7)	.005
Loneliness (University of California, Los Angeles Loneliness Scale)	43.2 (10.3)	44.6 (11.5)	−1.8 (−3.6 to −0.1)	.040

Note. CI = confidence interval.
[a]Estimate (95% CI) from analysis of covariance model adjusting for the outcome measured at baseline and cohort number.

significant with $p < .05$. However, the 24-week intervention effects presented in Table 3 were approximately 15% to 20% smaller because of imputation of baseline values of the psychosocial outcome measures (essentially amounting to zero 24-week change).

Discussion

One of the aims of the most recent stage of the WTW study was to determine whether a computer-based intervention could influence the psychosocial health of rural chronically ill women positively in an effort to help them to adapt more successfully to their conditions. It was expected that those women who participated in the WTW intervention would score significantly higher on measures of social support, self-esteem, and acceptance of illness and lower on measures of depression, loneliness, and stress than the women who did not engage in the intervention. Significant anticipated results were demonstrated for five of the six psychosocial scores, social support excepted. Although significant improvement was seen in the women's perceptions of the level of social support immediately after the conclusion of the intervention (Figure 3), the significance was not sustained, although some improvement was seen, at the more distant measurement at 24 weeks. At this point (24 weeks), however, statistically significant improvements continued to be demonstrated for self-esteem and acceptance of illness as did the lower scores for depression, stress, and sense of loneliness. Although these differences were statistically significant, they may be considered of only moderate clinical significance.

The effect size of the impact provides additional interpretation. The largest effect size was for depression, stress, and acceptance of illness, with a medium-sized impact on self-esteem and loneliness. Unexpected was the modest impact on social support, a variable that in the past was a larger component of the outcomes of the intervention (Hill, Weinert, & Cudney, 2006; Weinert, Cudney, & Hill, 2008). It was concluded that the overall aim of improving the women's psychosocial health in the areas measured was achieved.

The sensitivity analysis shed some light on who completed the intervention. Married women tended to stay with the study regardless of group. Divorced women were twice as likely to drop out, which may have been related to the lack of support that can be provided by a spouse and to the added respon-

sibilities a single person must shoulder that are ordinarily shared in a marriage. A counterintuitive finding was that women who were stay-at-home homemakers were twice as likely to drop out of the study. Just the opposite might have been anticipated because it was logical to expect that women who also worked outside the home would have less time to attend to study activities and thus drop out. Likewise, it could be argued that homemakers' opportunities to interact with others outside the home would be more limited than those who were employed; thus, it would seem they would be eager for the chance to engage with other women. However, these assumptions were not supported by the findings.

It was anticipated that women with a better support system going into the study would not have the need for or benefit as much from the social support offered by participation. This notion was supported because the women who scored higher on social support were more likely to drop out of the intervention. Similarly, it was anticipated that women who were lonely would find the virtual support group helpful. This idea was confirmed because more lonely women remained in the intervention.

The 15-year research journey of the WTW Project has led to the conclusion that key indicators for psychosocial adaptation to chronic illness can be influenced positively by a computer-based support and education intervention. Over time, the intervention was modified on the basis of the lessons learned from each phase, emerging technology, and refined thinking. In the most recent phase of the project, as reported here, we used a more user-friendly, less complex, more stand-alone intervention that has the potential to be adapted more readily clinically without sacrificing the capacity to impact psychosocial indicators positively.

Conclusion

Although one of the aims of the WTW study was to test the impact of a computer-based intervention on selected indicators of psychosocial adaptation, the successful results of which have been reported here, this information represents just one piece of the puzzle of the complex adaptation process as experienced by rural women living with chronic conditions. The analysis of the additional aims of the study is in process, including the examination of the impact of the intervention on self-management skills and quality of life. The concepts of the model (Figure 2) indicate that people are bombarded with environmental stimuli (such as chronic illnesses), evoking psychosocial responses that can be either a positive or a negative influence on the effectiveness of their illness management and quality of life. The results by this study will allow examination of these ideas and the patterns of interaction among the major constructs of the conceptual model. ▼

Accepted for publication September 28, 2010.

The Women to Women Conceptual Model for Adaptation to Chronic Illness was designed to guide the Women on Women Project–Phase III. The model was developed by Drs. Clarann Weinert, Wade Hill, Charlene Winters, Therese Sullivan, Lynn Paul, Deborah Haynes, Elizabeth Kinion, and Susan Luparell and Pat Oriet, BSN, Shirley Cudney, MA, and Amber Spring, MS.

Funding was received from the National Institutes of Health, the National Institute of Nursing Research (grant no. 2R01NR007908-04A1), and the NIH/National Center for Research Resources (grant no. UL1RR025014).

Corresponding author: Clarann Weinert, SC, PhD, RN, FAAN, College of Nursing, Montana State University, PO Box 173560, Bozeman, MT 59717 (e-mail: cweinert@montana.edu).

References

Bandura, A. (2004). Swimming against the mainstream: The early years from chilly tributary to transformative mainstream. *Behaviour Research and Therapy, 42*(6), 613–630.

Bond, G. E., Burr, R. L., Wolf, F. M., & Feldt, K. (2010).The effects of a Web-based intervention on psychosocial well-being among adults aged 60 and older with diabetes: A randomized trial. *Diabetes Educator, 36*(3), 446–456.

Brennan, P. F., Ripich, S., & Moore, S. M. (1991). The use of home-based computers to support persons living with AIDS/ARC. *Journal of Community Health Nursing, 8*(1), 3–14.

Buchanan, D. C., & Abram, H, S. (1975). Psychotic behavior resulting from a lateral ventricle meningioma· A case report. *Diseases of the Nervous System, 36*(7), 400–401.

Cagle, C. S. (2004). 3 themes described how self care management was learned and experienced by patients with chronic illness. *Evidence-Based Nursing, 7*(3), 94.

Carnegie Mellon University. (2007). *Stress contributes to range of chronic diseases, review shows.* ScienceDaily. Retrieved from http://www.sciencedaily.com /releases/2007/10/071009164122.htm

Centers for Disease Control and Prevention. (2010). *Chronic diseases and health promotion. Your online source for credible health information.* Retrieved from http://www.cdc.gov/chronicdisease/overview/index.htm

Chakraburtty, A. (2007). *Coping with chronic illnesses and depression.* Retrieved from http://www.webmd.com/depression/guide/chronic-illnesses-depression?page=2

Charmaz, K. (1983). Loss of self: A fundamental form of suffering in the chronically ill. *Sociology of Health & Illness, 5*(2), 168–195.

Cohen, S., Kamarck, T., & Mermelstein, R. (1983). A global measure of perceived stress. *Journal of Health and Social Behavior, 24*(4), 385–396.

Devine, G., & Orme, C. (1985). Center for Epidemiologic Studies Depression Scale. In D. J. Keyser & R. C. Sweetland (Eds.), *Test critiques* (Vol. 1, pp. 144–160). Kansas City, MO: Test Corp. of America.

Ernst, J. M., & Cacioppo, J. (1999). Lonely hearts: Psychological perspectives on loneliness. *Applied & Preventive Psychology, 8*, 1–22.

Falvo, D. R. (2005). *Medical and psychosocial aspects of chronic illness and disability.* Sudbury, MA: Jones and Bartlett.

Fox, S. (2007). *E-patients with disability or chronic disease. Pew Internet & American Life Project.* Retrieved from http://pewresearch.org/pubs/608/e-patients

Gray-Little, B., Williams, V. S. L., & Hancock, T. D. (1997). An item response theory analysis of the Rosenberg Self-esteem Scale. *Personality and Social Psychology Bulletin, 23*, 443–451.

Griffiths, F., Lindenmeyer, A., Powell, J., Lowe, P., & Thorogood, M. (2006). Why are health care interventions delivered over the Internet? A systematic review of the published literature. *Journal of Medical Internet Research, 8*(2), e10.

Hale, T. M., Cotten, S. R., Drentea, P., & Goldner, M. (2010). Rural-urban differences in general and health-related Internet use. *American Behavioral Scientist, 53*(9), 1304–1325.

Hall, M., & Havens, B. (1999). *The effects of social isolation and loneliness on the health of older women.* Winnipeg, Canada: Prairie Women's Health Center of Excellence.

Helgeson, V. S., & Reynolds, K. A. (2002). Social psychological aspects of chronic illness. In A. J. Christensen & M. H. Antoni (Eds.), *Chronic physical disorders: Behavioral medicine's perspective.* Malden, MA: Blackwell.

Hill, W., Weinert, C., & Cudney, S. (2006). Influence of a computer intervention on the psychological status of chronically ill rural women: Preliminary results. *Nursing Research, 55*(1), 34–42.

Juczynski, Z. (2001). *Evaluation tools in health promotion and psychology.* Warsaw, Poland: Pracownia Testow Psychologicznych.

Lorig, K. R., & Holman, H. (2003). Self-management education: History, definition, outcomes, and mechanisms. *Annals of Behavioral Medicine, 26*(1), 1–7.

Lorig, K., Holman, H., Sobel, D., Laurent, D., Gonzalez, V. M., & Minor, M. (2000). *Living a healthy life with chronic conditions* (2nd ed.). Boulder, CO: Bull Publishing Company.

Lorig, K. R., Ritter, P. L., Laurent, D. D., & Plant, K. (2006). Internet-based chronic disease self-management: A randomized trial. *Medical Care, 44*(11), 964–971.

Lyon, B. L. (2000). Stress, coping, and health: A conceptual overview. In V. H. Rice (Ed.), *Handbook of stress, coping, and health: Implications for nursing research, theory, and practice.* Thousand Oaks, CA: Sage.

Massie, R. K. (1984). The constant shadow: Reflections on the life of the chronically ill child. *Peabody Journal of Education, 61*(2), 16–27.

Norman, C. D. (2009). *Skills essential for ehealth. Health literacy, eHealth, and communication.* Retrieved from http://www.nap.edu/openbook.php?record_id=12474&page=10

Pollock, S. E., Christian, B. J., & Sands, D. (1990). Responses to chronic illness: Analysis of psychological and physiological adaptation. *Nursing Research, 39*(5), 300–304.

Rosenberg, M. (1965). *Society and the adolescent self-image.* Princeton, New Jersey: Princeton University Press.

Royer, A. (1998). *Life with chronic illness: Social and psychological dimensions.* Westport, CT: Praeger.

Rural Assistance Center. (2010). *Rural health disparities. Rural Health Disparities Resources.* Retrieved from http://www.raconline.org/info_guides/disparities/

Russell, D. W. (1996). UCLA Loneliness Scale (Version 3): reliability, validity, and factor structure. *Journal of Personality Assessment, 66*(1), 20–40.

Shaver, P. R., & Brennan, K. A. (1991). Measures of depression and loneliness. In J. P. Robinson, P. R. Shaver & L. S. Wrightsman (Eds.), *Measures of personality and social psychological attitudes. Measures of social psychological attitudes.* (Vol. 1, pp. 195–289). San Diego, CA: Academic Press.

Simon, G. E., Von Korff, M., & Lin, E. (2005). Clinical and functional outcomes of depression treatment in patients with and without chronic medical illness. *Psychological Medicine, 35*(2), 271–279.

Stuifbergen, A. K., Seraphine, A., & Roberts, G. (2000). An

explanatory model of health promotion and quality of life in chronic disabling conditions. *Nursing Research, 49*(3), 122–129.

Symister, P., & Friend, R. (2003). The influence of social support and problematic support on optimism and depression in chronic illness: A prospective study evaluating self-esteem as a mediator. *Health Psychology, 22*(2), 123–129.

van Belle, G., Fisher, L., Heagerty, P., & Lumley, T. (2004). *Biostatistics: A methodology for the health sciences* (2nd ed.). Hoboken, NJ: Wiley-Interscience.

Weinert, C. (2003). Measuring social support: PRQ2000. In O. Strickland & C. Dilorio (Eds.), *Measurement of nursing outcomes: Self care and coping* (Vol. 3, pp. 161–172). New York: Springer.

Weinert, C. (2009). *Rural chronically ill women: Online support network*. Unpublished raw data.

Weinert, C., Cudney, S., & Hill, W. G. (2008). Rural women, technology, and self-management of chronic illness. *Canadian Journal of Nursing Research, 40*(3), 114–134.

Weinert, C., Cudney, S., & Spring, A. (2008). Evolution of a conceptual model for adaptation to chronic illness. *Journal of Nursing Scholarship, 45*(4), 364–372. doi:10.1111/j.1547-5069.2008.00241.x

Weiss, R. (1969). The fund of sociability. *Transaction, 6,* 36–43.

White, N. E., Richter, J. M., & Fry, C. (1992). Coping, social support, and adaptation to chronic illness. *Western Journal of Nursing Research, 14*(2), 211–224.

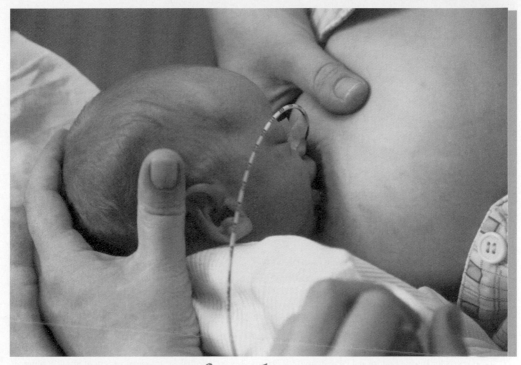

Rooting for the Breast:
Breastfeeding Promotion in the
NICU

Roberta Cricco-Lizza, PhD, MPH, RN

This study explored the structure and process of breastfeeding promotion in the neonatal intensive care unit (NICU). Mother's milk is particularly important for the health of premature and high-risk infants (American Academy of Pediatrics, 2005; Ip et al., 2007). Ingestion of breast milk in the NICU by low birth weight infants has been linked to beneficial health outcomes and enhanced cognitive development (Vohr et al., 2006). Breast milk provides protection against infections, sepsis, necrotizing enterocolitis, and retinopathy of prematurity (Furman, Taylor, Minich, & Hack, 2003; Hylander, Strobino, Pezzullo, & Dhannireddy, 2001; Schanler, Lau, Hurst, & Smith, 2005). The American Academy of Pediatrics recommends direct breastfeeding and/or use of mother's own pumped milk for high-risk infants; however, these reported rates are low for NICU babies (Espy & Senn, 2003). In addition to

129

Abstract

Purpose: This study explored the structure and process of breastfeeding promotion in the NICU.

Methods: An ethnographic approach was used with the techniques of participant observation, interviewing, and artifact assessment. This 14-month study took place in a level IV NICU in a Northeastern US children's hospital. General informants consisted of 114 purposively selected NICU nurses. From this group, 18 nurses served as key informants. There was an average of 13 interactions with each key informant and 3.5 for each general informant. Audiotaped interviews, feeding artifacts, and observational notes were gathered for descriptions of breastfeeding promotion. Data were coded and analyzed for recurring patterns. NUD*IST-aided data management and analysis.

Findings: There were three main findings: (1) organizational and human resources were developed to create a web of support to promote breastfeeding in the NICU; (2) variations in breastfeeding knowledge and experience within the nursing staff, marketing practices of formula companies, and insufficient support from other health professionals served as sources of inconsistent breastfeeding messages; and (3) promotion of breastfeeding in this NICU is evolving over time from a current breast milk feeding focus to the goal for a future breastfeeding process orientation.

Clinical Implications: NICU nurses should advocate for organizational and human resources to promote breastfeeding in the unit. To decrease inconsistent messages, staff development should be expanded to all professionals, and formula marketing practices should be curtailed.

Keywords: Breastfeeding; NICU; Nurses; Promotion.

maternal and neonatal issues, staff and hospital factors also influence NICU breastfeeding rates (Lessen & Crivelli-Kovach, 2007; Merewood, Philipp, Chawla, & Cimo, 2003).

Maternity practices in the United States are often not evidence based and have been shown to impede breastfeeding (Centers for Disease Control and Prevention, 2008; DiGirolamo, Grummer-Strawn, & Fein, 2001). The World Health Organization (WHO) and the United Nations Children's Fund (UNICEF) (1992) launched the Baby-Friendly Hospital Initiative (BFHI) to protect, promote, and support breastfeeding in birth environments. The recommended practices in this Initiative have been linked to improved breastfeeding rates, but they generally pertain to routine births in hospitals and birthing centers (Kramer et al., 2001). Mothers of high-risk infants face unique challenges to the initiation and continuation of breastfeeding (Meier, 2001; Spatz, 2006). Hospitals must address these challenges to prepare the NICU staff to support breastfeeding families. However, mothers have reported problems with hospital routines and inadequate support for breastfeeding from nurses and physicians in the NICU (Cricco-Lizza, 2006). Hospitals with NICU breastfeeding promotion programs have positively influenced breastfeeding rates (Dall'Oglio et al., 2007; do Nascimento & Issler, 2005).

More research is needed about effective ways to promote breastfeeding in the NICU. Structures and processes in an organization can advance or can hamper the implementation of health promotion strategies, and much can be gained by exploring the context of everyday practices (Yano, 2008). This report is part of a larger qualitative study of NICU nurses and infant feeding. In a previous publication from this study, nurses' personal contexts of infant feeding outside of the NICU were examined. The nurses identified a formula feeding norm during their own childhoods and described limited exposure to breastfeeding in nursing school (Cricco-Lizza, 2009). The current article examines the structures and processes that were developed to promote breastfeeding in the NICU.

Methods

An ethnographic approach was used with the techniques of participant observation, interviewing, and artifact analysis. By combining these three techniques, multiple sources of information were obtained for a comprehensive view of breastfeeding promotion in the NICU. The sample consisted of 114 nurses who were considered "general informants," purposefully selected to provide a wide angle view of breastfeeding promotion, and 18 "key informants" chosen from that group who were followed more intensively for an in-depth view. Both key and general informants were selected for maximal variety of infant feeding and NICU clinical experiences. The 14-month study was conducted in a level IV NICU in a freestanding children's hospital in the Northeastern United States. This study was approved by the Human Subjects' Committees and study information was provided to the nurses through the intranet, staff meetings, and individual encounters in the NICU. Nurses who served as key informants for the study signed informed consent before formal interviews.

Sample

From 250 nurses employed in this NICU, 114 served as the general informants; 96 of these were White, 9 African American, 8 Asian, and 1 Hispanic. Only one was a male. About 30% of the general informants had taken a hospital breastfeeding course developed before this study was initiated. The age of the 18 key informants ranged from 22 to 51 (mean = 33). Of these, 17 were female; 16 were White and 2 were African American. Two had diplomas in nursing, 1 had an associate degree, 14 had a BSN, and 1 had a master's degree. The key informants were almost evenly divided among all four expertise levels of the clinical ladder, from novices to clinical experts. About half of these key informants had taken the hospital breastfeeding course and almost one-fourth were on the breastfeeding committee.

Data Collection
Participant Observation

Unobtrusive observations focused on the nurses' behaviors during interactions with babies, families, nurses, and other healthcare professionals throughout everyday NICU activities. Included in these observations were feedings and routine care, shift reports, breastfeeding committee meetings, nutrition meetings, psychosocial rounds, and nurse-run breastfeeding support groups for parents. There were 128 observation sessions, which took place for 1 to 2 hours

> Nurses who had taken the breastfeeding course said that it helped them feel "comfortable," "competent," and "prepared" to teach breast-feeding to families.

during varying days and times of the week. The investigator introduced herself as a nurse researcher who was interested in learning about NICU nurses' perspectives about infant feeding. The researcher role evolved from observation to informal interviews over time. The nurses were asked about breastfeeding promotion within the context of everyday nursing care in the NICU. The general informants were observed/informally interviewed an average of 3.5 times each (range 1-24) over the study period. All observational data and informal interview data were documented immediately after each session.

Artifact Analysis

Documents can serve as a resource for investigating social meaning and practice (Miller & Alvarado, 2005). Breastfeeding standards of care, teaching plans, and policies and procedures were purposefully gathered and reviewed early in the study. These documents provided insight into officially recognized standards of care for infant feeding in this NICU. They also served as a springboard for lines of inquiry that were further developed during observations and interviews. In addition, parent education materials, posters on the unit, and signs placed at the bedside provided other sources of data about breastfeeding promotion in this NICU.

Formal Interviewing

Each of the 18 key informants engaged in a formal, 1-hour, tape-recorded interview in a private room near the NICU. Open-ended interview questions probed nursing perspectives about breastfeeding promotion in the NICU. In addition to the formal interview, they were also informally interviewed and/or observed a total of 3 to 43 times each (mean of 13.1) over the entire study. The formal interviews were transcribed verbatim and the transcriptions and tapes were reviewed for accuracy.

Data Analysis and Verification

The data from formal and informal interviews, observations, NICU artifacts, and ongoing memos were analyzed concurrently with data collection. QSR NUD*IST was used to facilitate data management, retrieval, and analysis. The data were examined line-by-line in an iterative fashion and codes were inductively derived for meaning. These codes were restructured into categories and then analyzed for patterns. Ongoing contact with general and key informants facilitated pattern identification and verification. The findings were continuously verified through triangulation of interviewing, participant observation, and artifact assessment and this helped to decrease bias. A peer-review group of pre- and postdoctoral nurse researchers also provided oral and written critique throughout the course of the study.

Findings

Organizational and Human Resources Were Developed To Create a Web of Support To Promote Breastfeeding in the NICU
Organizational Resources

There was consistent evidence that organizational resources had been developed in the NICU to encourage breastfeeding. A general informant described how multidisciplinary NICU representatives had reviewed the state of the science on breastfeeding. She said that they used these findings to conceptualize *"a continuum from informed decision making, pump access with establishment and maintenance of milk supply, breast milk feeding, skin-to-skin care, nonnutritive sucking, transition to breast, to preparation for discharge."*

A review of unit documents demonstrated that breastfeeding standards of care and policies and procedures clearly communicated unit-approved statements supporting the use of human milk and breastfeeding in the NICU. Breastfeeding teaching plans and educational materials were observed to be readily available on the unit and examination of the content showed that these documents focused on the specific needs of families with high-risk infants. The general and key informants referred to these documents and discussed how they were used during interactions with parents. One nurse said, *"We try to give them information. We have booklets, printouts, whatever about breastfeeding."*

APPENDIX B

Another stated, *"We present them with breastfeeding information as soon as they come in the door."* The admission packet for parents described breastfeeding as a *"wonderful"* decision for the health of the baby.

Discussion with general and key informants revealed an understanding of the breast milk management system in this NICU. These breast milk handling procedures were generally followed by the nurses, although discussion between the nurses and mothers about milk supply was sometimes overlooked, and occasionally this information did not get transmitted in shift reports. Observations in the unit showed that pump rooms were easily accessible and used by NICU mothers. These spaces had high visibility and accessibility in a central location. Rolling breast pumps were also on hand for bedside pumping and a rental station was available to support breast pumping away from the NICU. Observations also revealed that current literature about medications and breast milk was on reserve in the NICU. All of these structures and processes provided a foundation to promote breastfeeding.

Interviews of general and key informants demonstrated that these organizational resources were initiated by the NICU lactation and nursing professionals in this NICU, and further developed through the combined actions of the NICU breastfeeding committee members. NICU nurses, along with the lactation staff, served on this committee and they met on a monthly basis to discuss any ongoing issues related to breastfeeding on the unit. Observations demonstrated that the nurses who served on this committee were the leaders in all phases of breastfeeding promotion on the unit. Specific activities observed during this study included conference planning, quality improvement studies, World Breastfeeding Week events, and skin-to-skin care promotion. These activities had ripple effects throughout the unit. For example, one key informant stated, *"We had posters all around for World Breastfeeding Week, and a mother read... about all the benefits... and said, 'you know because of that I'm breastfeeding my baby.'"* Observations also demonstrated that there was an increase in mothers asking about doing skin-to-skin care after the breastfeeding committee members placed skin-to-skin posters in the NICU.

Efforts were also expended beyond the NICU to strengthen intra- and extra-hospital support for breastfeeding promotion. The breastfeeding committee successfully lobbied the hospital foundation to remove a public display panel within the hospital corridors that promoted bottle feeding. This committee also designated annual awards to staff nurses who were most active in breastfeeding promotion. Furthermore, the committee members conducted an annual breastfeeding conference and they were observed sharing the latest research-based feeding practices with NICU nurses from the varied hospitals in this perinatal catchment area. In addition, they used conference gatherings as opportunities to encourage staff nurses to become politically active in support of statewide breastfeeding legislation.

Human Resources

Staff development factors were also important for breastfeeding promotion in the unit. The NICU had lactation consultants and a nursing clinical specialist who provided weekday support for mothers who wanted to breastfeed their NICU babies. Bedside staff nurse support was important for initial referral and continuing assistance of these mothers. All nurses in the NICU were required to complete a Web-based module about the handling, storage, and management of breast milk. General and key informants also talked about the additional 16-hour breastfeeding course that had been developed before this study took place, and had been offered over the past few years at this hospital. They said that this course included information about breastfeeding benefits, anatomy and physiology of lactation, and specific NICU issues of pumping, lactoengineering, skin-to-skin care, transition to the breast, test weights, and concerns related to the transfer of viruses and drugs. They stated that they also received clinical experience with assessment of positioning, latch, and breastfeeding. The nurses who completed this course identified that they learned important information for their NICU nursing practice. Some nurses said: *"A lot of the things were new to me"* and *"It was excellent, very informative."* Other nurses said that this course helped them feel *"comfortable," "competent,"* and *"prepared"* to teach breastfeeding to families. One new graduate nurse stated, *"I don't hesitate to...help the baby latch on...try different holds...try different techniques."* There was also evidence that the benefits of this course extended to personal experiences outside of the NICU setting. For example, one nurse said that this course was the biggest influence on her decision to breastfeed her own child. She stated, *"From working here and becoming educated [and] knowing all the benefits it has for the baby and for the mom... I just thought that it would be a good thing to do."*

The nurses who completed this breastfeeding course were expected to act as bedside breastfeeding supporters and some of them served on the breastfeeding committee or helped to coordinate the parents' breastfeeding support group. Observations in the NICU demonstrated that the nurses who had taken this course were very positive about breastfeeding promotion. In varied situations these nurses were observed encouraging mothers who had low supplies and educating them about steps to take to increase yield. In one particular situation on the night shift, a new graduate nurse worked closely supporting and teaching new parents how to assess intake. She said that she felt pleased with her ability to facilitate their infant feeding. Another nurse was heard telling parents *"We want to help you"* when the mother was discouraged with pumping.

Variations in Breastfeeding Knowledge and Experience Within the Nursing Staff, Marketing Practices of Formula Companies and Insufficient Support From Other Health Professionals Served as Sources of Inconsistent Messages for Breastfeeding

Breastfeeding Knowledge and Experience of the NICU Nurses

There were considerable variations in the breastfeeding knowledge and experience of the NICU nurses. The 16-hour breastfeeding course was a requirement for all orientees, but for the rest of the NICU staff, it was optional. One of the key informants said, *"There's no requirement"* for existing NICU staff members to take the breastfeeding classes. During the study there were about 45 nurses out of 250 who had completed these classes and all had been paid for their time in class. Another key informant stated that nurses who had not taken this course were *"not practicing based on evidence right now; they are practicing based on their beliefs."* The NICU nurses freely spoke about their education for infant feeding and whether or not they had taken the breastfeeding course. One of the NICU nurses who had chosen not to take the course stated, *"I feel like for me if there's certain stuff I need to know, I'd rather know how to give a kid a bolus and do different stuff like that than breastfeed. I'd rather grab somebody else you know, a resource nurse or lactation consultant."* Another nurse voiced similar reasons why she had decided not to take the breastfeeding course. She asserted, *"If you give me a list of 10 different things to pursue interest-wise, breastfeeding would be somewhere towards the bottom. It's not something that I have ever gone out of my way to get involved in."* She said, *"If I have to go to an in-service I will, but I don't go out of my way to pursue [breastfeeding] conferences."*

The nurses who had not completed the breastfeeding course were generally more detached from breastfeeding promotion activities. Observations throughout the study demonstrated that these nurses were more likely to miss opportunities for breastfeeding promotion during the work day. Nurses who had not taken this course sometimes treated breast milk and formula as equivalent or did not promote direct breastfeeding to pumping mothers. For example, a mother who was committed to breastfeeding expressed concern to her nurse over her baby's difficulty eating. She asked the nurse what the goal was for her child. This nurse said that she had to take a certain amount of *"p.o. feeds"* or the rest would be given by tube. When the mother asked the meaning of the term *"p.o. feeds,"* the nurse replied, *"all of the feeds by bottle."* This general

informant seemed unaware that she had dismissed breastfeeding.

Formula Company Marketing

The marketing practices of formula companies also presented challenges for breastfeeding promotion. The nurses frequently identified formula companies when they talked about infant feeding information that was perceived as educational. One key informant said, *"Formula reps come in and do a little lunch and do a little slideshow."* Many of the informants said that they attended these formula company-sponsored in-services and they talked confidently about the messages learned there. One nurse said that she was told that a certain formula *"is better for eye and brain development."* Another nurse stated that a particular formula company publishes *"a calendar every year with kids that have been on some of their different formulas, very specialized formulas, just to show you... how these kids have progressed [and] grown."* She said, *"They help them because they have these special formulas available."* One other nurse also went to these in-services and said that it helped in, *"finding ... what formulas [were] most like breast milk and really helped the baby with digestion."* Another nurse stated that the formula companies have an annual conference and the *"topics are non formula related so you can get a big audience of nurses to go, but in between the speakers it's almost commercial breaks for the product."* She said that they offer *"good topics and it's really reasonable and you get really good food... and you get contact hours for certification."* This nurse declared that the formula companies were *"trying to push the science of 'this is such a superior product' and that may catch the nurses."* One of the nurses who supported breastfeeding also sarcastically referred to *"the cutest lunch bags"* that the formula representative was giving to the staff.

Insufficient Support from other Healthcare Professionals

Other challenges for breastfeeding promotion included the varied feeding approaches of other professionals. Some of the nurses did not feel that the physicians promoted breastfeeding. One key informant said, *"The doctors here are more totally focused on the disease process, getting the baby better... getting the baby out of here. I don't think I've EVER heard... a doctor here question the mom about how she was planning to feed the baby. I think they're too busy. And it's just the LAST thing on their list of priorities."*

Observations at the bedside established that the lactation staff and nurses were the most likely to promote breastfeeding with the parents. Nurses' interactions with mothers and members of other disciplines were frequently observed. The physicians rarely mentioned breastfeeding. The speech/infant feeding therapists focused on bottle feeding and in one case, one of them made deprecating comments to the nurse and parents about the pumping advice of the lactation staff. Infant feeding instructions posted at the bedside by these therapists consistently described procedures for the use of pacifiers and bottles.

Promotion of Breastfeeding in This NICU Is Evolving Over Time From a Current Breast Milk Feeding Focus To the Goal for a Future Breastfeeding Process Orientation

The general and key informants identified that there had been significant changes in breastfeeding promotion in the NICU over the past 5 years. The NICU had not documented rates of breastfeeding or breast milk feeding prior to instituting their efforts to promote breastfeeding. However, one key informant repeated a common refrain when she said, *"We really have grown."* Another nurse described her individual growth and the changes that had occurred in the unit since she took the breastfeeding course. She said: *"I feel since I started here we have come a long way as far [as] educating nurses and I think people are a lot more comfortable now, educating families and mothers about breastfeeding. Although I was a new nurse and really hadn't been exposed that much to breastfeeding, I didn't know much about it. You know it was a little uncomfortable for me…because people asked me questions and I didn't know what to tell them or how to help them. But now that we've been educated, I think that it's a lot easier."*

> "I feel since I started here we have come a long way as far [as] educating nurses and I think people are a lot more comfortable now, educating families and mothers about breastfeeding."

There was general acknowledgement that support for breastfeeding still varied in the NICU. One nurse said, *"I think that more [nurses] are understanding the importance of breast milk but I don't think that 100% of them are."* This nurse felt that some nurses' *"lack of information"* and *"lack of awareness of its importance"* interfered with breastfeeding promotion. Another nurse said, *"I would say some nurses do a better job at trying to steer them [mothers] towards breastfeeding or pumping than other nurses."*

There were variations in the breastfeeding measures currently collected by the staff on the unit. During the study, monthly rates for percent of NICU babies ever receiving any human milk varied from 53% to 95% with an average of 71%. The nurses did not gather measures about any differences in the percentage of feeds of breast milk consumed or rates of transition to actual breastfeeding. In general, the nurses were more oriented to breast milk feeding than actual breastfeeding. Frequently, the nurses mentioned the scientific advantages of breast milk when they engaged in breastfeeding promotion. During the parents' breastfeeding support meetings, the nurses often used cards that listed varying science-based statements about the properties of breast milk. Likewise one of the breastfeeding promotion signs on the

unit was worded, *"Breast milk is more than nutrition. It is protection."* The focus was usually on breast milk as a scientific product rather than breastfeeding as human process between mother and baby.

Interviews and observations demonstrated that breast milk feeding was more widespread than actual breastfeeding. Overall one of the key informants said, *"We've come a long way here. More [babies] receive breast milk at this point than ever in our past."* Another key informant further clarified this. She said, *"We are trying to work on the notion that baby can go to breast for the first oral feed. It doesn't need to be the bottle. That's a hard notion."* Other nurses concurred that it was the *"transition to the breast"* that was the area most in need of improvement. During observations some of the nurses could be seen handing a defrosted bottle of breast milk to a mother instead of helping her to breastfeed. When one key informant was asked about this practice, she stated, *"It does get overlooked sometimes definitely…I know that plenty of time we feed the kid the bottle."* Another key informant spoke for many when she attributed this practice to: *"Doctors and nurses being uncomfortable with the breastfeeding, extra work for the nurses, getting the test weight scale, and making sure that the screens are up and appropriate. And just, you know, it IS a lot of extra work."*

There was also evidence that attempts to make the NICU more breastfeeding supportive occasionally took its toll on the staff. One general informant who was a member of the breastfeeding committee said that it was discouraging because one nurse helps with breastfeeding and the next one does not. A key informant described the continuing struggle to promote breastfeeding in the NICU. She said: *"But the difficult thing is trying to change culture and practice in this unit. It's very difficult…For instance with breastfeeding, we've made such headway in the last couple of years, but sometimes we have to stop and look back and say we are making headway because on a daily basis, at times, it doesn't feel that way because you are constantly struggling or you feel like that somebody is always trying to undo something that you've done."*

Nevertheless, the breastfeeding committee members remained committed to breastfeeding promotion and to changing the NICU culture to support high-risk families with this process. One of them reflected a common sentiment when she stated: "*I think we send the message that it's important…That we've made such a change in our culture and it's not 100% across the board, but there are enough of us that we are making a change happen. And* [it is one] *that moms really value.*" These nurses had a long term view of the change process in the NICU and decided to work together over time to overcome the hurdles. Another breastfeeding committee member said: "*It's really up to us. It's not fair if we don't provide the adequate education and be able to give the parents the proper information to make an informed decision…. And WE CAN, as NICU nurses, we can get there.*

> "It's really up to us. It's not fair if we don't provide the adequate education and … give the parents the proper information to make an informed decision….and WE CAN, as NICU nurses, we can get there."

Discussion/Clinical Nursing Implications

The BFHI has provided clear guidelines to promote breast feeding in birth settings; however, high-risk infants require special care to safeguard their need for breastfeeding. These infants face distinctive challenges related to their compromised physical states and their separation from their mothers, and many questions exist about how NICUs can support these vulnerable families. This study used an ethnographic approach to examine the organizational and human resource support for breastfeeding promotion in the NICU and detailed the multifaceted elements that should be considered in a high-risk setting.

The staff in this particular NICU had limited experience and exposure to breastfeeding during their formative years and in their nursing school education (Cricco-Lizza, 2009). This greatly increased the demand on the institution to develop resources to meet the needs for breastfeeding promotion. Leaders in lactation and nursing spearheaded the changes that initiated this still evolving process. They started a breastfeeding committee that actively involved the staff nurses in this evidence-based change process. As a group

they developed systems of support and material resources for pumping and breast milk management, and constructed wide ranging policy, procedure, and teaching materials as staff resources. This infrastructural support was highly visible for the staff and parents and clearly communicated the value of breastfeeding within the daily activities of the unit. The group also took these changes outside of the NICU into the hospital itself, the multiple hospitals in this perinatal catchment area and on to legislators in this state. In such a manner they built a multifaceted web of support. This web could be further enhanced by efforts to gather more detailed data about breast milk and breastfeeding rates. These rates could guide breastfeeding promotion efforts within the unit.

Development of human resources met with mixed success. The breastfeeding course was specifically geared for breastfeeding promotion in an acute care setting. The staff members who completed this 2-day session served as extensions of the lactation staff and as bedside sources of breastfeeding expertise. Siddell, Marinelli, Froman, and Burke (2003) demonstrated that a breastfeeding educational intervention significantly increased NICU nurses' breastfeeding knowledge and altered some attitudes about breastfeeding. The findings of this ethnographic study support this and showed that these nurses not only served as leaders on the unit, but some also took this knowledge back into their personal lives outside of the NICU. Jones, Shapiro, and Roshon (2007) determined that an organized team of experts coupled with training and continued troubleshooting could affect culture change in an acute care setting. During the time of the study, about 43 NICU nurses had fulfilled the course requirements to serve as these bedside supporters. These nurses promoted breastfeeding and acted as change agents in this NICU. Those nurses who did not take the course maintained a more detached stance in breastfeeding activities. In the demanding setting of the NICU, nurses without the breastfeeding training missed opportunities to promote and support breastfeeding. This uneven knowledge and skill with breastfeeding could serve as a source of inconsistent messages for families. This finding suggests that the time is right to implement the breastfeeding course for the entire staff. Breastfeeding training for all staff members is a requirement for birth hospitals for BFHI and is probably even more important for the vulnerable babies in non-birth hospital NICUs.

Nurses were also exposed to formula marketing messages in educational forums for NICU staff. Many of these nurses had not attended the breastfeeding course and identified these formula programs as sources for infant feeding

CLINICAL IMPLICATIONS

NICU nurses should:

❖ Develop organizational and human resources for breastfeeding promotion

❖ Provide breastfeeding education for all NICU staff

❖ Encourage multidisciplinary representation for breastfeeding committees and projects

❖ Limit formula marketing practices in the NICU to avoid inconsistent feeding messages

❖ Utilize in-house experts to provide staff education about infant feeding

❖ Gather specific breastfeeding and breast milk feeding rates to guide promotion efforts

education. Bernaix (2000) found that knowledge about breastfeeding was predictive of maternal child nurses' supportive behaviors for breastfeeding, and emphasized the need for accurate knowledge. The NICU nurses in this current study repeated some of the non-evidence-based formula company claims, and some accepted small gifts and lunches from the sales representatives. The American Academy of Pediatrics (2005) has identified formula marketing as an obstacle to breastfeeding. This study suggests that direct infant formula marketing to professionals by formula representatives also compromises clear messages about breastfeeding promotion in the NICU. Sponsored educational offerings, gifts, and meals can create conflicts of interest and serve as threats to professional integrity (Erlen, 2008; Hagen, Pijl-Zieber, Souveny, & Lacroix, 2008; Stokamer, 2003).

The nurses also perceived a lack of support for breastfeeding from other NICU healthcare professionals. The study findings demonstrated that there were inconsistent recommendations from health professionals in this NICU. Mothers have previously reported conflicting breastfeeding advice from professionals (McInnes & Chambers, 2008). do Nascimento and Issler (2005) found that a trained interdisciplinary team provided consistent information and attained a 94.6% rate for breast milk consumption at discharge from a Brazilian NICU. Multidisciplinary commitment is crucial for successful implementation of evidence-based practice in critical care units (Weinert & Mann, 2008).

This study also indicated that inconsistent messages can contribute to decreased morale and frustration for the nurses who do promote breastfeeding. The findings revealed that breastfeeding promotion in the NICU was not without its difficulties and that implementation occurred over time. Nevertheless, infrastructural and human resource development

set the foundation for breastfeeding promotion and helped to buffer some of the inconsistent messages generated by formula marketing and the lack of breastfeeding education among some nurses and health professionals. To ensure that messages are clear and consistent, education about breastfeeding should be required for all staff members who interact with NICU parents. In addition, NICUs should reconsider whether outside corporations should be allowed access to the unit to market their products to the hospital staff. NICU babies should receive care based on scientific evidence that is not conflicting with commercial interests. Feeding education could be easily provided by experts in nutrition from within the NICU.

This article focused on structure and processes of breastfeeding promotion. Future manuscripts will shed further light on the nurses' infant feeding beliefs and experiences and how these get expressed in the everyday demands of nursing in the NICU setting. ❖

Acknowledgments

The author acknowledges funding from the National Institute of Nursing Research/National Institutes of Health Grant to the University of Pennsylvania School of Nursing, Research on Vulnerable Women, Children and Families (T32-NR-07100) and the Xi Chapter of Sigma Theta Tau International Honor Society of Nursing. The author also thanks Drs. Janet Deatrick, Sandra Founds, Diane Spatz, and Frances Ward for support during this study.

Roberta Cricco-Lizza, PhD, MPH, RN, is associated with Center for Health Disparities Research, University of Pennsylvania School of Nursing, Philadelphia, PA. She can be reached via e-mail at rcricco@nursing.upenn.edu

The author has disclosed that there are no financial relationships related to this article.

References

American Academy of Pediatrics. (2005). Breastfeeding and the use of human milk. *Pediatrics, 115,* 496-506.

Bernaix, L. W. (2000). Nurses' attitudes, subjective norms, and behavioral intentions toward support of breastfeeding mothers. *Journal of Human Lactation, 16,* 201-209.

Centers for Disease Control and Prevention. (2008). Breastfeeding-related maternity practices at hospitals and birth centers—United States, 2007. *Morbidity and Mortality Weekly Review, 57,* 521-525.

Cricco-Lizza, R. (2006). Black non-Hispanic mothers' perceptions about the promotion of infant feeding methods by nurses and physicians. *Journal of Obstetric, Gynecologic and Neonatal Nursing, 35,* 173-180.

Cricco-Lizza, R. (2009). Formative infant feeding experiences and education of NICU nurses. *MCN The American Journal of Maternal Child Nursing.*

Dall'Oglio, I., Salvatori, G., Bonci, E., Nantini, B., D'Agostino, G., & Dotta, A. (2007). Breastfeeding promotion in neonatal intensive care unit: Impact of a new program toward a BFHI for high-risk infants. *Acta Paediatric 96,* 1626-1631.

DiGirolamo, A. M., Grummer-Strawn, L. M., & Fein, S. (2001). Maternity care practices: Implications for breastfeeding. *Birth, 28,* 94-100.

do Nascimento, M. B., & Issler, H. (2005). Breastfeeding the premature infant: Experience of a baby-friendly hospital in Brazil. *Journal of Human Lactation, 21,* 47-52.

Erlen, J. A. (2008). Conflict of interest: Nurses at risk! *Orthopedic Nursing, 27,* 135-139.

Espy, K. A., & Senn, T. E. (2003). Incidence and correlates of breast milk feeding in hospitalized preterm infants. *Social Science and Medicine, 57,* 1421-1428.

Furman, L., Taylor, G., Minich, N., & Hack, M. (2003). The effect of maternal milk on neonatal morbidity of very low-birth-weight infants. *Archives of Pediatrics Adolescent Medicine, 157,* 66-71.

Hagen, B., Pijl-Zieber, E. M., Souveny, K., & Lacroix, A. (2008). Let's do lunch? The ethics of accepting gifts from the pharmaceutical industry. *Canadian Nurse, 104,* (4), 30-35.

Hylander, M. A., Strobino, D., Pezzullo, J. C., & Dhanireddy, R. (2001). Association of human milk feedings in retinopathy of prematurity among very low birth weight infants. *Journal of Perinatology, 21,* 356-362.

Ip, S., Chung, M., Raman, G., Magula, N., DeVine, D., Trikalinos, T., et al. (2007). *Breastfeeding and maternal and infant health outcomes in developed countries* (Evidence Report/Technology Assessment No. 153). AHRQ Publication No. 07-E007. Rockville, MD: Agency for Healthcare Research and Quality.

Jones, A. E., Shapiro, N. I., & Roshon, M. (2007). Implementing early goal-directed therapy in the emergency setting: The challenges and experiences of translating research innovations into clinical reality in academic and community settings. *Academic Emergency Medicine, 14,* 1072-1078.

Kramer, M. S., Chalmers, B., Hodnett, E. D., Sevkovskaya, Z., Dzikovick, I., Shapiro, S., et al. (2001). Promotion of breastfeeding intervention trial (PROBIT): A randomized trial in the Republic of Belarus. *Journal of the American Medical Association, 285,* 413-420.

Lessen, R., & Crivelli-Kovach, A. (2007). Prediction of initiation and duration of breastfeeding for neonates admitted to the neonatal intensive care unit. *Journal of Perinatal Nursing, 21,* 256-266.

McInnes, R. J., & Chambers, J. A. (2008). Supporting breastfeeding mothers: Qualitative synthesis. *Journal of Advanced Nursing, 62,* 407-427.

Meier, P. P. (2001). Breastfeeding in the special care nursery: Prematures and infants with medical problems. *Pediatric Clinics of North America, 48* (2), 425-442.

Merewood, A., Philipp, B. L., Chawla, N., & Cimo, S. (2003). The baby-friendly hospital initiative increases breastfeeding rates in a US neonatal intensive care unit. *Journal of Human Lactation, 19,* 166-171.

Miller, F. A., & Alvarado, K. (2005). Incorporating documents into qualitative nursing research. *Journal of Nursing Scholarship, 37,* 348-353.

Schanler, R. J., Lau, C., Hurst, N. M., & Smith, E. O. (2005). Randomized trial of donor human milk versus preterm formula as substitutes for mothers' own milk in the feeding of extremely premature infants. *Pediatrics, 116,* 400-406.

Siddell, E., Marinelli, K., Froman, R. D., & Burke, G. (2003). Evaluation of an educational intervention on breastfeeding for NICU nurses. *Journal of Human Lactation, 19,* 293-302.

Spatz, D. L. (2006). State of the science: Use of human milk and breastfeeding for vulnerable infants. *Journal of Perinatal and Neonatal Nursing, 20,* 51-55.

Stokamer, C. L. (2003). Pharmaceutical gift giving: Analysis of an ethical dilemma. *Journal of Nursing Administration, 33,* 48-51.

Vohr, B. W., Poindexter, B. B., Dusick, A. M., McKinley, L. T., Wright, L. L., Langer, J. C., et al. (2006). Beneficial effects of breast milk in the neonatal intensive care unit on the developmental outcome of extremely low birth weight infants at 18 months of age. *Pediatrics, 118*(1), pp. e115-e123. Retrieved June 1, 2009, from http://pediatrics.aappublications.org/cgi/content/full/118/1/e115

Weinert, C. R., & Mann, H. J. (2008). The science of implementation: Changing the practice of critical care. *Current Opinion in Critical Care, 14,* 460-465.

World Health Organization and United Nations Children's Fund. (1992). Baby Friendly Hospital Initiative. Geneva: WHO/UNICEF.

Yano, E. (2008). The role of organizational research in implementing evidence-based practice: QUERI series. *Implementation Science, 3,* 29. Retrieved June 1, 2009, from http://www.pubmedcentral.nih.gov/articlerender.fcgi?tool=pubmed&pubmedid=18510749

Nursing Research • January/February 2010 • Vol 59, No 1S, S58–S65

A Nurse-Facilitated Depression Screening Program in an Army Primary Care Clinic

An Evidence-Based Project

Edward E. Yackel ▼ Madelyn S. McKennan ▼ Adrianna Fox-Deise

▶ **Background:** Depression, sometimes with suicidal manifestations, is a medical condition commonly seen in primary care clinics. Routine screening for depression and suicidal ideation is recommended of all adult patients in the primary care setting because it offers depressed patients a greater chance of recovery and response to treatment, yet such screening often is overlooked or omitted.

▶ **Objective:** The purpose of this study was to develop, to implement, and to test the efficacy of a systematic depression screening process to increase the identification of depression in family members of active duty soldiers older than 18 years at a military family practice clinic located on an Army infantry post in the Pacific.

▶ **Methods:** The Iowa Model of Evidence-Based Practice to Promote Quality Care was used to develop a practice guideline incorporating a decision algorithm for nurses to screen for depression. A pilot project to institute this change in practice was conducted, and outcomes were measured.

▶ **Results:** Before implementation, approximately 100 patients were diagnosed with depression in each of the 3 months preceding the practice change. Approximately 130 patients a month were assigned a 311.0 Code 3 months after the practice change, and 140 patients per month received screenings and were assigned the correct International Classification of Diseases, Ninth Revision Code 311.0 at 1 year. The improved screening and coding for depression and suicidality added approximately 3 minutes to the patient screening process. The education of staff in the process of screening for depression and correct coding coupled with monitoring and staff feedback improved compliance with the identification and the documentation of patients with depression. Nurses were more likely than primary care providers to agree strongly that screening for depression enhances quality of care.

▶ **Discussion:** Data gathered during this project support the integration of military and civilian nurse-facilitated screening for depression in the military primary care setting. The decision algorithm should be adapted and tested in other primary care environments.

▶ **Key Words:** decision algorithm · depression screening · evidence-based practice · military primary care clinic

Mental illness ranks first among morbidities that cause disability in the United States, Canada, and Western Europe, with the associated healthcare cost in the United States estimated at $150 billion in 2003 (Centers for Disease Control and Prevention [CDC], 2003). A psychometric comparison of military and civilian populations in primary care settings revealed no statistical difference in the prevalence of mood disorders (Jackson, O'Malley, & Kroenke, 1999). However, Waldrep, Cozza, and Chun (2004) found that the deployment of a spouse or parent can challenge the ability of a military family member to cope with a preexisting medical or mental health illness. These authors recommended that clinicians identify those family members who require additional services and suggested actions that might mitigate the impact of deployment on the family unit.

Depression is a common medical condition seen frequently in primary care clinics. Patients with depression who present to primary care clinics have a greater chance of responding to treatment and recovery if primary care providers screen for depression using a short self-administered questionnaire as part of a comprehensive disease management program (DMP). The role of nurses in the process of screening for depression has yet to be delineated, so this evidence-based practice (EBP) project was designed to develop, to implement, and to evaluate a standardized nursing procedure to improve the screening of family members for depression at a military family practice clinic located on a U.S. Army infantry post in Hawaii. This EBP project was based on the Veterans Administration/ Department of Defense Behavioral Health Clinical Practice Guideline (VA/DoD BHCPG, 2002) for screening and treatment of depression as the DMP to guide practice change.

The absence in this clinic of a systematic method to screen family members of deployed soldiers for depression and the inability to estimate rates of depression in this clinical population were the problem-focused triggers for this project. National standards and guidelines that call for the

Edward E. Yackel, MSN, RN, FNP-BC, is Lieutenant Colonel, U.S. Army Nurse Corps, McDonald Army Health Center, Fort Eustis, Virginia.

Madelyn S. McKennan, MSN, RN, FNP-BC, is Lieutenant Colonel, U.S. Army Nurse Corps, Schofield Barracks Army Health Clinic, Honolulu, Hawaii.

Adrianna Fox-Deise, RN, FNP, is Instructor, School of Nursing and Dental Hygiene, University of Hawaii at Manoa.

139

screening of all adults for depression in primary care settings, such as the VA/DoD BHCPG (2002) and the recommendations and rationale published by the U.S. Preventive Services Task Force (USPSTF, 2002), were the knowledge-focused triggers that guided practice change in this primary care clinic.

A multidisciplinary panel of stakeholders—advanced practice registered nurses (APRNs), physicians, certified nurse assistants (CNAs), registered nurses (RNs), psychologist, and clinic administrators—formed the EBP team. This team was led by a change champion (an APRN) and an opinion leader (a physician). The change champion was an expert clinician who had positive working relationships with other healthcare professionals and who was passionate and committed about screening for depression in primary care. Similarly, the opinion leader was viewed as an important and respected source of influence among his peer group, demonstrated technical competence, and excelled as a teacher and mentor on the subject of depression. The EBP team met to review both problem- and knowledge-focused triggers and determined that screening for depression was a priority for the organization. The EBP project received enthusiastic support throughout the organization and at the highest levels of nursing leadership.

Because of the relevance to the outpatient setting in taking into account clinical decision making, the clinician, and organizational perspectives (Titler et al., 2001), the Iowa Model of Evidence-Based Practice to Promote Quality Care (see the Titler and Moore editorial in this supplement) was chosen to guide an EBP improvement systematically in a military primary practice clinic.

Literature Review

The published medical and nursing literature was reviewed to identify studies evaluating the efficacy of screening for depression in primary care and methodological approaches to such screening. The MEDLINE, the Cochrane, and the Cumulative Index to Nursing and Allied Health Literature databases were searched for English-language articles using eight subject headings (primary care, clinical practice guidelines, mental health, depression instruments, depression screening, suicide screening, military healthcare, and deployment). In addition, bibliographies of the articles obtained were searched for relevant articles to generate additional references. Editorials were rejected, as were articles with data targeting pediatric populations exclusively. Two guidelines (graded as Level I), 3 Level I articles, 17 Level II articles, and 10 Level III articles were critiqued using USPSTF criteria by two APRNs, a physician, and a nurse researcher for inclusion in a literature synthesis. Level I articles included evidence obtained from at least one randomized controlled trial. Level II articles included evidence from well-designed controlled trials without randomization (classified as Level II-1), evidence from cohort or case–control analytic studies (Level II-2), and evidence from multiple time series with or without intervention (Level II-3). Level III articles included opinions of respected authorities that were based on clinical experience or descriptive studies and case reports (Harris et al., 2001). The literature synthesis (Table 1) facilitated the categorization of articles into three focus areas: (a) prevalence of depression in primary care populations; (b) depression management programs and evaluation of suicidal risk; and (c) depression screening instruments and their use in primary care settings.

Prevalence of Depression Depression is a common medical condition associated with high direct and indirect healthcare costs (Badamgarav et al., 2003; Valenstein, Vijan, Zeber, Boehm, & Buttar, 2001). Dickey and Blumberg (2002) analyzed data from the 1999 National Health Interview Survey and found that 6.3% or 12.5 million noninstitutionalized U.S. adults suffer from major depression. The prevalence of major depression in primary care settings is 5% to 9% among adults, with half of these unrecognized and untreated (Hirschfeld et al., 1997; Hunter, Hunter, West, Kinder, & Carroll, 2002; Simon & VonKorff, 1995). Depressive illness in primary care is less severe than in mental health settings; thus, the short-term prognosis, the chance of recovery, and the response to treatment are greater in primary care settings (Dickey & Blumberg, 2002; Pignone et al., 2002; Simon & VonKorff, 1995).

Within the next 20 years, depression is projected to be the second highest cause of disability in the world and to have a lifetime prevalence of 15% to 25% (Badamgarav et al., 2003). Depression has been shown to increase the morbidity and mortality associated with other chronic diseases, such as diabetes and cardiovascular disorders (Hunter et al., 2002; Pignone et al., 2002). Furthermore, family members of patients with depression have increased physical morbidity and psychopathology (Sobieraj, Williams, Marley, & Ryan, 1998). A majority of adult patients with mental health concerns such as depression will seek and receive care in primary care settings (Dickey & Blumberg, 2002; Pignone et al., 2002).

The lifetime suicide risk for all patients diagnosed with major depressive disorder has been estimated as 3.5% (Blair-West, Mellsop, & Eyeson-Annan, 1997). Harris and Barraclough (1997) found a 12- to 20-fold risk for suicide associated with depressive disorder using the general population for comparison. Suicide is the second-leading cause of death among those aged 25 to 34 years, accounting for 12.9% of all deaths annually (CDC, 2007). Luoma, Martin, and Pearson (2002) reviewed 40 studies examining rates of contact with primary care providers before suicide and found that approximately 45% of patients who committed suicide had contact with a primary care provider within 1 month of taking their lives, suggesting that screening for risk of suicide in patients with depression is important in primary care settings. Although the literature supports the efficacy of DMPs that include screening for depression, the USPSTF (2004) found insufficient evidence to recommend for or against screening for risk of suicide by primary care clinicians. Focusing on the detection and care of patients with depression who are at higher risk for self-harm and improving the ability of primary care providers to identify and to treat those at risk for suicide are suggested strategies for suicide prevention efforts (Luoma et al., 2002; Schulberg et al., 2005).

Depression Screening Instruments

A variety of self-administered questionnaires are available for assessing the severity of depression and risk of suicide in primary care. The Patient Health Questionnaire depression module (PHQ-9) and a two-item version of the PHQ depression module, the PHQ-2, provide primary care providers with valid and reliable measures to assess patients with depression in busy primary care settings (Kroenke, Spitzer, & Williams, 2001, 2003). The PHQ-9 is the self-administered

TABLE I. Selected Literature Synthesis

Focus area	Journal or source	Year	Description	Level of evidence
Prevalence of depression	General Hospital Psychiatry	1995	Literature review	Literature synthesis
	JAMA	2006	Population-based descriptive study	Level II-3
	Military Medicine	1999	Psychometric comparison: military vs. civilian	Level II-3
	Archives of Family Medicine	1995	Epidemiological study with 1- year follow-up	Level II-2
	Journal of the American Board Family Practice	2005	Descriptive study	Level III
	Military Medicine	2002	Comparative study: PHQ vs. progress notes	Level II-3
	Iraq War Clinicians Guide	2004	Opinion by respected authority	Level III
	American Journal of Psychiatry	2003	Meta-analysis	Level I
	National Mental Health Information Center	1999	Survey report	Level III
	JAMA	1997	Consensus statement	Level III
Depression management programs and evaluation of suicide risk	Annals of Internal Medicine	2002	Systematic literature review	Guideline/Level I
	General Hospital Psychiatry	1992	Abstract	Level III
	American Journal of Psychiatry	2002	Meta-analysis of descriptive studies/reports	Level III
	Journal of General Internal Medicine	1996	Structured interviews, comparison of three studies	Level II-1
	Annals of Family Medicine	2005	Randomized controlled trial	Level I
	British Journal of Psychiatry	1997	Meta-analysis	Level II-1
	Centers for Disease Control and Prevention	2007	Report/literature review	Level III
Depression screening instruments	American Journal of Managed Care	2004	Psychometric comparison of one-item depression screen versus PHQ	Level II-3
	Journal of General Internal Medicine	1997	Comparing validity of PHQ-2 to validity of other known measures	Level II-2
	Medical Care	2003	Survey, nonrandomized	Level II-2
	Psychotherapy and Psychosomatics	2004	Descriptive comparison of three questionnaires	Level II-3
	Journal of General Internal Medicine	2001	PHQ-9 compared with other measures/nonrandomized	Level II-2
	Department of Veterans Affairs	2000	Clinical practice guideline	Guideline/level I
	JAMA	1999	Criterion standard study: PRIME MD	Level I
	American Journal of Obstetrics and Gynecology	2000	Validity study of PHQ in obstetrician-gynecologist patients	Level II-2

Note. Level I articles included evidence obtained from at least one randomized controlled trial. Level II articles included evidence from well-designed controlled trials without randomization (classified as Level II-1), evidence from cohort or case–control analytic studies (Level II-2), and evidence from multiple time series with or without intervention (Level II-3). Level III articles included opinions of respected authorities that were based on clinical experience or descriptive studies and case reports (Harris et al., 2001).

depression module of the Primary Care Evaluation of Mental Disorders (a diagnostic instrument for common mental disorders designed for primary care providers to assess the cognitive and physical symptoms of depressive disorders; Hunter et al., 2002). Kroenke et al. (2001) examined the validity of the PHQ-9 by analyzing data from 6,000 patients aged 18 years or older who had completed the PHQ-9 in eight primary care clinics and seven obstetrics-gynecology clinics. Recent data show that the PHQ-9 has a sensitivity of 88% and a specificity of 88% for major depression, with excellent internal reliability (α = .89) and validity in measuring the severity of depression (Corson, Gerrity, & Dobscha, 2004; Kroenke et al., 2001). Lowe et al. (2004) compared the criterion validity of the PHQ-9 for diagnosing depressive episodes with two other well-established instruments and concluded that the PHQ-9 demonstrated a diagnostic advantage and had superior criterion validity when compared with the other instruments. The last item of the PHQ-9 assesses patients for suicidal risk, which is one of the diagnostic criteria for depressive disorders. Feeling suicidal predicts plans to attempt suicide with 83% sensitivity, 98% specificity, and 30% positive predictive value when asked as a single self-report item (Olfson, Weissman, Leon, Sheehan, & Farber, 1996). Corson et al. (2004) reported that use of the PHQ-9 death or suicide item identified one third (7%) of patients in a VA primary care clinic with active suicidal ideation who would not have been treated otherwise.

Shorter screening tests with questions about depressed mood and anhedonia (inability to have pleasurable feelings) appear to detect a majority of depressed patients (Pignone et al., 2002). The PHQ-2 is a self-administered questionnaire used to ascertain the frequency of depressed mood and anhedonia over the past 2 weeks. Kroenke et al. (2003) established the criterion validity of the PHQ-2 by comparing its operating characteristics with an interview by an independent mental health provider and reported a sensitivity of 83% and a specificity of 92%. Corson et al. and Kroenke et al. reported 97% sensitivity and 91% specificity for depression when using the PHQ-2 to screen for this disorder in a VA primary care setting. Thus, the literature provides strong evidence for the validity of the PHQ-2 as a brief screening measure that facilitates the diagnosis of major depression. However, it is recognized as an initial step in a DMP that requires further assessment and implementation to care for patients with major depression (Corson et al., 2004; Kroenke et al., 2003; USPSTF, 2002).

The VA/DoD BHCPG (2002) for screening and treatment of depression is an example of a DMP that includes screening for depression and suicide. The guideline is designed for use by providers who care for patients with depression in military primary care clinics. The VA/DoD BHCPG DMP describes (a) the screening and recognition of depression and suicidal ideation; (b) the assessment of physical and mental status; (c) the diagnostic criteria and assessment of risk factors; (d) a treatment plan that includes suggestions for managing medications, counseling, and referral criteria; (e) patient and family education; and (f) the monitoring and documentation of follow-up. The VA/DoD BHCPG is designed for the primary care setting and describes the role of primary care providers, but it does not explicate the role of nursing staff in implementing the process.

Evidence has been found that screening improves the identification of depressed patients and that effective follow-up and treatment of depressed adults decrease clinical morbidity in primary care settings (USPSTF, 2002). Evidence-based guidelines, patient education, collaborative and multidisciplinary care, and monitoring are used in DMPs to provide comprehensive care for patients with chronic diseases such as depression (Badamgarav et al., 2003). The DMPs that include screening for depression are more effective than the programs that are focused on depression screening alone (Bijl,

van Marwijk, de Haan, van Tilburg, & Beekman, 2004; Pignone et al., 2002). Badamgarav et al. (2003) systematically reviewed the published medical literature evaluating the effectiveness of DMPs for chronic conditions such as depression and found that disease management improves the detection and care of patients with depression. Similarly, a systematic review and a meta-analysis of randomized controlled trials of DMPs for depression concluded that the costs of depression programs are within the cost range of other public health improvements and that enhanced quality of care is possible (Neumeyer-Gromen, Lampert, Stark, & Kallischnigg, 2004). Primary care providers play a vital role in DMPs to improve the detection and care of patients with depression. Notably absent from the literature are descriptors of nursing processes that facilitate screening for depression and the role that nurses play in the DMPs. The purpose of this EBP project was to implement and to evaluate the change process methodology involved in screening family members of military active duty soldiers for depression.

Setting

The setting for this EBP project was a military family practice clinic with an enrollment of 14,322 family members and approximately 175 daily patient visits. Before implementation of the project, only female family members were screened routinely for depression (at well-woman visits), and nurses did not participate in screening for depression. This process resulted in 100 cases of depression being captured a month. Family members of military active duty soldiers older than 18 years who could read, write, and communicate in English were screened. Patient care was documented in a hard-copy medical record or in the military's electronic medical record, the Armed Forces Health Longitudinal Technology Application (AHLTA). The selection of the screening process for the EBP project was based on the VA/DoD BHCPG for screening and treatment of depression and similar patient populations studied by other investigators (Kroenke et al., 2003; Olfson et al., 1996). All military family members have open access to mental health services. Patients who require inpatient psychiatric care are referred by their primary care provider or mental health provider to a regional military medical center.

Implementation: Decision Algorithm

Two questions from the PHQ-2 ("During the past month, have you often been bothered by feeling down, depressed or hopeless?" and "During the past month, have you often been bothered by little interest or pleasure in doing things?") and one question from the PHQ-9 ("Do you have thoughts that you would be better off dead or hurting yourself in some way?") were selected for use in the project. The decision algorithm for nurses (Figure 1) integrates the PHQ-2 and the PHQ-9 questions as steps in the depression screening process. The first step of the depression screening process prompts nursing staff to ask the PHQ-2 questions in an effort to determine the presence of depressed mood or anhedonia. A negative response to the PHQ-2 questions concludes the depression screening process, and the primary care provider addresses the patient's primary complaint. The second step of the screening process directs nurses to ask the PHQ-9 question (suicidal ideation) when a positive response is given to

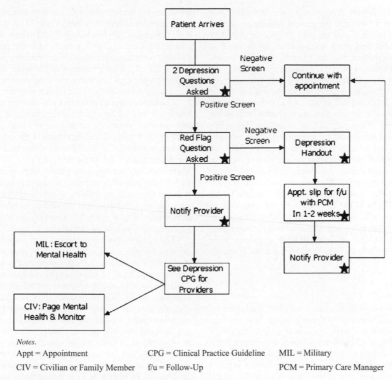

FIGURE 1. A decision algorithm for nurses.

either of the PHQ-2 questions. A patient who denies suicidal ideation is given a depression handout listing behavioral health support services, locations of clinics, and contact numbers. Subsequently, the patient is offered a follow-up appointment in 1 or 2 weeks with the primary care provider to discuss assessment and treatment of depression. The patient's appointment continues after the nurse reports the results of the depression screening to the primary care provider. A patient who responds positively to the PHQ-9 (*red flag*) question is referred immediately to a mental health professional for further evaluation. Documentation of the depression screening process is completed by nurses in the AHLTA system. Primary care providers are encouraged to use the VA/DoD BHCPG to assess and to treat patients with depression.

Piloting the Change
Creating an environment for a practice change to occur is an important element in the EBP process; therefore, a pilot project was undertaken to identify barriers in implementing the decision algorithm. A physician, a CNA, and two RNs (a nurse researcher and a research assistant) from the EBP team were selected to model the change in clinical practice over a 3-day period. The experienced nurse researcher instructed the CNA on depression, depression screening, and integra-

tion of the EBP decision algorithm into existing screening practices by providing verbal education and written materials. The CNA was required to verbalize and to demonstrate the use of the decision algorithm before starting the pilot. All patients meeting the inclusion criteria were screened for depression using the decision algorithm. The experienced nurse researcher and research assistant observed screening practices during the pilot to evaluate the process and outcomes and to make recommendations aimed at improving the process.

Instituting the Change in Practice
Feedback from all participants in the pilot project was used to formulate six recommendations aimed at minimizing barriers in implementing the decision algorithm and in instituting the change in practice: (a) integrate the PHQ-2 and the PHQ-9 depression screening questions into both the hard-copy medical record and the AHLTA system to add continuity during unscheduled computer downtime; (b) educate staff (providers and nurses) on the decision algorithm and the documentation process for both hard-copy and electronic medical records; (c) provide depression awareness education by a mental health professional to increase the nursing staff's comfort when asking questions about depression; (d) post the decision algorithm at the nursing team center to foster recognition and

comprehension; (e) display depression posters prominently in patient care areas to sensitize the patient population to this common mental health condition; and (f) educate providers (physicians, APRNs, and physician assistants) on the need to document and use the International Classification of Diseases, Ninth Revision (ICD-9) Code 311.0 (depressive disorder, not otherwise specified) consistently to simplify data retrieval from military medical databases. Forty staff members (RNs, LPNs, CNAs, APRNs, PAs, and MDs) were educated in using the decision algorithm and the documentation process for both the hard-copy and the electronic medical record by the family practice clinic head nurse (EBP team member). A psychologist provided depression education to 17 nurses (RN, LPN, or CNA). This included the definition of depression, how to approach asking questions on depression, and role playing the depression screening process. Thirteen of the family practice clinic providers (100%) were educated by the opinion leader on the use of Code 311.0 to document the diagnosis of depression. Depression posters were displayed in patient care areas, the decision algorithm was displayed at the nursing team center, and the PHQ-2 and the PHQ-9 questions were integrated into the hard-copy and the AHLTA medical record.

Results

Outcome Measures

Four measures were used to assess the success of implementing the EBP decision algorithm in the family practice clinic: (a) number of patients diagnosed with depression; (b) satisfaction of providers and nurses; (c) compliance in documentation (measured via random chart audits); and (d) time–motion evaluation of the patient screening process. Data collection began 3 months after implementation of the decision algorithm by the RN researcher.

An assessment of the numbers of patients diagnosed with depression was based on data gathered from a military medical database to establish the number of family members diagnosed with depression in the family practice clinic using the ICD-9 Code 311.0 before and after the practice change. With nurses administering the depression screening to all adult patients (not just females) and providers using Code 311.0 to identify those with depression, approximately 130 patients a month were assigned a Code 311.0 3 months into the practice change and 140 patients a month at 1 year after the practice change (Figure 2). A possible correlation between deployment of soldiers to Iraq and increase in the number of family members presenting for treatment of depression was not examined.

The satisfaction of providers and nursing staff was measured at 3 and 12 months after the change in practice using one question answered on a 4-point Likert scale: "Implementing depression screening enhances the quality of care in the family practice clinic." Participants rated their level of agreement from 1 (*strongly disagree*) to 4 (*strongly agree*). Three months after implementation, 64% of the nurses and 45% of the providers strongly agreed that screening for depression enhanced the quality of care in the clinic. At 1 year after the implementation of the decision algorithm, 95% of nurses and 54% of providers strongly agreed that screening for depression enhanced the quality of care.

The nurse researcher evaluated staff compliance in documenting the process of screening for depression using a standardized audit form to review systematically selected (every fourth record from 11 providers) electronic medical records. Thirty records that met selection criteria were audited at 3 months, and 30 different records were audited at 6 months after the practice change was implemented. The number of records to audit was determined on the basis of patient visits per day and the rate of major depression in primary care (5–9%) obtained from the literature review. Three months into the practice change, 26 (87%) of 30 reviewed charts showed evidence of documentation for depression screening; 7 (27%) of 26 charts verified that patients screened for depression were positive for depressed mood or anhedonia without suicidal ideation. Six months after the practice change, evidence of documentation for depression screening was shown in 29 (97%) of the 30 charts, and patients who were screened for depression were positive for depressed mood or anhedonia without suicidal ideation in 10 (33%) charts. The

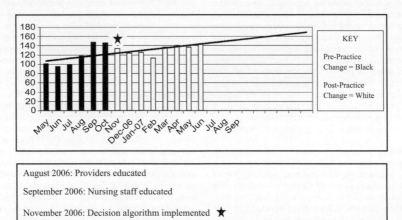

FIGURE 2. Number of depression cases before and after practice change.

nurse researcher was unable to determine the compliance of nursing staff in documenting notification of a mental health provider, given that no cases of suicidal ideation were identified in the audited charts. An important facet of compliance with documentation throughout the institutionalization of the decision algorithm was continual education and feedback to both providers and nurses on requirements.

Time–motion data were collected for the length of time it took to screen patients. The screening process included greeting the patient, obtaining weight and vital signs, escorting the patient into an examination room, reviewing demographic data, reviewing the screening questions on depression and suicide, and entering data into the AHLTA system. Variability among the nurses in the process for screening patients during the first month of the project initially resulted in a time variance of 11 minutes, with a range of 5 to 30 minutes for each screening. The clinic head nurse standardized the screening process by asking the nurses to enter data into the AHLTA in the examination rooms instead of returning to the team center. This resulted in a mean time reduction of 4 minutes, 58 seconds after the practice change. The mean time added per patient encounter after the practice change was 2 minutes, 53 seconds.

Discussion

Data gathered during the EBP project support the relevance of a nurse-facilitated program to screen for depression in a primary care setting. The VA/DoD BHCPG is designed for primary care and describes the role of primary care providers in the DMP but it does not describe the role of nurses in the depression screening process. The decision algorithm was a valuable tool defining the steps to be followed by nurses when screening patients for depression. More important, incorporating nurses into the depression screening process accomplished the first step of the VA/DoD BHCPG in a multidisciplinary effort consistent with recommendations found in the literature.

Nurses can be instrumental in depression screening in the primary care setting, leading to appropriate referral for further care. The prevalence, the morbidity, and the mortality associated with depression necessitate that nurses be involved integrally in this process as part of the healthcare team. In this pilot project, one provider, a CNA, and two RNs identified barriers in implementing the decision algorithm into the business practices of the family practice clinic. Although procedural barriers to the implementation of the decision algorithm were addressed, incorporating the process of screening for depression into existing screening practices was not clearly defined. The wide range seen in screening times during the first month of the project was most likely related to procedural differences in whether nursing staff entered vital signs and questionnaire data into the electronic medical record (the AHLTA) during or after seeing the patient. Standardization of the time of data entry improved screening times. A mandatory program for reconciling medications was implemented during the EBP project and may have affected the outcome of the time–motion study because the effects of implementing both screening for depression and medication reconciliation might have been measured.

A majority of staff members strongly agreed that screening for depression is a quality component of clinical practice, despite both providers and nurses acknowledging an increased workload because of the EBP project. The decision algorithm was designed to allow primary care providers the option of implementing the VA/DoD BHCPG upon notification of screening results by nurses. The hope was that if the nursing staff followed the procedural steps outlined in the decision algorithm, the need for providers to intercede in the process of screening for depression would be mitigated. However, clinical assessment of the presenting illness and trends in patients' healthcare utilization may have affected how providers responded to the screening results. Some providers were not comfortable with the process of screening for depression, which may have played a role also in how they responded to patients who reported anhedonia or depressed mood. Conversely, nurses who were comfortable with screening for depression were more likely to respond that such screening enhanced the quality of patient care. The difference between nurse and provider levels of comfort may have been the result of the difference in the educational offerings presented to each group. Nurses were offered depression awareness training and repeated education on the decision algorithm and documentation requirements, whereas providers were educated only on the management of depression in primary care and implementation of the decision algorithm. Standardization of educational offerings for all members of the healthcare team is recommended to provide consistent information and continuity of care and to foster trust in the depression screening process.

Both providers and nurses considered depression screening beneficial to family members of deployed soldiers. One year after the practice change, 10 providers were asked to reflect on how many patients had a positive screening for suicidal ideation that required immediate referral to a behavioral health specialist. These providers estimated that approximately 36 patients reported suicidal ideation who would not otherwise have been detected. Although no data were obtained on the relationship between the deployment of soldiers and reports of depression and suicidal ideation by family members, further study on the relationship between these variables is recommended.

Implications for Practice and Research

The integration of a nurse-facilitated depression screening program into the business practices of a busy military family practice clinic was viewed by providers, nursing staff, and nursing leadership as a quality component of clinical practice that benefited the population served. The Iowa Model of Evidence-Based Practice to Promote Quality Care (Titler et al., 2001) and the decision algorithm for nurses were essential tools in implementing practice change and appear to have great utility in the primary care setting. The use of an EBP model provides a systematic method for nurses to evaluate critically, to define, and to implement changes in practice. The decision algorithm for nurses was a valuable tool in the depression screening process and should be tested in other primary care settings. In addition, further study is warranted to determine whether having nurses screen for depression influences the practice patterns of primary care providers when implementing a DMP such as the VA/DoD BHCPG. ▼

Accepted for publication September 30, 2009.

This project was funded by an award from the TriService Nursing Research Program, grant no. N03-P18. The Uniformed Services University of the Health Sciences (USUHS), 4301 Jones Bridge Rd., Bethesda, MD 20814-4799, is the awarding and administering office.

This project was sponsored by the TriService Nursing Research Program, Uniformed Services University of the Health Sciences; however, the information or content and conclusions do not necessarily represent the official position or policy of, nor should any official endorsement be inferred by, the TriService Nursing Research Program, Uniformed Services University of the Health Sciences, the Department of Defense, or the U.S. Government.

The following people contributed to the study: Nathan DeWeese, MD; Ms. Renee Latimer, RN, MPH; Mrs. Charlotte Grant, NA; Mr. Wesley Grant, NA; Richard Schobitz, PhD; and Mr. Adrian Santos, RN, BSN.

The authors thank LTC Debra Mark and LTC Mary Hardy, who were responsible for implementation of the Evidence-Based Practice Training Program at Tripler Army Medical Center, and CAPT Patricia Kelley, without whom we could not have conducted this project.

The views and opinions expressed in this article are solely those of the authors and do not reflect the policy or position of the Department of the Army, the Department of Defense, or the U.S. Government.

Corresponding author: Edward E. Yackel, MSN, RN, FNP-BC, U.S. Army Nurse Corps, McDonald Army Health Center, Fort Eustis, VA 23604 (e-mail: Ed.yackel@us.army.mil).

References

Badamgarav, E., Weingarten, S. R., Henning, J. M., Knight, K., Hasselbald, V., Gano, A. Jr., et al. (2003). Effectiveness of disease management programs in depression: A systematic review. *American Journal of Psychiatry, 160*(12), 2080–2090.

Bijl, D., van Marwijk, H. W., de Haan, M., van Tilburg, W., & Beekman, A. J. (2004). Effectiveness of disease management programmes for recognition, diagnosis and treatment of depression in primary care. *European Journal of General Practice, 10*(1), 6–12.

Blair-West, G. W., Mellsop, G. W., & Eyeson-Annan, M. L. (1997). Down-rating lifetime suicide risk in major depression. *Acta Psychiatrica Scandinavica, 95*(3), 259–263.

Centers for Disease Control and Prevention. (2003). *Healthy people 2010: Progress review focus area 18.* Retrieved July 5, 2006, from http://www.cdc.gov/nchs/about/otheract/hpdata2010/focusareas/fa18-mentalhealth.htm

Centers for Disease Control and Prevention. (2007). *Suicide: Facts at a glance.* Retrieved July 22, 2007, from http://www.cdc.gov/injury

Corson, K., Gerrity, M. S., & Dobscha, S. K. (2004). Screening for depression and suicidality in a VA primary care setting: 2 items are better than 1 item. *American Journal of Managed Care, 10*(11 Pt. 2), 839–845.

Dickey, W. C., & Blumberg, S. J. (2002). *Prevalence of mental disorders and contact with mental health professionals among adults in the United States, National Health Interview Survey, 1999.* Retrieved July 5, 2006, from http://mentalhealth.samhsa.gov/publications/allpubs/SMA04-3938/Chapter08.asp

Harris, E. C., & Barraclough, B. (1997). Suicide as an outcome for mental disorders. A meta-analysis. *British Journal of Psychiatry, 170,* 205–228.

Harris, R. P., Helfan, M., Woolf, S. H., Lohr, K. N., Mulrow, C. D., Teutsch, S. M., et al. (2001). Current methods of the US Preventive Services Task Force: A review of the process. *American Journal of Preventive Medicine, 20*(Suppl. 3), 21–35.

Hirschfeld, R. M., Keller, M. B., Panico, S., Arons, B. S., Barlow, D., Davidoff, F., et al. (1997). The National Depressive and Manic-Depressive Association consensus statement on the undertreatment of depression. *JAMA, 277*(4), 333–340.

Hunter, C. L., Hunter, C. M., West, E. T., Kinder, M. H., & Carroll, D. W. (2002). Recognition of depressive disorders by primary care providers in a military medical setting. *Military Medicine, 167*(4), 308–311.

Jackson, J. L., O'Malley, P. G., & Kroenke, K. (1999). A psychometric comparison of military and civilian medical practices. *Military Medicine, 164*(2), 112–115.

Kroenke, K., Spitzer, R. L., & Williams, J. B. (2001). The PHQ-9: Validity of a brief depression severity measure. *Journal of General Internal Medicine, 16*(9), 606–613.

Kroenke, K., Spitzer, R. L., & Williams, J. B. (2003). The Patient Health Questionnaire-2: Validity of a two-item depression screener. *Medical Care, 41*(11), 1284–1292.

Lowe, B., Grafe, K., Zipfel, S., Witte, S., Loerch, B., & Herzog, W. (2004). Diagnosing ICD-10 depressive episodes: Superior criterion validity of the Patient Health Questionnaire. *Psychotherapy and Psychosomatics, 73*(6), 386–390.

Luoma, J. B., Martin, C. E., & Pearson, J. L. (2002). Contact with mental health and primary care providers before suicide: A review of the evidence. *American Journal of Psychiatry, 159*(6), 909–916.

Neumeyer-Gromen, A., Lampert, T., Stark, K., & Kallischnigg, G. (2004). Disease management programs for depression: A systematic review and meta-analysis of randomized controlled trials. *Medical Care, 42*(12), 1211–1221.

Olfson, M., Weissman, M. M., Leon, A. C., Sheehan, D. V., & Farber, L. (1996). Suicidal ideation in primary care. *Journal of General Internal Medicine, 11*(8), 447–453.

Pignone, M., Gaynes, B. N., Rushton, J. L., Mulrow, C. D., Orleans, C. T., Whitener, B. L., et al. (2002). *Screening for depression: Systematic evidence review no. 6.* Prepared by the Research Triangle Institute, University of North Carolina Evidence-Based Practice Center under Contract No. 290-97-0011. Rockville, MD: Agency for Healthcare Research and Quality.

Schulberg, H. C., Lee, P. W., Bruce, M. L., Raue, P. J., Lefever, J. J., Williams, J. W. Jr., et al. (2005). Suicidal ideation and risk levels among primary care patients with uncomplicated depression. *Annals of Family Medicine, 3*(6), 523–528.

Simon, G. E., & VonKorff, M. (1995). Recognition, management and outcomes of depression in primary care. *Archives of Family Medicine, 4*(2), 99–105.

Sobieraj, M., Williams, J., Marley, J., & Ryan, P. (1998). The impact of depression on the physical health of family members. *British Journal of General Practice, 48*(435), 1653–1655.

Titler, M. G., Kleiber, C., Steelman, V. J., Rakel, B. A., Budreau, G., Everett, L. Q., et al. (2001). The Iowa Model of Evidence-Based Practice to Promote Quality Care. *Critical Care Nursing Clinics of North America, 13*(4), 497–509.

United States Preventive Services Task Force. (2002). Screening for depression: Recommendations and rationale. *Annals of Internal Medicine, 136*(10), 760–764.

United States Preventive Services Task Force. (2004). Screening for suicide risk: Recommendation and rationale. *Annals of Internal Medicine, 140*(10), 820–821.

Valenstein, M., Vijan, S., Zeber, J. E., Boehm, K., & Buttar, A. (2001). The cost-utility of screening for depression in primary care. *Annals of Internal Medicine, 134*(5), 345–360.

Veterans Administration/Department of Defense. (2002). *Management of major depressive disorder (MDD) in adults in the primary care setting, initial assessment and treatment.* Retrieved January 25, 2006, from http://oqp.med.va.gov/cpg/cpg.htm

Waldrep, D. A., Cozza, S. J., & Chun, R. S. (2004). XIII. The impact of deployment on the military family. From the National Center for Post-Traumatic Stress Disorder. *Iraq War Clinician Guide.* Retrieved August 29, 2006, from http://www.ptsd.va.gov/professional/manuals/manual-pdf/iwcg/iraq_clinician_guide_ch_13.pdf

Nursing Research • July/August 2009 • Vol 58, No 4, 274–282

Why Do Elders Delay Responding to Heart Failure Symptoms?

Corrine Y. Jurgens ▾ Linda Hoke ▾ Janet Byrnes ▾ Barbara Riegel

▶ **Background:** Elders with heart failure (HF) are at risk for frequent hospitalizations for symptom management. Repeated admissions are partly related to delay in responding to HF symptoms. Contextual factors such as prior illness experiences and social/emotional factors may affect symptom interpretation and response. The Self-Regulation Model of Illness guided this study as it acknowledges the dynamic nature of illness and influence of contextual factors and social environment on the interpretation and response to symptoms.

▶ **Objective:** The purpose of this study was to describe contextual factors related to symptom recognition and response among elders hospitalized with decompensated HF.

▶ **Methods:** A mixed-methods design was used. The HF Symptom Perception Scale (physical factors), Specific Activity Scale (functional performance), and Response to Symptoms Questionnaire (cognitive/emotional factors) were administered to participants aged ≥65 years. Symptom duration and clinical details were collected by interview and chart review. Open-ended questions addressing the symptom experience, including the context in which symptoms occurred, were audiotaped, transcribed, analyzed, and compared across cases to inform the quantitative data.

▶ **Results:** The convenience sample (n = 77) was 48% female, 85.7% were non-Hispanic White, and mean age was 75.9 years (SD = 7.7 years). Functional performance was low (81% class III/IV). The most frequently reported symptoms were dyspnea, dyspnea on exertion, and fatigue. Median duration of early symptoms of HF decompensation was 5 to 7 days, but dyspnea duration ranged from 30 minutes to 90 days before action was taken. Longer dyspnea duration was associated with higher physical symptom distress (r = .30) and lower anxiety (r = −.31). Sensing and attributing meaning to early symptoms of HF decompensation were problematic.

▶ **Discussion:** The physical symptom experience and the cognitive and emotional response to HF symptoms were inadequate for timely care seeking for most of this older aged sample.

▶ **Key Words:** delay · elders · heart failure · symptom management

Heart failure (HF) is the most common admission diagnosis in the United States for persons over 65 years of age (Thomas & Rich, 2007), with readmission often occurring within 60 days of discharge (Moser, Doering, &

Chung, 2005). Among Medicare beneficiaries, there were 673,600 discharges for HF in 2003 at a cost of $4.4 billion (Rosamond et al., 2008). These frequent hospitalizations are costly and contribute to poor-quality life for patients with HF (Rodriguez-Artalejo et al., 2005). Hospital admission typically is due to escalating symptoms of fluid overload. In one study, it was estimated that as many as 57% of admissions are potentially preventable with adequate self-care, which includes medication adherence and monitoring for symptom changes (Schiff, Fung, Speroff, & McNutt, 2003).

Part of the reason for repeated admissions is that patients delay responding to their HF symptoms. This delay may be related to poor symptom recognition. Various contextual factors such as prior illness experience, social situations, or the environment where symptoms are experienced may influence symptom response. Therefore, the purpose of this study was to describe contextual factors related to symptom recognition and response among elders hospitalized with decompensated HF.

A factor complicating symptom monitoring is the physical subtlety of early-warning symptoms of HF decompensation. Early symptoms, such as fatigue and dyspnea with activity, are typically ambiguous, nonspecific, and insidious, which may impede their recognition as significant and related to HF. Elders, in particular, are known to discount the early symptoms of decompensated HF, such as fatigue or shortness of breath, as normal aging (Leventhal & Prohaska, 1986; Miller, 2000; Patel, Shafazand, Schaufelberger, & Ekman, 2007). The interpretation and response to symptoms also are known to be affected by the social and emotional context in which they occur (Burnett, Blumenthal, Mark, Leimberger, & Califf, 1995; Horowitz, Rein, & Leventhal, 2004).

Symptom Recognition as a Component of Self-Care

Self-care has been defined as a naturalistic decision-making process involving the choice of behaviors that maintain

Corrine Y. Jurgens, PhD, RN, ANP-BC, FAHA, is Clinical Associate Professor, Stony Brook University, New York, and John A. Hartford Postdoctoral Fellow, University of Pennsylvania, Philadelphia.

Linda Hoke, PhD, RN, APN-BC, CCNS, CRRN, is Clinical Nurse Specialist, Hospital of the University of Pennsylvania, Philadelphia.

Janet Byrnes, MS, RN, ANP, is Assistant Director of Nursing, Stony Brook University Medical Center, New York.

Barbara Riegel, DNSc, RN, FAAN, FAHA, is Professor, University of Pennsylvania, Philadelphia.

147

physiologic stability (*maintenance*) and the response to symptoms when they occur (*management*; Riegel et al., 2004). Symptom recognition is key to effective self-care. Patient education is the primary intervention used to promote symptom recognition, as most investigators assume that failed self-care is due to a lack of knowledge. Patients are taught to monitor their symptoms daily with the assumption that they will notify the provider for a sudden weight gain or take other definitive actions (e.g., an extra diuretic) to avoid hospitalization. Unfortunately, few patients monitor their symptoms routinely, and those who do often are unsure about how to interpret them (Carlson, Riegel, & Moser, 2001; Ni et al., 1999).

Patients' perceptions of symptoms have been correlated with the decision to seek care, to self-manage the symptoms, or to do nothing (Cameron, Leventhal, & Leventhal, 1993; Horowitz et al., 2004; Leventhal & Prohaska, 1986). Symptoms perceived to be less serious or those that incur little anxiety are more likely to result in delay of timely medical attention (Burnett et al., 1995; Dracup & Moser, 1997; Horowitz et al., 2004). Studies of patients hospitalized with decompensated HF suggest that patients typically endure increasing symptoms over days or weeks before seeking care (Evangelista, Dracup, & Doering, 2000, 2002; Friedman, 1997; Goldberg et al., 2008; Jurgens, 2006). Prior research has shown that in persons with HF, the factors associated with longer delay are younger age, male gender, African American race, multiple presenting symptoms, presenting with dyspnea and edema, a gradual onset of symptoms, higher symptom distress, absence of HF history, symptom onset between 12 midnight and 6 a.m., care by a primary care physician, and higher or worse New York Heart Association (NYHA)

class (Goldberg et al, 2008; Evangelista et al., 2000, 2002; Jurgens, 2006).

A hospitalization for HF in the prior 6 months increases the risk of cardiovascular-related death or HF hospitalization by 73% (Pocock et al., 2006). As yet, there are no published reports as to whether delay in seeking care for decompensated HF also negatively affects morbidity and mortality; however, we assume that appropriate self-care leading to early intervention in the course of an exacerbation may avert hospitalization. Furthermore, to the best of our knowledge, there are no published studies specifically examining contextual factors affecting elders hospitalized with decompensated HF.

Conceptual Framework

The Self-Regulation Model of Illness guided this study as it describes symptoms in a manner beyond a simple physical experience (Cameron et al., 1993; Cameron & Leventhal, 2003). Symptoms are multidimensional with physical, cognitive, and emotional components that translate into how individuals variably feel, think, and emotionally respond when symptoms arise (Figure 1). The Self-Regulation Model of Illness also incorporates the physical symptom experience within the context of an individual's experience both past and present including the social environment or situation in which it occurs. The model thus acknowledges the dynamic nature of illness, care seeking, and the influence of contextual factors and the social environment on the interpretation and response to symptoms.

According to the Self-Regulation Model of Illness, the response to illness occurs as a result of a person's perceptions of his/her illness or symptoms. Furthermore, response to illness is influenced by one's abstract knowledge or semantic

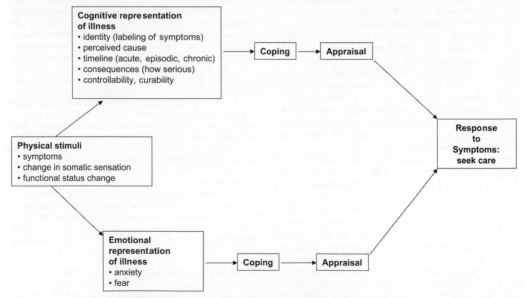

FIGURE 1. Self-regulation model of illness.

memory about the illness (such as risk for illness), previous experiences with comorbid or episodic illness, and beliefs about the consequences and controllability of the illness. As such, prior illness experience provides a source of contextual knowledge with which one can begin to label symptoms.

Illness perceptions are developed via two parallel pathways (cognitive and emotional). A cognitive representation is the assessment of a health threat and is embedded in the personal and social context in which one lives. Forming a cognitive representation includes determining the identity (labeling), perceived cause(s), timeline (is it acute or chronic?), consequences (how serious), and controllability/curability of the symptom or illness. The cognitive representation begins when one is first aware of a change in somatic state. Sensing symptoms or declining functional status prompts the assessment of possible causes. An emotional representation is the affective response to the change in somatic sensation and its subsequent cognitive representation. The intensity of the emotional response like anxiety or fear affects the response to symptoms and coping with the threat of illness. Coping could involve waiting to see what happens and delaying seeking care or calling for help. Professional and social relationships influence the way one copes with illness. Potential resources for help could include either medical or lay (e.g., family members or friends) consultation. Lastly is the evaluation phase in which the health threat and the effect of the coping plan is assessed.

We propose that delay in seeking care is due to the difficulty that HF patients experience in discerning the quality and meaning of their symptoms. Heart failure causes a multitude of symptoms, and comorbid conditions add to the number of symptoms experienced. Hypertension, coronary artery disease, chronic lung disease, and depression are common (Ceia et al., 2004; Dahlstrom, 2005; Masoudi & Krumholz, 2003). In addition, various contextual factors such as prior illness or symptom experience, social situation, or environment where the symptoms are experienced may affect symptom interpretation. The influence of contextual factors on recognition and response to acute HF symptoms is as yet unknown. Therefore, the specific aims of this study were to (a) describe the experience of and the cognitive and emotional response to the symptoms of decompensated HF, (b) determine the influence of sociodemographic, clinical, cognitive, emotional, and social contextual factors on symptom duration during this time, and (c) describe self-care behaviors prior to seeking care for decompensated HF.

Methods

A mixed-methods design with an emphasis on the quantitative data (QUANT/qual) was used to address the specific aims. In the quantitative component, an exploratory descriptive design was used to examine the duration of those symptoms before care seeking, patient responses to symptoms of decompensated HF, and self-care behaviors. Qualitative methods were used to elicit narrative accounts of the symptom perception process and to explore the contextual factors that influenced the process, thereby enhancing the quantitative data.

Sample

A convenience sample of adult men and women hospitalized in an emergency department or as inpatients with a diagnosis of decompensated HF was recruited at tertiary care hospitals in Philadelphia and New York. In addition to conducting a power analysis to determine sample size, the feasibility of conducting a mixed-method study (QUANT/qual) was considered. Guidelines for sample size vary from 15 (Stevens, 1996) to approximately 40 (Cohen & Cohen, 1983) participants per predictor for multiple regression analysis. The exploratory nature of the study, together with the ability to meet the aims, was factored into the determination of the sample of 77 participants.

Participants were enrolled if they were 65 years of age or older, cognitively intact, medically stable, able to read or understand English fluently, and provided written informed consent. The diagnosis of HF was confirmed using the Framingham criteria (Ho, Anderson, Kannel, Grossman, & Levy, 1993). The Framingham criteria use the presence of two major criteria (e.g., neck vein distention, rales, and S3 gallop) or one major and two minor criteria (e.g., extremity edema, dyspnea on exertion, and pulmonary vascular congestion by chest x-ray) to diagnose HF. Participants were enrolled within 3 days of admission to limit problems with ability to recall their illness experience. Participants also had to be living independently in the community and able to manage their illness by self-care. The study protocol was reviewed and approved by the institutional review boards at Stony Brook University and the University of Pennsylvania. All participants signed an informed consent agreement.

Procedure and Measures

Heart Failure Somatic Perception Scale   The Heart Failure Somatic Perception Scale was used to assess perceived symptom distress associated with the current hospitalization for HF (Jurgens, Fain, & Riegel, 2006). The scale, derived from the Framingham Diagnostic Criteria (Ho et al., 1993) and the literature, has 17 items that address symptom occurrence and perceived symptom severity on a 4-point Likert scale ranging from 0 = "not at all" to 3 = "extremely, could not have been worse" (possible range 0–51). The scale items are summative; higher scores indicate higher perceived distress.

The original questionnaire consisted of 12 items. Content validity was confirmed by nurse scientists in HF and expert HF nurse clinicians. Theta reliability for nonparallel items was 0.71 (Jurgens et al., 2006). Five additional items were added for this study; two items target the HF symptoms of nocturia and increased abdominal girth. Also, as patients often decrease their activity to accommodate escalating symptoms, making these symptoms difficult to capture, additional alternate items measuring dyspnea, fatigue, and dyspnea on exertion were added. For example, dyspnea on exertion was addressed by asking about difficulty with usual activities because of shortness of breath. The added alternate item asks if getting dressed made it hard to breathe. In consideration of the addition of more than one item assessing the symptoms cited above, items were no longer discrete and Cronbach's α was used to assess reliability. In the current study, the Cronbach's α for the 17-item version was .80.

Response to Symptoms Questionnaire   The Response to Symptom Questionnaire (revised; Dracup & Moser, 1997) was used to assess cognitive, emotional, and social contextual factors affecting symptom response. The questionnaire addresses the following variables from the conceptual model: (a) the context in which the symptoms occurred, (b) affective or emotional response to symptoms, (c) cognitive response to symptoms (e.g., symptom appraisal), (d) response of others to the symptoms, and (e) the perceived severity of the symptoms in general. Instrument authors evaluated content validity, but reliability has not been reported (Dracup & Moser, 1997). The questionnaire was developed using single items to assess various contextual factors affecting response to acute myocardial infarction symptoms (Burnett et al., 1995). It was modified for use in patients with HF by the primary author. Questions on the process of seeking care were deleted (e.g., where they were when the symptoms were first noticed, who was with them, and self-care attempts). These were written as open-ended questions for the qualitative interview. Wording was changed from *heart attack* to *heart failure* as appropriate. The revision was evaluated for content validity by nursing experts in cardiac research and clinical practice. The items use a 5-point Likert scale to address how patients responded cognitively, emotionally, or behaviorally to their symptoms (e.g., 1 = "not at all anxious" to 5 = "extremely anxious"). Theta reliability, appropriate for questionnaires with discrete nonparallel items (Carmines & Zeller, 1979), was 0.72 for the 15 items used in the current study.

NYHA Functional Class and Specific Activity Scale Functional status can be affected by symptom burden and was measured in two ways. The NYHA functional class (range = class 1 to 4) on the day of admission was determined from review of the medical record or by interview if it was not documented in the admission physical examination. A higher class indicates worse functional ability. In addition, the participant's typical functional level when not acutely ill was measured using the Specific Activity Scale (Goldman, Hashimoto, Cook, & Loscalzo, 1981). This scale produces metabolic units based on common daily activities. Similar to the NYHA classes, this scale categorizes patients into one of four classes, with higher class indicating worse functional ability.

Charlson Comorbidity Index To examine potential differences in symptom distress related to comorbid illnesses at the time of enrollment, the Charlson Comorbidity Index was assessed (Katz, Chang, Sangha, Fossel, & Bates, 1996). Responses were weighted and indexed into one of three comorbidity categories (low, moderate, or high) according to the published method. Scores can range from 0 to 34, although every patient in this study had a score of at least 1 because they were all diagnosed with HF. Validity of the scale was demonstrated by the instrument authors when comorbidity category was shown to predict mortality, complications, healthcare resource use, length of hospital stay, discharge disposition, and cost (Charlson, Pompei, Ales, & MacKenzie, 1987; Katz et al., 1996).

Interview Sociodemographic and clinical data were collected through interview and review of the medical record. The content of the interview is outlined in Table 1. Symptom duration before hospitalization was used as a measure of

the time taken to assess and respond to the symptoms of HF decompensation. Symptom duration was calculated in hours from the time a participant was first aware of symptoms until arrival at the hospital. The precise time of symptom onset was determined by participants with a use of calendar to assist recall. Once a particular time frame such as a weekend, social event, appointment, or holiday was identified, symptom duration was explored in relation to that day and time. Although this technique is subject to recall bias, Dempsey, Dracup, and Moser (1995) found that with careful questioning, patients are able to pinpoint the time of onset quite specifically. Prodromal or subacute symptoms were quantified in addition to the symptoms that were more acute in nature. Chronic symptoms were quantified from the time they increased in severity over the participant's baseline. Omnipresent chronic symptoms that did not vary in severity were recorded as present, but the duration was not quantified for the analysis. Participation in an HF clinic was documented to assess for ongoing disease management and access to information and support.

Upon completion of preliminary demographic and clinical data collection, open-ended questions were used to identify contextual factors affecting the process and decision to seek care. Individuals were asked to describe factors including but not limited to social/situational factors such as location when symptoms were noticed; contact with and response of family, friends, or health providers; and self-care

TABLE 1. Content of Interview

Sociodemographic data	Occupation
	Marital status
	Living arrangement
	Education
	Income level
History related to HF	Year of HF diagnosis
	Number of previous HF-related hospitalizations
	Use of emergency medical services
	Medication history
	Participation in HF clinic
Symptoms	Symptom presence, duration, severity
	Symptom pattern (gradual or sudden onset)
	Decision to seek care (self or other person)
Factors affecting decision to seek care	Open-ended questions
	"Tell me more about the time leading up to this hospitalization."
	"What did you do when you first noticed your symptoms?"
	"What did you think was causing your symptoms?"

Note. HF = heart failure.

behaviors. All interviews were conducted in the participant's hospital room and averaged an hour in duration. The audio-taped sessions were transcribed verbatim and augmented with field notes and participant observations.

Data Analysis

The relationship between duration of HF symptoms, perceived symptom distress, and cognitive and emotional factors was explored using Pearson correlations. Hierarchical regression was used to identify predictors of duration of dyspnea in three steps. A priori predictors of interest included age, gender (male = 1, female = 0), and perceived symptom severity. The HF Somatic Perception Scale score was used to reflect the physical symptom experience as depicted in the Self-Regulation Model of Illness. Contextual factors in the regression included the cognitive (perceived seriousness of symptoms) and emotional (anxiety) response to symptoms. Gender and age were entered in the first step, followed by perceived symptom distress. Anxiety and perceived seriousness were entered together in the last step. Logarithmic transformation was used to normalize the distribution of symptom duration for analysis. Median duration versus the mean is reported as extreme outliers skew interpretation of the data.

To assess for multicollinearity, correlations between the predictor variables were inspected. The highest correlation was between anxiety and perceived seriousness ($r = .635$). Although high, the correlation did not meet the cut-point for multicollinearity, predetermined as a linear correlation of greater than .8 (Allison, 1999). Tolerance for each independent variable ranged from .527 to .974, which is above the point of .40 considered problematic when assessing multicollinearity (Allison, 1999). Quantitative data were analyzed using the Statistical Package for the Social Sciences software version 14.0 (Chicago, Illinois).

Over 1,000 pages of qualitative data were analyzed using content analysis with Atlas.ti version 5.0.67 (Berlin, Germany) to identify cognitive, emotional, and contextual factors affecting the process and decision to seek care (Ayres, Kavanaugh, & Knafl, 2003; Denzin & Lincoln, 2000). First, data were analyzed using a priori codes based on the Self-Regulation Model of Illness (physical stimuli, cognitive appraisal, emotional response, and social factors). Voluntary explanations from explorations of self-care behaviors before admission and the Response to Symptoms Questionnaire were described. Repetitive themes were clustered into subgroups, labeled into meaningful categories and discussed with a coinvestigator. Then, across-case comparison analysis was conducted between those participants with and without a previous HF-related hospitalization by constructing a matrix of common experiences among the participants. This analysis was an iterative process whereby the researcher moved back and forth between individual cases and across cases to track variability of themes (Ayres et al., 2003). The final step in the data analysis was integration of the quantitative and qualitative data.

Methodological rigor of the qualitative analysis was maintained through an audit trail, periodic debriefing with a coinvestigator, and discussions with colleagues knowledgeable about HF self-care and mixed-methods research techniques. An audit trail of process and analytic memos

and coding books was maintained to support the credibility of the study.

Results

Study Sample

Participants ($n = 77$; Table 2) were enrolled over a 19-month period from October 2004 until May 2006. A prior HF-related

TABLE 2. Sociodemographic and Clinical Characteristics ($n = 77$)

Variable	n (%)
Gender	
Men	40 (51.9)
Women	37 (48.1)
Race/Ethnicity	
Non-Hispanic White	66 (85.7)
Black	9 (11.7)
Hispanic	1 (1.3)
Other	1 (1.3)
Marital status	
Married	37 (48.1)
Widowed	34 (44.2)
Divorced, separated, never married	6 (7.8)
Education	
Less than 12 years	18 (23.4)
High school diploma	34 (44.2)
Some college/associate degree	7 (9.1)
Baccalaureate degree	10 (13)
Graduate degree	8 (10.4)
Total household income in past year	
Less than $10,000	10 (13)
$10,000–$24,999	24 (31.2)
$25,000–$39,999	10 (13)
$40,000–$54,999	7 (9.1)
$55,000 or greater	12 (15.6)
Do not know	12 (15.6)
Declined to answer	2 (2.6)
Comorbid illness	
Coronary artery disease	54 (70.1)
Hypertension	55 (72)
Diabetes	31 (40.3)
Charlson comorbidity category	
Low	36 (46.8)
Moderate	33 (42.9)
High	8 (10.4)
Specific Activity Scale—functional performance	
Class 1	1 (1.3)
Class 2	14 (18.2)
Class 3	39 (50.6)
Class 4	23 (29.9)

hospital admission was reported by 72% of the sample, with a median duration since diagnosis of 5 years (SD = 5.2 years). Functional capacity was low, with 81% of the participants classified as class 3 or 4 on the Specific Activity Scale. All participants completed the quantitative and qualitative procedures, although 13 tapes were unusable because of errors in the recording process (e.g., incorrect tape speed and equipment malfunction). Nineteen potential participants declined enrollment, citing reasons such as not wanting to sign a consent, not wanting to take the time, or lack of interest. Those who declined did not differ significantly from the 77 participants on any demographic or clinical characteristic.

Physical Stimuli: Symptoms

Dyspnea, dyspnea on exertion, and fatigue were the most frequently reported symptoms (Table 3). Dyspnea duration had a range of 30 minutes to 90 days, with nearly half reporting dyspnea for greater than 3 days before admission. Only a minority of participants (n = 8; 11.8%) reported experiencing dyspnea for longer than 2 weeks before admission. Mean perceived symptom (Table 4) was significantly correlated with dyspnea duration (r = .30, p = .013). There were no significant differences in symptom distress scores in relation to age, gender, or Charlson Comorbidity category. Most participants (79%) made the decision themselves to seek care in response to their symptoms rather than being encouraged by others to do so.

Cognitive Response to Symptoms

Analysis of the Response to Symptoms Questionnaire revealed that over half of the sample did not know the symptoms of HF (56%) or realize their importance. Nearly 87% of the sample believed their symptoms to have some degree of seriousness, but most (80%) waited for the symptoms to go away. The correlation of dyspnea duration and perceived seriousness approached significance (r = −.23, p = .06). Slightly over half (50.6%) were reluctant to trouble anyone for help. Interestingly, 54% believed that they had little to no control over their symptoms.

Qualitative analysis revealed that over half had no idea what was causing their symptoms. Approximately a third misattributed their symptoms to conditions unrelated to their heart (e.g., upper respiratory infections, travel, arthritis, and emotional stress). "I knew I was getting short of breath. I had

TABLE 4. Mean Scores of Physical, Cognitive, and Emotional Response Measures (n = 77)

	Mean (SD)
Symptom distress	
Heart Failure Somatic Perception Scale	19.6 (8.5)
Cognitive responses	
Seriousness of symptoms	2.92 (1.24)
Perceived control related to symptoms	2.36 (1.22)
Emotional responses	
Anxiety related to symptoms	2.84 (1.28)
Fear of consequences of seeking help	1.79 (1.24)
Embarrassment related to seeking help	1.35 (.91)

no idea that this had anything to do with the heart. I thought it was the lungs." For some, the accumulation of additional HF symptoms triggered care seeking but not necessarily the identification of their symptoms as HF related. A 68-year-old woman had symptoms of increasing dyspnea, fatigue, and edema before seeking care, stating:

> It had gone on for a few months where I just couldn't do some of the physical things I used to do. Like, um, walk a mile…. When I got these shortness of breath attacks, I would attribute it more to anxiety than to the heart. I was slower than my usual self. My feet were swollen, too, but that's been going on for years. This time my abdomen was swollen too. On Friday, I couldn't get out of my car so I called a friend [to take her to the hospital].

Among those with a previous HF-related admission (n = 53), a group one might assume would be more knowledgeable, 10 participants had no idea as to what was causing their symptoms. Further analysis of this subgroup identified comorbid illness such as chronic lung disease and obesity, incorrect symptom attribution (e.g., a cold or physical exertion), and a gradual progression of symptom severity as factors hampering the identification of their HF symptoms. An 82-year-old man with dyspnea and fatigue gradually increasing over a 2- to 3-month period said he used a treadmill daily. The number of steps on the treadmill had recently decreased, but he was not concerned. The change in his functional status lacked meaning for him in relation to his heart, and his wife initiated care seeking. Other participants did not recognize or define their physical decline as valid symptoms. One participant stated, "Fatigue is not a symptom," and another said, "I'm not tired, I'm just slowing down." Interestingly, attribution of symptoms specifically to advanced age was not a common theme in this older aged sample.

Emotional Response to Symptoms

Emotional response to symptoms was measured using items from the Response to Symptoms Questionnaire. The duration of the early symptoms of HF (dyspnea on exertion, fatigue, edema, and weight gain) was unrelated to anxiety or fear at their onset. Dyspnea (vs. dyspnea on exertion) and anxiety

TABLE 3. Symptom Frequency and Duration Before Hospital Admission (n = 77)

Symptoms	n (%)	Median duration (days)
Dyspnea	68 (88)	3
Dyspnea on exertion	59 (77)	5
Fatigue	52 (68)	7
Edema	33 (43)	7
Orthopnea	27 (35)	3.4
Weight gain	26 (34)	9
Chest pain	25 (32)	1

were significantly related once dyspnea became more omni-present; dyspnea and anxiety were inversely related ($r = -.31$, $p = .012$), indicating that a longer duration of dyspnea before hospital admission was associated with lower anxiety. Weight gain and fear produced a similar relationship ($r = -.63$, $p = .001$). There was no significant relationship between dyspnea duration and fear ($r = .03$, $p = .80$). A single item rating general symptom intensity on a scale of 0 ("no symptoms") to 10 ("worst symptoms experienced") was weakly correlated with fear ($r = .28$, $p = .012$). Only 28 (36.3%) participants experienced fear in relation to their symptoms, with 76.6% reporting no fear or being mildly fearful. The narrative accounts were consistent with the quantitative findings. Participants cited a variety of reasons for lack of fear or anxiety regarding their symptoms. A 69-year-old man stated, "I have shortness of breath 'cause I've had a heart attack and bypass, so a lot of problems… I wasn't alarmed by it." A 66-year-old man was not fearful about his several days of dyspnea until he noticed leg swelling.

Social Factors and Response to Symptoms

Social factors, as assessed with the Response to Symptoms Questionnaire, were not a predominant influence on symptom response; 84% denied feeling embarrassed to seek care. Likewise, 87% denied that social plans factored into their decision to delay or seek care. Few (19%) reported delaying care because they were waiting for family to arrive, and less than one third reported delaying care because of wanting to avoid hospitalization.

The qualitative data offered explanations for delay in care seeking. Participants reported not wanting to inconvenience, disturb, or communicate their symptoms to their family or friends: "I didn't want to alarm my wife." "I didn't want to 'wake/bother' my daughter." As a result of these reasons, some participants who were acutely short of breath waited until morning to call for help. Among those who wished to avoid hospitalization, various reasons cited included caregiver responsibilities, prior negative hospital experiences, and financial concerns. One participant with outstanding medical bills reported, "I'm not anxious to come to the hospital because it's very expensive. I want to leave something to my children."

The influence of family factored into care-seeking decisions in approximately 25% of the sample. In some cases, participants were unaware of their symptoms of dyspnea or decreased activity tolerance and their family initiated seeking care. For example, one family noticed that the participant was short of breath with activity for 2 weeks before hospitalization. This 81-year-old woman was unaware of her dyspnea until 5 days before admission, when it was increasingly severe. Her daughter observed her distress and made the decision to seek care, saying, "Momma, do you know you're not breathing well?" Another participant reported not knowing why he was in the hospital and said, "If my wife went out and bought some groceries, and she wanted me to carry them into the house, I would carry them and start puffing. I wasn't helping around the house lately, so my wife called the doctor and moved up the appointment." A gradual increase in symptom severity, followed by adaptation by pacing activities, impeded some patients in recognizing the importance of their symptoms until their families intervened.

Influence of Contextual Factors on Dyspnea Duration

The hierarchical regression model explained 29% of the variance in duration of dyspnea before seeking care (Table 5). Three of the five predictors contributed significantly ($p \le .03$) to the explained variance. Male gender, higher symptom distress, and lower anxiety were associated with a longer duration of dyspnea. Older age approached significance, with a $p = .053$.

Self-Care Management Behaviors

The qualitative data revealed the use of alternative strategies than those routinely suggested to HF patients. Few ($n = 4$) took an extra dose of their diuretic. One explained, "I'm already on medication." Others described energy conservation measures such as resting, sitting up, or sleeping in a recliner as temporarily sufficient for improving symptoms. "I control my symptoms by not going up and down stairs." Several participants tried various medications not typically used for treating symptoms of HF, including aspirin, sublingual nitroglycerin, acetaminophen, inhalers, cold remedies, and higher doses of oxygen. Some simply took deep breaths, tried to calm themselves, or prayed. None of the participants reported decreasing their sodium or fluid intake in response to escalating symptoms.

Discussion

Sensing and attributing meaning to the early symptoms of HF decompensation were problematic for participants in this older aged sample. Many participants interpreted their symptoms in the context of a less threatening condition or illness and were not alarmed enough to seek care. Poor symptom recognition resulted in nearly half of the participants experiencing dyspnea for 3 days or more before hospitalization for decompensated HF, a finding consistent with those of others (Evangelista et al., 2000, 2002; Friedman, 1997; Goldberg et al., 2008; Jurgens, 2006). Symptoms increased gradually, generating little anxiety or fear, and participants were hesitant to bother others about their symptoms. According to the Self-Regulation Model of Illness, responding to symptoms is an iterative process. The process begins with *sensing* a somatic change in physical status, which

TABLE 5. Hierarchical Regression Predictors for Duration of Dyspnea ($n = 68$)

Predictor	B	SE	Standard β	p
Age	0.056	0.028	.235	.053
Gender	1.141	0.427	.311	.01
Physical factor				
Symptom distress	0.074	0.024	.347	.003
Cognitive factor				
Seriousness	−0.061	0.234	−.039	.795
Emotional factor				
Anxiety	−0.464	0.215	−.323	.035

$R = .539$, $R^2 = .29$.

initiates an attempt to label the sensation, assessing its cause, applying a coping strategy, and evaluating the effect of the strategy. If the strategy is ineffective, the symptom or sensation is relabeled or the cause is reevaluated and another coping strategy is tried. In this study, some participants were physically unaware of their escalating symptoms, which may be an important factor in symptom response. There is growing evidence that HF is associated with changes in cognitive function, which may impair symptom perception and the ability to make self-care decisions (Alves et al., 2005; Woo, Macey, Fonarow, Hamilton, & Harper, 2003). The physical symptom experience is clearly an insufficient stimulus for a timely process of seeking care.

The cognitive representation or labeling of HF symptoms was also problematic and negatively affected timely care seeking in this sample. Congruent with prior HF studies of both inpatients and outpatients (Horowitz et al., 2004; Patel et al., 2007), the cognitive representation of symptoms was either absent or incorrect for many participants trying to *interpret* the meaning of their symptoms. Resources for identifying and interpreting current symptoms (lay sources, family, and healthcare providers) were inadequate for timely care for many of the participants.

Most striking was the lack of an emotional response (e.g., anxiety) to the early symptoms of HF decompensation, which further compromised an effective response. One explanation may be that patients with HF view symptoms individually as opposed to being related to one another. As such, symptoms such as dyspnea with activity and fatigue are unlikely to cause concern and are more easily dismissed as unimportant or unworthy of medical attention. Patients also appear to decrease activity to accommodate symptoms such as dyspnea associated with walking. Elders who lead generally sedentary lives may not perform activities that incur dyspnea or fatigue, making these nonspecific symptoms less noticeable.

Similar to previous studies (Friedman, 1997; Jurgens, 2006), prior experience with an HF-related hospital admission did not assure accurate labeling of symptoms or timely self-care. Although a definition of what constitutes delay in treatment for decompensated HF has not been established, these elders waited long enough that emergency hospitalization was necessary for symptom management. Few intentionally ignored their symptoms or avoided hospitalization, but knowledge about HF and symptom recognition abilities were poor. Those most likely to delay seeking care were men, those with higher symptom distress, and those with lower anxiety.

Confirming the study by Patel et al. (2007), the social influence of family had both positive and negative outcomes in relation to timely medical attention. Several participants reported reluctance to disturb family members despite significant respiratory distress. In other cases, the family members were instrumental in initiating access to treatment. Educating both patient and family regarding the significance and necessity of early intervention for escalating symptoms is important.

Study Strengths and Limitations

The results of the study are strengthened by the mixed-methods design. Detailed narrative accounts of the symptom perception process added depth to the analysis and interpretation of the results by illustrating the highly variable and often incorrect interpretations of the meaning of symptoms. The complexity of the contextual factors affecting the process that patients with HF use to make self-care decisions would be overlooked if the analysis was based on quantitative data alone.

Limitations to the generalizability of these results include the relatively small and largely White sample. The sample size was robust for the qualitative data but was limited for the quantitative analysis. The richness of the qualitative data was limited by interviewing and equipment use skills of the research assistants in some cases. Lastly, the quantitative analysis of emotional factors such as fear, anxiety, and embarrassment in relation to symptom duration was limited by the use of single items from the Response to Symptoms Questionnaire. Although summated scores from multiple-item scales are commonly used for such analyses (e.g., to measure anxiety), single-item scales are reported to generate valid measures and are, in some cases, superior to multiple-item scales (Gardner, Cummings, Dunham, & Pierce, 1998).

Conclusion

The window of opportunity to treat the early symptoms of HF decompensation is hampered by the difficulty that patients experience in sensing and interpreting the meaning of these symptoms. The lack of an emotional response to symptoms decreases the likelihood of instituting timely self-care management strategies or seeking medical guidance. Educating patients in HF self-care might be more effective if the meaning of their symptoms were clearer. Strategies for helping patients to evaluate their symptoms are in need of further study. ▼

Accepted for publication January 30, 2009.

Funding for this study was provided by the John A. Hartford Foundation Building Academic Geriatric Nursing Capacity Scholarship Program.

The authors gratefully acknowledge the scholarly support of Dr. Neville Strumpf and the faculty of the University of Pennsylvania's Hartford Center of Geriatric Nursing Excellence.

Corresponding author: Corrine Y. Jurgens, PhD, RN, ANP-BC, FAHA, School of Nursing, Stony Brook University, HSC L2-223, Stony Brook, NY 11794-8240 (e-mail: corrine.jurgens@stonybrook.edu).

References

Allison, P. D. (1999). *Multiple regression: A primer.* Thousand Oaks, CA: Pine Forge Press.

Alves, T. C., Rays, J., Fraguas, R. Jr., Wajngarten, M., Meneghetti, J. C., Prando, S., et al. (2005). Localized cerebral blood flow reductions in patients with heart failure: A study using 99mtc-hmpao spect. *Journal of Neuroimaging, 15,* 150–156.

Ayres, L., Kavanaugh, K., & Knafl, K. A. (2003). Within-case and across-case approaches to qualitative data analysis. *Qualitative Health Research, 13,* 871–883.

Burnett, R. E., Blumenthal, J. A., Mark, D. B., Leimberger, J. D., & Califf, R. M. (1995). Distinguishing between early and late responders to symptoms of acute myocardial infarction. *American Journal of Cardiology, 75,* 1019–1022.

Cameron, L., Leventhal, E. A., & Leventhal, H. (1993). Symptom representations and affect as determinants of care seeking in a community-dwelling, adult sample population. *Health Psychology, 12,* 171–179.

Cameron, L. D., & Leventhal, H. (Eds.). (2003). *The self-regulation of health and illness behavior.* London: Routledge.

Carlson, B., Riegel, B., & Moser, D. K. (2001). Self-care abilities of patients with heart failure. *Heart & Lung, 30,* 351–359.

Carmines, E. G., & Zeller, R. A. (1979). *Reliability and validity assessment.* Beverly Hills, CA: Sage Publications.

Ceia, F., Fonseca, C., Mota, T., Morais, H., Matias, F., Costa, C., et al. (2004). Aetiology, comorbidity and drug therapy of chronic heart failure in the real world: The EPICA substudy. *European Journal of Heart Failure, 6,* 801–806.

Charlson, M. E., Pompei, P., Ales, K. L., & MacKenzie, C. R. (1987). A new method of classifying prognostic comorbidity in longitudinal studies: Development and validation. *Journal of Chronic Diseases, 40,* 373–383.

Cohen, J., & Cohen, P. (1983). *Applied multiple regression/correlation analysis for the behavioral sciences* (2nd ed.). Hillsdale, NJ: Lawrence Erlbaum Associates.

Dahlstrom, U. (2005). Frequent non-cardiac comorbidities in patients with chronic heart failure. *European Journal of Heart Failure, 7,* 309–316.

Dempsey, S. J., Dracup, K., & Moser, D. K. (1995). Women's decision to seek care for symptoms of acute myocardial infarction. *Heart & Lung, 24,* 444–456.

Denzin, N., & Lincoln, Y. (Eds.). (2000). *Handbook of qualitative research* (2nd ed.). Thousand Oaks, CA: Sage Publications.

Dracup, K., & Moser, D. K. (1997). Beyond sociodemographics: Factors influencing the decision to seek treatment for symptoms of acute myocardial infarction. *Heart & Lung, 26,* 253–262.

Evangelista, L. S., Dracup, K., & Doering, L. V. (2000). Treatment-seeking delays in heart failure patients. *Journal of Heart and Lung Transplantation, 19,* 932–938.

Evangelista, L. S., Dracup, K., & Doering, L. V. (2002). Racial differences in treatment-seeking delays among heart failure patients. *Journal of Cardiac Failure, 8,* 381–386.

Friedman, M. M. (1997). Older adults' symptoms and their duration before hospitalization for heart failure. *Heart & Lung, 26,* 169–176.

Gardner, D. G., Cummings, L. L., Dunham, R. B., & Pierce, J. L. (1998). Single-item versus multiple-item measurement scales: An empirical comparison. *Educational and Psychological Measurement, 58,* 898–915.

Goldberg, R. J., Goldberg, J. H., Pruell, S., Yarzebski, J., Lessard, D., Spencer, F. A., et al. (2008). Delays in seeking medical care in hospitalized patients with decompensated heart failure. *American Journal of Medicine, 121,* 212–218.

Goldman, L., Hashimoto, B., Cook, E. F., & Loscalzo, A. (1981). Comparative reproducibility and validity of systems for assessing cardiovascular functional class: Advantages of a new specific activity scale. *Circulation, 64,* 1227–1234.

Ho, K. K. L., Anderson, K. M., Kannel, W. B., Grossman, W., & Levy, D. (1993). Survival after the onset of congestive heart failure in Framingham heart study subjects. *Circulation, 88,* 107–115.

Horowitz, C. R., Rein, S. B., & Leventhal, H. (2004). A story of maladies, misconceptions, and mishaps: Effective management of heart failure. *Social Science & Medicine, 58,* 631–643.

Jurgens, C. Y. (2006). Somatic awareness, uncertainty, and delay in care-seeking in acute heart failure. *Research in Nursing & Health, 29,* 74–86.

Jurgens, C. Y., Fain, J. A., & Riegel, B. (2006). Psychometric testing of the heart failure somatic awareness scale. *Journal of Cardiovascular Nursing, 21,* 95–102.

Katz, J. N., Chang, L. C., Sangha, O., Fossel, A. H., & Bates, D. W. (1996). Can comorbidity be measured by questionnaire rather than medical record review? *Medical Care, 34,* 73–84.

Leventhal, E. A., & Prohaska, T. R. (1986). Age, symptom interpretation, and health behavior. *Journal of the American Geriatric Society, 34,* 185–191.

Masoudi, F. A., & Krumholz, H. M. (2003). Polypharmacy and comorbidity in heart failure. *BMJ, 327,* 513–514.

Miller, C. L. (2000). Cue sensitivity in women with cardiac disease. *Progress in Cardiovascular Nursing, 15,* 82–89.

Moser, D. K., Doering, L. V., & Chung, M. L. (2005). Vulnerabilities of patients recovering from an exacerbation of chronic heart failure. *American Heart Journal, 150,* 984.e7–984.e13.

Ni, H., Nauman, D., Burgess, D., Wise, K., Crispell, K., & Hershberger, R. E. (1999). Factors influencing knowledge of and adherence to self-care among patients with heart failure. *Archives of Internal Medicine, 159,* 1613–1619.

Patel, H., Shafazand, M., Schaufelberger, M., & Ekman, I. (2007). Reasons for seeking acute care in chronic heart failure. *European Journal of Heart Failure, 9,* 702–708.

Pocock, S. J., Wang, D., Pfeffer, M. A., Yusuf, S., McMurray, J. J., Swedberg, K. B., et al. (2006). Predictors of mortality and morbidity in patients with chronic heart failure. *European Heart Journal, 27,* 65–75.

Riegel, B., Carlson, B., Moser, D. K., Sebern, M., Hicks, F. D., & Roland, V. (2004). Psychometric testing of the self-care of heart failure index. *Journal of Cardiac Failure, 10,* 350–360.

Rodriguez-Artalejo, F., Guallar-Castillon, P., Pascual, C. R., Otero, C. M., Montes, A. O., Garcia, A. N., et al. (2005). Health-related quality of life as a predictor of hospital readmission and death among patients with heart failure. *Archives of Internal Medicine, 165,* 1274–1279.

Rosamond, W., Flegal, K., Furie, K., Go, A., Greenlund, K., Haase, N., et al. (2008). Heart disease and stroke statistics—2008 update: A report from the American Heart Association statistics committee and stroke statistics subcommittee. *Circulation, 117,* e25–e146.

Schiff, G. D., Fung, S., Speroff, T., & McNutt, R. A. (2003). Decompensated heart failure: Symptoms, patterns of onset, and contributing factors. *American Journal of Medicine, 114,* 625–630.

Stevens, J. (1996). *Applied multivariate statistics for the social sciences* (2nd ed.). Mahwah, NJ: Lawrence Erlbaum.

Thomas, S., & Rich, M. W. (2007). Epidemiology, pathophysiology, and prognosis of heart failure in the elderly. *Clinics in Geriatric Medicine, 23,* 1–10.

Vinson, J. M., Rich, M. W., Sperry, J. C., Shah, A. S., & McNamara, T. (1990). Early readmission of elderly patients with congestive heart failure. *Journal of the American Geriatric Society, 38,* 1290–1295.

Woo, M. A., Macey, P. M., Fonarow, G. C., Hamilton, M. A., & Harper, R. M. (2003). Regional brain gray matter loss in heart failure. *Journal of Applied Physiology, 95,* 677–684.

Care Transition Experiences of Spousal Caregivers: From a Geriatric Rehabilitation Unit to Home

Qualitative Health Research
XX(X) 1–17
© The Author(s) 2011
Reprints and permission:
sagepub.com/journalsPermissions.nav
DOI: 10.1177/1049732311407078
http://qhr.sagepub.com
⑤SAGE

Kerry Byrne,[1] Joseph B. Orange,[2]
and Catherine Ward-Griffin[2]

Abstract

The purpose of this study was to develop a theoretical framework about caregivers' experiences and the processes in which they engaged during their spouses' transition from a geriatric rehabilitation unit to home. We used a constructivist grounded theory methodology approach. Forty-five interviews were conducted across three points in time with 18 older adult spousal caregivers. A theoretical framework was developed within which reconciling in response to fluctuating needs emerged as the basic social process. Reconciling included three subprocesses (i.e., navigating, safekeeping, and repositioning), and highlighted how caregivers responded to the fluctuating needs of their spouse, to their own needs, and to those of the marital dyad. Reconciling was situated within a context shaped by a trajectory of prior care transitions and intertwined life events experienced by caregivers. Findings serve as a resource for scientists, rehabilitation clinicians, educators, and decision makers toward improving transitional care for spousal caregivers.

Keywords

aging, caregivers / caregiving; grounded theory; health care; rehabilitation; relationships; relationships, primary partner; theory development

Recent initiatives in care for older persons with disabilities include geriatric rehabilitation units (GRUs). Care transitions into and out of GRUs involve both the older person/patient and his or her family members (Fredman & Daly, 1998). Several researchers have called for the inclusion of family caregivers and their goals (e.g., knowledge of and access to services) in GRU assessment and rehabilitation programs (Aminzadeh et al., 2005; Bradley et al., 2000; Demers, Ska, Desrosiers, Alix, & Wolfson, 2004; Hills, 1998). When family caregivers agree with recommendations made for their relatives during geriatric assessments, adherence to the recommendations is more likely to occur (Bogardus et al., 2004). Despite a primary focus on the older adults in the GRU, their family caregivers often require their own health-related support in addition to information about how best to care for their relatives (Demers et al.; Hills); however, little is known about how family caregivers experience their relative's transition from the GRU to home, and about the processes engaged in during care transitions.

Current models and theories of family caregiving (Lazarus & Folkman, 1984; Pearlin, Mullan, Semple, & Skaff, 1990; Schumacher, 1995; Skaff, Pearlin, & Mullan, 1996) and

transitions (Chick & Meleis, 1986; Meleis, Sawyer, Im, Hilfinger Messias, & Schumacher, 2000; Schumacher, Jones, & Meleis, 1999) include, in part, concepts and processes related to caregiving during transitions from hospital to home settings. However, none focus on the processes enacted by caregivers during the experiences of their relative's transition from a GRU to home. As a result, rehabilitation researchers, clinicians, and policy makers have few conceptual resources to help them understand how caregivers experience the transition of their husband or wife from a GRU hospital based setting to home or, moreover, what caregivers actually "do" during these transitions. The purpose of our study was to develop a theoretical framework illustrating how spousal caregivers experience the transition

[1]University of British Columbia, Vancouver, British Columbia, Canada
[2]University of Western Ontario, London, Ontario, Canada

Corresponding Author:
Kerry Byrne, University of British Columbia Department of Sociology, 1314-6303 N.W. Marine Drive, Vancouver, British Columbia, V6T 1Z1, Canada
Email: Kerry.Byrne@ubc.ca

157

of their husband or wife from a GRU hospital-based setting to the home.

Literature Review

Spousal Caregiving

Spouses, more than any other caregiver, are likely to provide care during periods of disability and illness, and are likely to continue doing so even as their own health declines (Chappell, 1992; Hess & Soldo, 1985). A study commissioned by Health Canada (2002) found that family caregivers are most likely to provide care to a spouse or partner (38%). Spousal caregivers experience adverse emotional and physical health, caregiving burden, and challenges with the role of caregiving (Braun, Mikulincer, Rydall, Walsh, & Rodin, 2007; Connell, Janevic, & Gallant, 2001; Jacobi et al., 2003). Fredman and Daly (1998) reported that 46% of caregivers are the spouses of individuals who are discharged from GRUs. Given the extent to which spouses engage in caregiving and the difficulties they encounter during transitional care, the present study focused specifically on spousal caregivers.

Transitional Care

Transitional care is defined as "a set of actions designed to ensure the coordination and continuity of health care as patients transfer between different locations or different levels of care within the same location" (Coleman, Boult, & American Geriatrics Society Health Care Systems Committee, 2003, p. 556). The study of transitional care is crucial to optimize quality care for older adults with complex care needs (Coleman et al.). Coleman and Williams (2007) proposed several key elements of a research agenda designed to improve the quality of transitions out of hospitals for older adults. They called for greater recognition of the integral role of family caregivers during care transitions. Older adults and their family caregivers encounter numerous difficulties during care transitions (from acute care to home and into long-term care), such as not feeling prepared for the transition, a lack of communication with health care providers, difficulty obtaining needed information (e.g., medical aspects of care), and access to resources (Bull, 1992; Bull, Maryuyama, & Luo, 1995; Davies & Nolan, 2003, 2004; Grimmer & Moss, 2001). These difficulties contribute to family caregivers' negative experiences of care transitions.

Current definitions of and approaches to transitional care (Coleman et al., 2003; Holland & Harris, 2007) focus on patients' experiences of moving between and among a range of health care settings. Unfortunately, caregivers' experiences often are not highlighted in definitions and current approaches. In several recent interventions aimed at improving care transitions, caregivers' experiences, their characteristics, and outcomes during transition were not reported and/or distinguished from patients' perspectives and experiences (Naylor, 2002; Naylor et al., 2007, Parry, Kramer, & Coleman, 2006). Although patients' perspectives of care transitions obviously are critically important, grouping patient and caregiver perspectives makes it very difficult to discern concerns specific to each group. The blending clouds our understandings of caregivers' experiences of their relatives' transitions to and from health care settings. A recent exception is the study by Shyu, Chen, Chen, Wang, and Shao (2008), in which the investigators examined the outcomes of a caregiver-oriented care transition intervention for family caregivers of individuals who had suffered a stroke. They found that their intervention resulted in higher self-evaluations of preparation and better satisfaction of discharge needs in comparison to a control group who received only routine care.

Caregiving During Care Transitions From Hospital-Based Settings to Home

Several investigators have demonstrated that caregiver needs, concerns, relationships, and burdens are salient and change throughout the transition from hospital to home for caregivers of older adult care recipients (e.g., Bull, 1990; Grimmer, Falco, & Moss, 2004; Kane, Reinardy, Penrod, & Huck, 1999; Naylor, Stephens, Bowles, & Bixby, 2005; Shyu, 2000a). Many of these authors identified "issues" that occur during transitions from hospital to home, but few identified how caregivers respond to the difficulties, changes, and unmet needs that arise during the transition. Notable exceptions include five studies that explored processes engaged in during care transitions from hospital to home (Bull, 1992; Bull & Jervis, 1997; Li & Shyu, 2007; Shyu, 2000a, 2000b, 2000c), and whose authors put forth theoretical frameworks (Bull, 1990; Li & Shyu; Shyu, 2000b) to understand what caregivers are "doing" during periods of transitional care.

The published articles reporting on these studies offer useful findings; however, they provide limited information about how spousal caregivers experience their husband's or wife's transition. First, none of the authors considered the transition from a GRU unit to home. GRUs are an increasingly common type of health care setting for older adults, and differ from acute care settings, where the majority of care transition work has been completed. Second, the majority of studies group experiences of spousal caregivers with other types of caregivers (e.g., adult children, daughters-in-law, siblings), even though research findings suggest that spouses experience caregiving differently (Barnes, Given, & Given, 1992; Frederick & Fast, 1999; George & Gwyther, 1986; Hayes, Zimmerman, & Boylstein, 2010; Navon & Weinblatt, 1996). The grouping reduces our ability to understand fully the issues specific to spousal caregivers' experiences of care transitions. Third, the experiences of spousal caregivers aged 65 years and older are underrepresented. For instance, the average age of caregivers in studies that identified "how" they manage transitions are always below 60 years (Bull, 1992; Bull & Jervis, 1997; Li & Shyu, 2007; Shyu, 2000b, 2000c). Finally, the experiences of caregivers prior to the discharge of their relative from a hospital-based setting were addressed only by Shyu (2000b, 2000c). Despite the important collective efforts of these investigators, we are left with little knowledge about how spousal caregivers prepare for the transition home from a GRU.

Recent attempts to describe transitions to care for family caregivers of older adults have yielded no theoretical or conceptual framework that specifically addresses older adult spousal caregivers' experiences of their relative's transition from a GRU to home. Such a framework would help guide education, research, and practice in rehabilitation settings. The aim of our study was to develop a theoretical understanding of the processes engaged in by spousal caregivers during the transfer of their husband/wife from a GRU to home. We gathered the perspectives of spousal caregivers who cared for older adult husbands or wives with and without cognitive impairment or dementia.

Methodology

A constructivist grounded theory methodology was used because it emphasizes the examination of processes and the creation of interpretive understandings (Charmaz, 2006). Ontologically, a constructivist approach highlights how the processes enacted during transition for caregivers are viewed as both individually experienced and socially constructed via interactions with other people. Grounded theory is an ideal methodology to understand actions and processes through transitions (Morse, 2009), and has been used by qualitative researchers to study processes engaged in by patients (Grant, St John, & Patterson, 2009) and family caregivers (Bull & McShane, 2008; Holtslander & Duggleby, 2009).

Sampling and Recruitment

A 36-bed inpatient GRU housed within a larger long-term care hospital in Ontario, Canada served as the recruitment site. The first author (Byrne) contacted spousal caregivers only after they indicated to a GRU team member who was not affiliated with the study that they were willing to participate. Spousal caregivers participated in three interviews (i.e., 48 hours prior to discharge, 2 weeks postdischarge, and 1 month postdischarge). In keeping with grounded theory methodology, both initial and theoretical sampling techniques were used to guide data collection

(Charmaz, 2006; Cutcliffe, 2000). Initial sampling criteria included spousal caregivers returning home with their husband or wife, and spouses (both men and women) caring for their partner who did or did not have cognitive impairment or dementia.

Participants

Eighteen caregivers participated in the study (9 men, 9 women). Caregivers' mean age was 77.4 years (range 65 to 89). They were married, on average, 47 years (range 8 to 60). Four caregivers were in a second marriage (M =19.5 years, range 8 to 36), and 14 were in their first marriage (M = 54.9 years, range 44 to 60). Eleven caregivers reported receiving home care services, and 5 did not receive any home care services. Two caregivers were not available for followup postdischarge (see below). Care recipients' mean age was 78.7 years (range 65 to 90). Five care recipients had a diagnosis of dementia, 4 had other cognitive impairments (e.g., delirium, mild cognitive impairment), and 9 had no identified cognitive issues. The mean length of stay on the GRU for care recipients was 41 days (range 22 to 77). Reasons for admission to the GRU included deconditioning (some from acute care), hip fracture, hip replacement, stroke, and knee joint replacement.

Data Collection

The first author conducted 45 face-to-face interviews with 18 spousal caregivers on the GRU and in their homes. Interviews lasted between 35 and 120 minutes. Fifteen of 18 caregivers were interviewed more than once (i.e., across time); of these 15, total interview time per participant ranged from 1.5 to 5 hours.

Sensitizing concepts, based on previous research on caregiving and transitions (e.g., Grimmer et al., 2004; Kneeshaw, Considine, & Jennings, 1999; Showalter, Burger, & Salyer, 2000) such as changes in relationship and social supports, were used as points of departure for the interview guide and also guided the initial analysis. As recommended by Charmaz (2006), these concepts were incorporated into specific questions in the initial interview guide and were used as tentative tools to develop ideas about the processes in our data. For instance, participants were asked how they would describe their relationship with their spouse currently (at the time of interview) in comparison to before they were admitted to the GRU, and about who had been especially helpful to them in caring for their spouse. We were particularly attuned and sensitive to these concepts during initial coding and debriefing, as well.

Three time points for data collection were planned: 48 hours prior to discharge from the GRU, 2 weeks postdischarge, and 4 to 6 weeks postdischarge. These time periods were based on previous research on care transitions (Bull, 1992; Bull & Jervis, 1997; Lin, Hung, Liao, Sheen, & Jong, 2006; Naylor, 2000). Minor changes to the initial intended time points were made for several participants because of loss to follow up and scheduling conflicts. Twelve caregivers were interviewed at all three time points. Three caregivers were interviewed at two points in time ($n = 1$ at 2 weeks and 1 month postdischarge; $n = 2$ prior to discharge and 2 weeks postdischarge); of these, 1 caregiver was not available prior to discharge, 1 did not want to be followed up for a third interview, and 1 could not be reached for a third interview. Three caregivers were interviewed only once ($n = 2$ prior to discharge; $n = 1$ at 2 weeks post discharge); of these, 2 were not discharged as planned and so could not be followed up, and 1 was not available at the other points in time (i.e., prior to discharge or 1 month postdischarge). First interviews were conducted between 72 and 48 hours prior to discharge ($n = 12$) and 1 to 6 days postdischarge ($n = 6$). Second interviews occurred between 14 and 21 days postdischarge (one of the second interviews was conducted 29 days postdischarge because of scheduling conflicts). Third interviews were conducted between 28 and 64 days postdischarge. Data collection began September 2006 and continued until November 2007.

In accordance with theoretical sampling, the categories noted to be relevant to the development of the emerging theoretical framework guided the sampling process rather than particular sample characteristics such as demographics. For example, as we tried to understand how and when caregivers "shifted the boundaries" (an element in the theoretical framework), it emerged that this experience might be different for men caregivers. Therefore, the last few caregivers who were interviewed were deliberately men so that elements of how and when they shifted the boundaries and how this differed from the experiences that emerged for women caregivers could be explored.

Interviews were digitally audio-recorded by the first author, transcribed verbatim by an experienced transcriptionist, and verified by the first author. In keeping with grounded theory methodology, data generation and data analysis occurred simultaneously, which supported follow-ups with participants about emergent codes and categories.

Observations

Observations of interactions between spouses and care recipients were made prior to, during, and after interviews, and were recorded in a field notebook (guided by Charmaz, 2006; Morse & Field, 1995). Specific observation times were not established a priori. The interviewer (first author) was "finely tuned in" to look for interactions that would help elucidate processes and categories emerging from the

data (Charmaz). Throughout the duration of the study, an electronic field notebook was used to record observations, reflexive journal entries, audit trail details, and field notes about each interview.

Care recipient spouses were included in observations but were not interviewed. We wanted spousal caregivers to be able to speak candidly about their relationships, and thus provided the option for them to be interviewed either without partners present or outside of their homes. If care recipients were present, we did not want to miss the opportunity to observe interactions; thus, we included an observational component and included the care recipient in this method of data collection. This approach proved to be fruitful, as the interviewer was able to "see" the actions engaged in by caregivers during the interviews in which partners were present.

Analysis

The first author engaged in line-by-line coding. As data collection and analysis progressed, all authors contributed to focused coding, followed by theoretical coding (Charmaz, 2006) using the constant comparative method with all units of data. For example, in the early stages of data collection and analysis, we noticed that caregivers continually used the phrase "I don't know," and thus an open code by this name was created to capture this aspect of the data. As data collection and analysis proceeded, we engaged in focused coding using the term *knowing/not knowing* to reflect these instances in the data. The following comment by Marie,[1] was coded as knowing/not knowing, but through theoretical coding was understood to be part of the process of navigating:

I don't know how long it [medication for dementia] will last, I can't find out. I've asked different doctors and nurses and they don't know, don't say how long it'll, but I hope it's years. You know, asked those questions. Why and how long do they think, maybe they can't tell, I don't know, how long do they think that they can give it to him?

To develop this category further, caregivers were asked how they became informed and what helped or did not help them to do so. We began to understand how navigating was critical to safekeeping (theoretical coding). Constant comparison entailed comparing incident to incident and comparing incidents over time between and within participants. Charmaz (2006) encouraged looking for implicit actions and meanings, comparing statements at one point, and comparing incidents at different points in time. Tables were created to compare instances across time. Once the theoretical code of navigating was identified, quotations from participants that reflected the various elements of this process (such as negotiating paths) were put into a table so we could examine the change in processes across time.

Moving from line-by-line coding to focused coding was not a linear process. As we engaged with the data, we returned to the data collected to explore new ideas and conceptualizations of codes. The simultaneous actions of collecting and analyzing data supported the discovery of gaps in the data, which were then filled by going back to existing participants and conducting interviews with new participants.

When a code was raised to the level of a category, the first author created a memo describing the category, the elements contained in the category, illustrative quotes that reflected the category, and further ideas on which to follow up to ensure theoretical saturation of the category. These memos were shared and discussed among authors. This process continued until we had no new elements to add to a category. To foster theoretical sensitivity, memos focused on actions and processes, and gradually incorporated relevant literature (e.g., theoretical perspectives on transition; Charmaz, 2006). We used diagramming (Lofland, Snow, Anderson, & Lofland, 2006) throughout data generation and analysis to help us understand the relationships between and within the emerging processes.

Criteria for Rigor

The criteria and techniques we used to evaluate the rigor of this study were a combination of those deemed to be important for (a) qualitative research in general, (b) constructivist approaches, and (c) grounded theory methodology. Techniques to establish reflexivity, transparency, authenticity, and credibility (Ballinger, 2004; Beck,1993; Charmaz, 2006; Chiovitti & Piran, 2003; Guba & Lincoln, 1989) included peer debriefing, reflexive journal entries, postinterview notes, an audit trail, theoretical sampling, memoing, constant comparison methods, triangulation, and member checking.

The paradigm of our research was constructivist, and assumed multiple realities; consequently, the repeatability of the research itself was not relevant (Sandelowksi, 1993). However, techniques traditionally associated with repeatability and confirmability, such as triangulation and member checks, were used and conceptualized according to a constructivist perspective. Our use of member checking facilitated a fuller understanding of the experiences of participants. The preliminary theoretical framework was shared with five caregivers (who had participated in earlier interviews) to explore whether or not their experiences of transition were reflected in the emergent framework. Caregivers reported being able to "see" their own experience of transition in the processes presented. In addition, the framework was further refined to reflect the

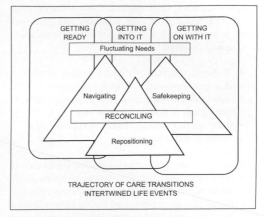

Figure 1. Theoretical framework of reconciling

feedback from these participants. For example, the phase of getting ready was focused on largely relative to the physical and environmental preparations that must be made throughout transition; however, during reflections about the findings presented, caregivers discussed the need to be mentally and emotionally prepared during the phase of getting ready. On returning to the data generated for the study and considering participant experiences, emotional aspects of this phase and the framework in general were explored more fully and included in the final theoretical framework. Similarly, we used triangulation not to confirm existing data, but rather to enhance completeness (Redfern & Norman, 1994). This was achieved through our use of in-depth interviews, observations, and detailed field notes.

The University of Western Ontario Ethics Board for Health Sciences Research Involving Human Subjects (HSREB) and the hospital ethics board at the GRU approved the procedures for interviewing and consent. Participants received a detailed letter of information (LOI) and were informed that they had the right to withdraw from the study at any time. Direct and clear wording in the LOI indicated that participant information would be treated confidentially and used only for the purposes of the study. Participants were informed that there would be no identifiable individual data in published findings, and participants' names and other identifying demographic information would be altered to ensure participants' anonymity.

Findings

Overall Framework: Reconciling

The findings from this study describe the basic social process of reconciling (see Figure 1) enacted by caregivers to integrate and merge the dissonance between their past and present knowledge, skills, roles, relationships (e.g., marital relationships), beliefs, routines, and life circumstances. Reconciling occurred

- Within a context shaped by a trajectory of prior care transitions and intertwined life events
- Across three overlapping phases: getting ready, getting into it, and getting on with it
- Through three subprocesses: navigating, safe-keeping, and repositioning

Reconciling captures spousal caregivers' interactions with their husband's or wife's health care providers, families, and friends, and advances a theoretical understanding of the strategies caregivers used during their relative's transition from the GRU to home. The following excerpt from Eileen, who cared for her husband with dementia, illustrates the basic social process of reconciling:

> But you adjust somehow. It's amazing what you can adjust to, it's amazing how you can say, "Well, this is the way it is." I'm not a person that goes around feeling bitter or down or depressed or anything like that, you just deal with what you got dealt, as they say. So it's just getting, my getting used to somebody who moves differently. I mean it takes him a long time to get up out of his chair, and to get to the bathroom or to the bedroom. And I have to allow for that. I can't operate mentally in the same way that I used to because it ain't going to happen. It's different now.

Why did caregivers engage in reconciling? They did so in response to fluctuating needs, including the physical, medical, emotional, and social needs of the caregivers themselves, their spouse, and the marital dyad. Caregivers' needs included information, skills, and directives about medications and medical aspects of care (e.g., how to use a condom catheter); exercise regimes; cognitive impairment; dementia; transportation options; services in the community (e.g., how to "get out" in public with their spouse and the walker; caregiver respite; how to connect with other caregivers); food preparation (e.g., how to prepare low-sodium food); how to work through their own emotions of anxiety, guilt, and feeling unappreciated; and finally, their own social needs and those of their partner. Needs fluctuated for a variety of reasons. Prior to leaving the GRU, during the phase of getting into it, several caregivers did not discuss a lot of needs; however, once caregivers were home with their husband or wife and were getting into it, needs surfaced and caregivers realized they were missing essential knowledge required to care for their spouse or themselves. In some cases, changing circumstances, such as declining function or increased

depression, necessitated the need for information about the decline or how to cope with the psychological changes caregivers were observing.

Understanding the Context That Shapes the Process of Reconciling

As depicted in Figure 1, reconciling from the GRU to home was embedded within (a) a trajectory of prior care and resultant health care setting transitions, and (b) the context of ongoing intertwined life events that were often the result of the caregivers' own aging-related experiences.

Reconciling within the context of a trajectory of care transitions. During the first interview (generally 48 hours prior to the discharge of their spouse) it became apparent that even though caregivers were in the midst of preparing to take their spouse home from the GRU, they were still coping with issues that occurred in other health care settings. For instance, Tony spent much time reflecting on his experiences during the time his wife was in acute care. During this period he was told that his wife would likely not survive, but that if she did she would require long-term care. Although neither of these scenarios materialized, during the first interview with Tony, he was still reconciling these experiences:

> The rough time, the really, really rough time was when she was at [acute care unit], when she was really sick. That was the rough time. I mean, many a time I'd come home crying, and I would just lay in bed and just let it go.

Similarly, to understand how Marie experienced the GRU-to-home transition, it was critical to understand the context of the multiple care settings from which she and her husband had emerged. A year before Marie's first interview, her husband was admitted to acute care and then discharged to a long-term care facility under the following circumstances, as explained by Marie:

> Yeah because they wouldn't do nothing [at acute care]. And then they, the bed come up at [nursing home], which I didn't want but you can't say no. They said you have no say, if a bed comes and you refuse it you pay for the hospital bed. And I couldn't refuse it, I had nothing to say, he had to go. Wherever they said, what they come up with. So I had to sign and let him go there.

Marie worked steadily from that point forward to get her husband home, and part of that work was getting him into the GRU. She explained her struggle:

> Well there's a lot in the family that didn't want me to bring him, but I said, "No, he's coming home."

He's not staying. Why would he have to stay in there," I said? It's not for him. All the while he's okay, he's got his mind now, why would I put him in there to stay? I wanted him home with me, I really missed him. So I would never ask her [sister], or anyone else. I'd have to figure it out myself, that's the only way you can do things. You can't rely on anyone. I can't. I can't depend on anyone. I have people tell me I'm selfish. Do you think I'm selfish for wanting to bring him home?

Marie's decision to work toward having her husband at home influenced her experience of reconciling during the transition from the GRU to home, namely the lack of support she received from her family, who did not think she should be caring for her husband at home. Consequently, her experience of reconciling from the GRU to home was shaped by a lack of support, a feeling of isolation, and her decision not to rely on anyone. Understanding the process of reconciling for caregivers is a matter of placing the GRU-to-home transition within the context of where they have come "from."

Reconciling within the context of intertwined life events. It was not only the multiple care transitions that were most salient in shaping the process of reconciling; rather, caregivers were reconciling within a context of ongoing, intertwined life events (i.e., intertwined with GRU-to-home transitions). These interwoven life events often involved larger life transitions such as relocating their home to new living circumstances (e.g., downsizing to an apartment or condominium); coping with their own health issues, illnesses, and transitions within their own marriage; and other family and friend relationships. Individual caregiving circumstances meant that some caregivers were relocating to new living circumstances, coping with an alcoholic partner or the death of a child, and handling adverse relationships with other family members. These intertwined life events served to facilitate or undermine reconciling. For several years prior to the interview Jessica had been dealing with her husband, who was an alcoholic. This "dealing with" influenced tremendously her experience of reconciling. Jessica revealed what it was like to be home with her husband after the admission to the GRU:

Well it's probably a lot calmer. See, I haven't told you [that] the initiating problem here was acute alcoholism, and so life hasn't been very peaceful. And now he's been off it for four months, and he's also been on antidepressants, so he's not as he was, so he's not as difficult and cranky to deal with. He's much calmer. Certainly so that makes it easier, yeah. So however, it's nice to see him sober for a change.

Relocating to smaller living arrangements was paramount for several caregivers. Some caregivers were in the process of relocating while their spouses were on the GRU, whereas others had moved just prior to the GRU admission. In addition, caregivers were reconciling within a context shaped by their own ongoing health and illness experiences. Declines in the their own health and function were a very real worry, because many knew that if something happened to them, their spouse would end up in long-term care. Sean expressed his worry: "The only concerns that I got right now, dear, is if I stay healthy. That's my biggest concern." A detailed examination of contextual forces shaping the process of reconciling enabled us to increase our understanding of the meanings of past forces on transitions. In the next sections we describe the three phases of reconciling.

Three Phases of Reconciling

Each of the three phases of reconciling (getting ready, getting into it, getting on with it) was differentiated by (a) the saliency of each subprocess (i.e., navigating, safekeeping, and repositioning) within a phase, and (b) the patterns among the subprocesses engaged in within each phase across time. The three phases, though not mutually exclusive on a time scale, corresponded approximately to spousal caregivers' experiences prior to discharge home (i.e., getting ready), the first 2 to 3 weeks home postdischarge (i.e., getting into it), and several weeks postdischarge (i.e., getting on with it). The phases were not necessarily linear, but rather overlapped one another. Movement from one phase to another was subtle, particularly the shift between getting into it and getting on with it.

The first phase of reconciling, getting ready, was characterized by spousal caregivers' multifaceted preparations, including physical, emotional, and environmental, which were aimed at optimizing the care provided for their spouses. Tony explained:

There's getting ready emotionally, getting ready physically, and then getting the house ready. 'Cause a lot of people coming out of [the GRU], you have to make a lot of changes to the house. So to me, getting ready can be multifaceted.

For the most part, caregivers were pleased to be taking their spouse home. However, they also were aware of how difficult it would be and aware of the need to prepare themselves emotionally. Jack revealed how, in some ways, it was easier for him to have his wife on the GRU: "I didn't have to worry about caring for her [at home] . . . so actually going to the hospital was easier for me, because I didn't have to look after her." In the getting-ready phase, spousal caregivers were juggling numerous pieces of information and were meeting with a range of health care providers. This occurred while they prepared themselves emotionally for their spouse to return home and made needed physical changes to their home to ensure safety (e.g., installed wheelchair ramps, grab bars, and so forth).

The second phase of reconciling, getting into it, began when husbands or wives were discharged home and spousal caregivers assumed the majority of care. The preparations and knowledge gleaned (or not) influenced caregivers on a day-to-day basis. The getting-into-it phase was the busiest of the three phases for caregivers, during which time they coped with multiple demands surrounding care for their spouse.

Movement from the second phase of getting into it to the third phase of getting on with it was relatively insidious. The third phase of reconciling, getting on with it, represented a subtle shift from a focus that included GRU-related issues, such as illness and impairments, to a focus on striving for predictability, enabling the social health of their spouse and shifting the care boundaries that caregivers set previously for themselves. The phase of getting on with it was demarcated by the focus of caregivers on not just the medical aspects of care, but rather on a distinct attention to facilitate and enable opportunities for social participation both within and outside of the home for themselves, their spouse, and them as a couple. The three phases, and the second and third in particular, are best explained and understood through an exploration of the various subprocesses enacted by spouses during this care transition.

Subprocesses Enacted Across Phases of Reconciling

Caregivers were reconciling through the three phases by enacting three interdependent subprocesses including navigating, safekeeping, and repositioning. These three subprocesses encompassed a range of strategies that changed over time, in response to the fluctuating needs of caregivers, the needs of their spouse, and their marriage. A brief overview of each subprocess and associated strategies is provided in the following section; however, a more detailed discussion of these subprocesses can be found in Byrne (2008), and will be the topic of forthcoming articles.

Navigating. Navigating emerged as a subprocess whereby caregivers were locating, evaluating, creating, and integrating past and current sources of knowledge. Through navigating, caregivers were reconciling previous knowledge with new knowledge needed to care for their spouse, themselves individually, and as a couple. Navigating was accomplished through three strategies, including negotiating paths to knowledge formulation, maneuvering obstacles, and making decisions. Caregivers negotiated paths that were merging, connecting, and diverging toward the formulation of the knowledge base they needed. A merging path resulted when caregivers used knowledge and skills gleaned from previous experiences with health care providers and/or providing care for their spouse.

Connecting paths resulted when caregivers received much-needed new knowledge to meet the needs of their spouse, themselves, and the marital dyad. Kathleen explained:

> Yeah, that you got all, because usually when you leave the hospital they give you your list of prescriptions to get filled and everything. But I think if your husband isn't walking great, well, you have to have a walker and things; for the bathroom to sit on, he's got a higher seat to sit on, and he's got a seat in the bathtub for when he's getting a bath. He doesn't have to stand all the time, and he has safety bars all around the shower to hold on to. But they did ask me at the GRU what I had and what I didn't have, to make sure I had everything.

Divergent paths, conversely, resulted when caregivers did not receive needed knowledge. Paths were divergent when knowledge for caregivers was absent, incorrect, difficult to understand, conflicting, or when it is was provided at the wrong time:

> But just somebody to say, "How are you doing? How are things going? Is there anything you need that you're not getting?" and just like I could use somebody, I mean, somebody to come in and help with the housework, to clean, and but, just some support for caregivers, that's what you need, and I don't think it's available, to get it in terms of your, of your needs for your client. But there's no support for the caregiver. Does that make sense? Yeah, like this is what I did when I had this, or has anybody got any suggestions for that, or just a time to have a cup of coffee with somebody that's going through the same thing.

In response to these diverging paths, caregivers maneuvered obstacles by taking actions such as sorting multiple sources of knowledge, looking for directions, and learning through experiences. Jessica explained:

> And here's CCAC [community care access center], and everybody was coming in to his room at once. And um, so I came home and I had to sit down immediately and make out huge charts of, especially his medication chart, and uh, who was coming when, and try to sort out all this information that I got, that last day, which might have been perhaps a good idea to have had that a couple days before he went home, so I'd have time to work it out. But anyway I got it straightened away.

Caregivers made decisions based on the information and services that were available, and based on what was perceived as best for their husband or wife or themselves. Several caregivers turned down services they were offered because the services did not meet their specific needs, or they felt that the services were not needed. Deborah commented on her decision to not accept help from Meals on Wheels (an organization that provides home-delivered meals):

> And the social worker said what about Meals on Wheels, and I said oh no, I'm not going to sit and wait for somebody, if it's snowing. Well last week there was no Meals on Wheels, nobody got meals, it stopped. So I said, Meals on Wheels, I says no, I said I'm quite capable. So we eat when we want to, not because we have to. No, no, no they did send somebody down and were insisting on home, Meals on Wheels, and somebody to do your laundry. And I thought God's sake, no—I'd be sitting here waiting for somebody, I'd have it done.

Elements of navigating changed over time across phases. For example, during the phase of getting ready, caregivers most often faced an absence of sources of knowledge related to how their spouse would progress once discharged from the GRU, and which types of services would be received in the home. However, during the phase of getting into it, caregivers often did not have information about medications, dietary restrictions, and home care services, among other service-related information. It was only once their spouse was discharged home, and care was placed squarely on the shoulders of the caregivers, that the caregivers then realized the extent of what they did not know.

Safekeeping. Safekeeping, the second subprocess of reconciling, highlights how caregivers protected, promoted, and enhanced the emotional, physical, and social health of their spouse. Caregivers engaged in safekeeping when there was a risk or perceived threat to their spouse's safety, or to the maintenance of or improvement in physical, emotional, or social health and well-being. Three strategies were used by caregivers during safekeeping, including advocating, shielding, and enabling physical and social health. Caregivers advocated on behalf of their spouse by challenging health care providers or other family members to ensure that their spouse received proper care and requisite services. Sean discussed how he felt the home care services were not meeting his wife's needs, and how he was handling the situation:

> Yeah, they do, some of them are pretty good, but there's more of them that are just, I don't know. They, they come in and they just, sometimes I wonder if they, see they're supposed to brush her teeth, they're supposed to comb her hair, they're supposed to give her a, a sponge bath if she doesn't get in the

tub, and they're supposed to give her a bath twice a week, and I got after them last week. She had two baths last week, but I got after them because I wanted her, her bathed twice a week at least, a sponge bath. A sponge bath is not the same as a shower or baths, is it, eh? They're not doing, there's a couple of them there is not doing their job, I'll tell you that right now, and one of these days I'm going to get mad. I don't get mad, but when I do . . . .

In addition, caregivers, particularly for individuals with cognitive impairment or dementia, shielded the emotional health of their spouse. During interviews, caregivers did not want to discuss aspects of dementia while their spouse was present, stating that they did not talk about the "memory problems" or use the word *dementia* in front of him or her. For instance, while interviewing Marie, she stated,

> Yeah, well I'm hoping the Aricept [medication] will keep on working. And they're always coming out with new drugs [lowers her voice and looks at husband who is sitting across the room]. I don't talk to him too much about it, so . . . .

Observations revealed that caregivers shielded their partners from the interview process itself. This manifested, for example, as whispering or speaking in lowered, hushed tones during the interview. Enabling emerged as a strategy by which caregivers promoted, demanded, facilitated, or encouraged courses of action to benefit the physical and/or social health of their spouse and themselves. Jack explained:

> And it's quite easy to say, well, the caregiver to say, well the heck with the exercises, why bother? Or well, I'm going out, I'll bring someone in to look after you, and don't push, or let's go ourselves. You got to do a lot of pushing to get the person going. That's another thing I think a lot of people find difficult.

Enabling was intended to keep partners safe, to serve as a limit on caregivers' own worry and anxiety, and to meet the social needs of both their spouse and themselves. Several instances of enabling were observed while the first author was present in caregivers' homes. For instance, Patrick instructed his wife to uncross her legs, whereas Nicholas demonstrated to his wife how and when she should keep the brakes on her walker. Enabling health was affected by the knowledge barriers faced by caregivers. Kevin explained how not knowing influenced his ability to enable the physical health of his wife:

> I don't know when to push her. She gets out here and takes her walker and walks to the end of the

driveway and back, and then she says, "I'm tired." I don't know whether to say, "Do it again." Who am I to say that when she says she's tired? Unless I knew what I was doing, and I don't, I can't say that to her. I said, "Honey, leave it up to the day hospital. Whatever they tell you, that's what you should be doing."

Safekeeping manifested differently across phases depending on the strategy employed by caregivers. For instance, one of the major differences between the phases of getting into it and getting on with it was that spousal caregivers shifted from a focus of enabling physical health to a focus on enabling social health. Once caregivers mastered enabling physical health they began enabling social health for their spouse and themselves by engaging in social outings.

Repositioning. Repositioning, the third subprocess, was used by caregivers to alter, shift, and modify either temporarily or permanently their geographical space and place, relationships, and social positions. Positions for caregivers included locations, roles, beliefs, and attitudes, and encompassed geographical, emotional, and social aspects. Caregivers engaged in repositioning to reconcile the dissonance between past and present beliefs, and roles regarding, for example, what their marriages "used to be like" in relation to what their relationship was currently like. Repositioning strategies included vowing to care, anticipating, shifting the boundaries, and striving for predictability. The strategy of vowing to care was permeated with beliefs that providing care was part of the duty to the couple's relationship. Sean talked about caring for his wife with dementia:

Well, I, I, geez, that's, why do I do it? Why do I do it? Well, the way I look at it is, I've been married to her now for 52 years. I love the woman, and that's probably why I do it. I got, I don't find no other reason to do it, that's just, that's the reason, that's the reason why I do it, because I don't want to see nothing happen to her, or anything like that, as far as that, at least I hope not. And if I could do anything for her I'd gladly do it, if I could help her in any way, even if I can help her, you know, get rid of this dementia or Alzheimer's [disease], but I can't do that. The only one that can do that is the one up above. I can't do that. I just got to do the best I can and live with it.

In some cases, caregivers discussed how they repositioned their relationship from that as husband and wife to that of parent and child or brother and sister. Caregivers described power differentials that developed within their

relationship, role reversals, absent sexual relationships, and the need to learn how to operate as a single person. Changes to the spousal relationship, despite vowing to care, were not always viewed positively, but as an occurrence that had to happen out of necessity. It was difficult for caregivers to accept and cope with changing marital relationships from emotional perspectives. Irene explained: "I think because now he's become sort of like the child and I'm the parent. And I don't like that situation. I'd like to be an equal partner."

Anticipating emerged as a second strategy whereby caregivers envisioned immediate and long-term situations. Anticipating was critical to the entire process of reconciling, because it "paved the way" for merging and integrating past, present, and potential future circumstances. Anticipating was related to several other processes. As examples, caregivers anticipated what types of safekeeping they would engage in once home. They anticipated what kinds of activities they would enable once home. They anticipated the need for routines, and used anticipation as a strategy for maneuvering barriers (e.g., planning or waiting to look for directions). Without the proper sources of knowledge, or without understanding of information received, caregivers had a difficult time anticipating. For example, caregivers were unsure as to how their spouse would progress once home, and without information about potential progress once home from GRU team members it was difficult to anticipate what the coming situations (i.e., at home with their spouse) would entail.

Shifting the boundaries emerged as a third strategy of setting and shifting limits for "self" based on beliefs, feelings, and comfort levels. Caregivers adjusted their own activities outside of the home for fear that something bad would happen while they were gone, and/or for fear that their spouse would feel neglected if left on his or her own. During the phase of getting on with it, men and women differed in their responses relative to the strategy of shifting the boundaries, particularly for their own activities and participation. Men expressed the desire and the need for their own social life outside the marriage. Kevin illustrated how, although he wanted to participate in activities with his wife, he still needed to have his own life within the marriage:

We are definitely going to go to join something. I think it would be beneficial for my wife and could be beneficial for me to meet some people. What I gather is that the men go off and play darts and the women play euchre [game] or whatever they do. I think it's kind of necessary for caregivers and their spouses to get a little separate time from each other. My wife has always been insecure. If I go anywhere, she wants to come with me. If I am going to Canadian Tire she'll say, can I come? Sometimes I would like to go to be by myself. Part of my wife's being hospitalized, I would take walks by myself around the grounds of the hospital. I miss a lot of the male comradeship now, just don't have time for it really.

For women, however, guilt persisted about leaving their husband alone, even as time since discharge progressed. One month postdischarge, Phyllis explained:

Because it sort of hurts and it's an effort he doesn't want to particularly do it, so. Like for instance, he said, well my daughter asked us out for New Year's. [He said], "I couldn't go out again, I just, I'm not gonna go. You go." But uh, whether I'll go or not, I don't know, cause I'll feel badly leaving him. So I might go for a couple of hours or something.

Striving for predictability emerged as the fourth strategy, which included integrating predictable courses of action into day-to-day life. Caregivers were striving for predictability in response to the need for order and routine.

While spouses were on the GRU, most caregivers took daily trips to the hospital as a means of maintaining normalcy and providing emotional comfort for their spouse and for themselves. Once home, caregivers strove for predictability to integrate previous daily patterns, with the need to establish new patterns such as incorporating exercise regimes and new diets or, for some caregivers, making their spouse incorporate their assistive devices (e.g., walkers) into their life. Deborah commented, "But I have a routine that keeps me going," and Irene said, "But it's just to try and get some predictability in my routine, to know what, what's happening."

Discussion

Consistent with the aims of constructivist theorizing (Charmaz, 2006), the framework developed in this study provides a plausible account of the processes experienced by spousal caregivers during transition; highlights patterns and connections not previously considered; and provides new ways of thinking about the processes engaged in by spousal caregivers' to inform rehabilitation clinicians, researchers, and policy makers. This investigation is the first to explore the processes enacted by spousal caregivers during the transition of their relative from a GRU to home. Prior research describing the processes engaged in by family members during their relatives' hospital-to-home transition included processes directed mainly at medical aspects (Bull, 1992; Bull & Jervis, 1997) and, in a select few studies, the emotional and relational processes

involved in providing care (Bull, 1992; Shyu, 2000b, 2000c). However, none of the authors of the resulting articles mentioned the social aspects of providing care, such as enabling social health of the care recipients, or setting and shifting boundaries for their own social participation, as was identified in our findings. Reconciling was not simply about integrating past and present medical care routines or engaging in the more medical and physical aspects of caregiving, but rather reflected a strong emotional and social component, as well. This has not been addressed adequately in prior research. The needs, processes, and strategies engaged in by spousal caregivers highlight the medical, physical, emotional, and social elements of reconciling, and the biopsychosocial nature of care transitions as experienced by spousal caregivers.

Furthermore, in a theory of transition developed by Meleis and colleagues (2000), several patterns of transition, including single, multiple, sequential, simultaneous, related, or unrelated, are discussed. These patterns characterize the potential multiplicity and complexity of transitions as identified in their theory. Our framework supports the multidimensional and complex nature of transitions put forth by Meleis et al., and our findings show the influence of multiple sequential (health care setting transitions) and simultaneous (relocating, declining health of caregiver, changing spousal relationship) transitions on the experience of the transition from hospital to home (i.e., process of reconciling). It is the patterns among all of these different transitions that support a comprehensive understanding of the hospital-to-home transition itself, and elucidate the complexity of the process of reconciling. For example, Phyllis' experience of reconciling from hospital to home was influenced by her own declining health as she was feeling depressed about her health while simultaneously caring for her spouse and meeting his physical needs. Trying to come to terms with the present situation was complicated by her concerns about her own physical and emotional health.

Although the present study incorporated only a single care transition (i.e., from GRU to home), it highlights how experiences during prior health care setting trajectories influenced caregivers' engagement in the process of reconciling. This was particularly salient for caregivers who almost lost their spouse in acute care health settings, or who had particularly stressful experiences in acute care.In a study exploring caregivers' experiences of transition to long-term care, Reuss, Dupuis, and Whitfield (2005) reported that many of the families in their study (including spousal caregivers) experienced multiple transfers between different settings prior to their relatives' placement in a long-term care facility. They called for longitudinal research to explore the experiences of multiple transitions for families and their relatives. Our study supports this contention, and provides insight into one of the many potential care transitions (hospital to home) that can precede caregivers' experiences of the transfer of their relative to long-term care.

The process of reconciling identified in the present study was influenced not only by a range of caregiving contexts, but also by caregivers' experiences of intertwined life events. For example, in our findings, the death of a family member, marital discord, and conflicts with other family members influenced caregivers' experiences of reconciling. Intertwined life events share similarities with the concept of "linked lives" in Elder's life course theory, which addresses the interdependent nature of social life and relationships (Elder, 1998; Elder & Johnson, 2003). The emergence of the influence of intertwined life events during the transition from the GRU has important implications for the need to explore the experiences of older adults (65 and older) providing care during their older adult relatives' transition from hospital to home. Older adult caregivers are an underrepresented group of caregivers in other studies of hospital-to-home transitions. Spousal caregivers were experiencing transitions in other aspects of life that are common to aging individuals, such as relocation (Firbank & Johnson-Lafleur, 2007). Intertwined life events influenced the transition. For example, if caregivers had relocated recently, then they had greater difficulty reconciling, particularly with regard to striving for predictability. In addition, anticipating the need for relocation was perceived as stressful for some caregivers, especially if it involved the placement of their spouse in long-term care. Declining self-health was another key consideration regarding the process of reconciling for older adult caregivers, because they worried about whether or not their health status would allow them to provide care for their husband or wife. Moreover, the older adult caregivers worried about who would care for their husband or wife if they could not do so in the future because of their own declining health. Our study, unlike other research about care transitions, emphasized these unique aspects of care transitions experienced by older adult spousal caregivers.

Our findings contribute to the growing body of literature aimed at demonstrating the importance of needs assessments for family caregivers (Guberman, Keefe, Fancey, & Barylak, 2007; Nolan, Lundh, Grant, &Keady, 2003) by illustrating the fluctuating medical, physical, emotional, and social needs of spousal caregivers during the transition of their relative from the GRU to home. However, in addition to assessing caregiver needs, the strategies engaged in during hospital-to-home transitions might be an important part of a comprehensive caregiver assessment, and could be amenable to intervention (e.g., when caregivers were informed, they were able to enable physical health). Whereas the assessment of "needs" is

critical, recognizing that caregivers are engaging in multiple strategies to meet these needs during the transition from hospital to home also is essential. In addition to the changing types of needs of caregivers over time (Bull, 1990; Grimmer et al., 2004; Shyu, 2000b), our findings highlight how needs fluctuate in intensity over time. Several caregivers reported low levels of need prior to leaving the GRU, but once they returned home with their spouse their needs intensified. Thus, whereas the GRU is an ideal place in the continuum of care to ascertain caregiver needs, the process of needs assessment itself needs to be ongoing, not a one-time endeavor.

Aside from shielding, which caregivers to spouses with CI or dementia engaged in more frequently than other caregivers, the types of processes enacted by spousal caregivers to individuals with CI or dementia were relatively similar to those engaged in by caregivers to individuals without CI or dementia. However, the intensity of the need to engage in the processes differentiated these two groups. Caregivers of individuals with dementia often discussed more unknowns, particularly around the disease progression and disease-related medications. These caregivers required increased efforts to navigate, and needed to create a knowledge base that was much more diverse than that required of the other caregivers. These two findings are consistent with the broader caregiving–dementia literature which highlights that caregiving for those with dementia often is more demanding than caring for individuals without dementia (Ory, Hoffman, Yee, Tennstedt, & Schulz, 1999). The care recipients in this study who had dementia were in the mild-to-moderate clinical stages, as is the case for the majority of those on geriatric rehabilitation units (Wells, Seabrook, Stolee, Borrie, & Knoefel, 2003). Therefore, different experiences for those caring for individuals with and without CI or dementia might not be as salient within the context of this study.

Although gender differences are not identified in transitional care literature, research in the broader caregiving literature suggests that for caregiving wives, the exchange of emotional support with their care recipient husbands is related to decreased caregiver burden and higher levels of marital satisfaction, and that wife caregivers are more depressed and report higher levels of burden (Pruchno & Resch, 1989; Wright & Aquilino, 1998). In our study, both men and women discussed changes to their relationships; however, women were more apt to comment on the loss of conversation, missing how "life used to be," were more apt to discuss power differentials that developed within their relationship, and were more likely to identify shifts from partnership in marriage to dependency (e.g., Eileen, who described her relationship as akin to a parent–child relationship). This finding is similar to those of Jansson, Nordberg, and Grafstrom (2001), who reported that spousal caregivers undergo a transition from being an equal partner in marriage to "caregiver," requiring caregivers to sacrifice their own time to take care of their husband or wife. These findings point to a need for health care professionals to work with both husband and wife caregivers, paying careful attention to the emotional and relationship needs of caregiving wives, and ensuring that both men and, particularly women spousal caregivers, are assisted in shifting the boundaries they set for themselves around their own activities and participation.

Two prominent care-transition interventions for patients (Coleman et al., 2004; Naylor et al., 2004; Parry, Coleman, Smith, Frank, & Kramer, 2003) have demonstrated promising results for patient (e.g., positive perception of quality of care) and health care system outcomes (decreased rehospitalization). Whereas family caregivers were identified as integral to the success of both interventions, and were involved in the implementation of these interventions, their experiences with the transition intervention and their outcomes were not included. The effectiveness of these interventions for influencing caregiver experiences or outcomes during the transition of relatives from hospital to home is not known. Coleman and Williams (2007) proposed an approach to involve caregivers in transitional care that defined the type and intensity of roles that caregivers play; namely, the types of contributions caregivers make, including financial, advocacy, care coordination, emotional support, and direct care provision (creating the acronym FACED). Acknowledging the role of caregivers, and providing information to health care providers about the contributions of caregivers, is important to transitional care. What has not been emphasized adequately in this approach is how the care transition and potential transition interventions influence outcomes specific to caregivers, such as their own feelings of preparation and physical, psychological, and social health. Caregivers have their own unmet needs that occur during transition. A focus for future studies might include how to fulfill caregivers' needs, and to help them engage in the strategies they are using to care for their spouse, themselves, and the marital dyad. Such a focus would be critical to the design of interventions aimed at improving caregiver-specific outcomes.

Shyu and colleagues (2008) designed a caregiver-oriented transition intervention that included individualized health education, follow-up phone calls, and home visits for family caregivers following the discharge of their relative from a hospital setting. They demonstrated how focusing on caregiver-specific needs resulted in better self-evaluations of preparation, and better satisfaction of discharge needs after the intervention. Our theoretical framework might be useful to inform the development of future caregiver-oriented interventions during transition from a GRU to home, aimed at helping caregivers with what they are "doing" during transitions. For instance, interventions aimed at helping caregivers to navigate, safekeep, and reposition, with a focus on ways to enhance and improve the strategies engaged in by caregivers, would provide meaningful and useful skills and approaches.

Although the purpose of the present study was to highlight the experiences of spousal caregivers through transition from a GRU to home, a potential limitation is that the care recipient spouse was not interviewed. Changes in the nature of the relationship between caregivers and care recipients during the transition from hospital to home have been identified in previous studies (Shyu, 2000b, 2000c). In addition, our limited consideration of the complexity of social networks—in particular how the social interactions between spousal caregivers; care recipients and other family members (e.g., adult children); friends; and formal care providers might shape the phases and processes of reconciliation—is a limitation. Future research should expand the focus to include other individuals in the social networks of spousal caregivers to understand better the complexity of interactions and processes involved during care transitions. Our research provides insight into the importance of considering the trajectory of multiple care transitions experienced by caregivers. However, further research is needed that incorporates a longitudinal perspective whereby caregivers are recruited in acute care settings and followed through multiple care transitions across the care continuum. Another limitation, and an implication for future research, is that our study did not include caregivers from a range of cultural backgrounds, thereby limiting a consideration of how the experiences and processes might be different for caregivers in non-Western cultures (Li & Shyu, 2007).

The theoretical framework developed in this study provides a means of understanding the relationships and patterns among the processes engaged in by caregivers during the period of their relative's transition from a GRU to home. Helping caregivers to reconcile and meet their transitional-based needs will require a commitment on the part of both GRU team members and community health care professionals. The theoretical framework provides a resource to health care scientists, health care clinicians, educators, and decision makers regarding how they must work together to improve transitional care for spousal caregivers.

Acknowledgments

We thank the caregivers, GRU clinicians, and research team for their invaluable contributions to the study. The guidance and support of Ingrid Connidis and Margaret Cheesman is also acknowledged. We thank Catherine Craven for her help with the preparation of this article.

Authors' Note

Portions of this article were presented at the Canadian Association on Gerontology conference, October, 2008, London, Canada, and the British Society of Gerontology conference, September 2009, Bristol, United Kingdom.

Declaration of Conflicting Interests

The authors declared no conflicts of interest with respect to the authorship and/or publication of this article.

Funding

The authors disclosed receipt of the following financial support for the research and/or authorship of this article: Dr. Byrne was funded by a doctoral award from the Social Sciences and Humanities Research Council of Canada, and a Graduate Research Award from the Alzheimer Society of London Middlesex.

Note

1. All participant names are pseudonyms.

References

Aminzadeh, F., Byszewski, A., Dalziel, W. B., Wilson, M., Deane, N., & Papahariss-Wright, S. (2005). Effectiveness of outpatient geriatric assessment programs: Exploring caregiver needs, goals, and outcomes. *Journal of Gerontological Nursing, 31*(12), 19-25. Retrieved from http://www.jognonline.com/view.asp?rid=4673

Ballinger, C. (2004). Writing up rigour: Representing and evaluating good scholarship in qualitative research. *British Journal of Occupational Therapy, 67*, 540-546. Retrieved from http://www.ingentaconnect.com/content/cot/bjot/2004/00000067/00000012/art00004

Barnes, B., Given, C., & Given, B. (1992). Caregivers of elderly relatives: Spouses and adult children. *Health and Social Work, 17*, 282-289. Retrieved from http://www.ncbi.nlm.nih.gov/pubmed/1478554

Beck, C. T. (1993). Qualitative research: The evaluation of its credibility, fittingness and auditability. *Western Journal of Nursing Research, 15*, 263-266. doi:10.1177/019394599301500212

Bogardus, S. T., Jr., Bradley, E. H., Williams, C. S., Maciejewski, P. K., Gallo, W. T., & Inouye, S. K. (2004). Achieving goals in geriatric assessment: Role of caregiver agreement and adherence to recommendations. *Journal of the American Geriatrics Society, 52*, 99-105. doi:10.1111/j.1532-5415.2004.52017

Bradley, E. H., Bogardus, S. T., Jr., van Doorn, C., Williams, C. S., Cherlin, E., & Inouye, S. K. (2000). Goals in geriatric assessment: Are we measuring the right outcomes? *Gerontologist, 40*, 191-196. doi:10.1093/geront/40.2.191

Braun, M., Mikulincer, M., Rydall, A., Walsh, A., & Rodin, G. (2007). Hidden morbidity in cancer: Spouse caregivers. *Clinical Oncology, 25*, 4829-4834. doi:10.1200/JCO.2006.10.0909

Bull, M. J. (1990). Factors influencing family caregiver burden and health. *Western Journal of Nursing Research, 12*, 758-770. doi:10.1177/019394599001200605

Bull, M. J. (1992). Managing the transition from hospital to home. *Qualitative Health Research, 2*, 27-41. doi:10.1177/104973239200200103

Bull, M. J., & Jervis, L. L. (1997). Strategies used by chronically ill older women and their caregiving daughters in managing posthospital care. *Journal of Advanced Nursing, 25*, 541-547. doi:10.1046/j.1365-2648.1997.1997025541

Bull, M. J., Maruyama, G., & Luo, D. (1995). Testing a model for posthospital transition of family caregivers for elderly persons. *Nursing Research, 44*, 132-138. Retrieved from http://journals.lww.com/nursingresearchonline/Abstract/1995/05000/Testing_a_Model_for_Posthospital_Transition_of.2.aspx

Bull, M. J., & McShane, R. E. (2008). Seeking what's best during the transition to adult day health services. *Qualitative Health Research, 18*, 597-605. doi:10.1177/1049732308315174

Byrne, K. (2008). *Spousal caregivers' during their husbands'/wives' transition from a GRU to home.* (Unpublished doctoral dissertation). University of Western Ontario, London, ON, Canada.

Chappell, N. L. (1992). *Social support and aging.* Toronto, ON, Canada: Butterworths.

Charmaz, K. (2006). *Constructing grounded theory: A practical guide through qualitative analysis.* Thousand Oaks, CA: Sage.

Chick, N., & Meleis, A. I. (1986). Transitions: A nursing concern. In P.L. Chinn (Ed.), *Nursing research methodology: Issues and implementation* (pp. 237-257). Rockville, MD: Aspen.

Chiovitti, R. F., & Piran, N. (2003). Rigour and grounded theory research. *Journal of Advanced Nursing, 44*, 427-435. doi:10.1046/j.0309-2402.2003.02822

Coleman, E. A., Boult, C., & American Geriatrics Society Health Care Systems Committee. (2003). Improving the quality of transitional care for persons with complex care needs. *Journal of the American Geriatrics Society, 51*, 556-557. doi:10.1046/j.1532-5415.2003.51186

Coleman, E. A., Smith, J. D., Frank, J. C., Min, S. J., Parry, C., & Kramer, A. M. (2004). Preparing patients and caregivers to participate in care delivered across settings: The care transitions intervention. *Journal of the American Geriatrics Society, 52*, 1817-1825. doi:10.1111/j.1532-5415.2004.52504

Coleman, E. A., & Williams, M. V. (2007). Executing high-quality care transitions: A call to do it right. *Journal of Hospital Medicine, 2*, 287-290. doi:10.1002/jhm.276

Connell, C. M., Janevic, M. R., & Gallant, M. P. (2001). The costs of caring: Impact of dementia on family caregivers. *Journal of Geriatric Psychiatry, 14*, 179-187. doi:10.1177/089198870101400403

Cutcliffe, J. R. (2000). Methodological issues in grounded theory. *Journal of Advanced Nursing, 31*, 1476-1484. doi:10.1046/j.1365-2648.2000.01430

Davies, S., & Nolan, M. (2003). 'Making the best of things': Relatives' experiences of decisions about care-home entry. *Ageing & Society, 23*, 429-450. doi:10.1017/S0144686X03001259

Davies, S., & Nolan, M. (2004). Making the move: Relatives' experiences of transition to a care home. *Health and Social Care in the Community, 12*, 517-526. doi:10.1111/j.1365-2524.2004.00535

Demers, L., Ska, B., Desrosiers, J., Alix, C., & Wolfson, C. (2004). Development of a conceptual framework for the assessment of geriatric rehabilitation outcomes. *Archives of Gerontology and Geriatrics, 38*, 221-237. doi:10.1016/j.archger.2003.10.003

Elder, G. H., Jr. (1998). The life course and human development. In R. M. Lerner (Ed.), *Handbook of child psychology: Volume 1. Theoretical models of human development* (pp. 939-991). New York: Wiley.

Elder, G. H., Jr., & Johnson, M. K. (2003). The life course and aging: Challenges, lessons, and new directions. In R. A. Setterson, Jr. (Ed.), *Invitation to the life course: Toward new understandings of later life* (pp. 48-81). Amityville, NY: Baywood.

Firbank, O. E., & Johnson-Lafleur, J. (2007). Older persons relocating with a family caregiver: Processes, stages, and motives. *Journal of Applied Gerontology, 26*, 182-207. doi:10.1177/0733464807300224

Frederick, J., & Fast, J. (1999). Eldercare in Canada: Who does how much? *Canadian Social Trends, 53*, 26-32. Retrieved from http://www.statcan.gc.ca/pub/11-008-x/1999002/article/4661-eng.pdf

Fredman, L., & Daly, M. P. (1998). Enhancing practitioner ability to recognize and treat caregiver physical and mental consequences. *Topics in Geriatric Rehabilitation, 14*, 36-44.

George, L., & Gwyther, L. (1986). Caregiver well-being: A multidimensional examination of family caregivers of demented adults. *Gerontologist, 26*, 253-259. doi:10.1093/geront/26.3.253

Grant, S., St John, W., & Patterson, E. (2009). Recovery from total hip replacement surgery: "It's not just physical." *Qualitative Health Research, 19*, 1612-1620. doi:10.1177/1049732309350683

Grimmer, K., Falco, J., & Moss, J. (2004). Becoming a carer for an elderly person after discharge from an acute hospital admission. *Internet Journal of Allied Health Sciences & Practice, 2*(4). Retrieved from http://ijahsp.nova.edu/articles/vol2num4/grimmer-carer%20issues.pdf

Grimmer, K., & Moss, J. (2001). The development, validity and application of a new instrument to assess the quality of discharge planning activities from the community perspective. *International Journal for Quality in Health Care, 13*, 109-116. Retrieved from http://intqhc.oxfordjournals.org/cgi/reprint/13/2/109

Guba, E., & Lincoln, Y. (1989). *Fourth generation evaluation.* Beverly Hills, CA: Sage.

Guberman, N., Keefe, J., Fancey, P., & Barylak, L. (2007). 'Not another form!': Lessons for implementing carer assessment in health and social service agencies. *Health and Social Care in the Community, 15*, 577-587. doi:10.1111/j.1365-2524.2007.00718.x

Hayes, J., Zimmerman, M., & Boylstein, C. (2010). Responding to the symptoms of Alzheimer's disease: Husbands, wives, and the gendered dynamics of recognition and disclosure. *Qualitative Health Research, 20*, 1101-1115. doi:10.1177/1049732310369559

Health Canada. (2002). *National profile of family caregivers in Canada—Final report.* Retrieved from http://www.hc-sc.gc.ca/hcs-sss/pubs/home-domicile/2002-caregiv-interven/index-eng.php

Hess, B. B., & Soldo, B. J. (1985). Husband and wife networks. In W. J. Sauer & R. T. Coward (Eds.), *Social support networks and the care of the elderly: Theory, research and practice* (pp. 67-92). New York: Springer.

Hills, G. A. (1998). Caregivers of the elderly: Hidden patients and health team members. *Topics in Geriatric Rehabilitation, 14*, 1-11.

Holland, D. E., & Harris, M. R. (2007). Discharge planning, transitional care, coordination of care, and continuity of care: Clarifying the concepts and terms from the hospital perspective. *Home Health Care Services Quarterly, 26*(4), 3-19. doi:10.1300/J027v26n04_02

Holtslander, L. F., & Duggleby, W. D. (2009). The hope experience of older bereaved women who cared for a spouse with terminal cancer. *Qualitative Health Research, 19*, 388-400. doi:10.1177/1049732308329682

Jacobi, C. E., van den Berg, B., Boshuizen, H. C., Rupp, I., Dinant, H. J., & van den Bos, A. M. (2003). Dimension-specific burden of caregiving among partners of rheumatoid arthritis patients. *Rheumatology, 42*, 1226-1233. doi:10.1093/rheumatology/keg366

Jansson, W., Nordberg, G., & Grafstrom, M. (2001). Patterns of elderly spousal caregiving in dementia care: An observational study. *Journal of Advanced Nursing, 34*, 804-812. Retrieved from http://www3.interscience.wiley.com/cgi-bin/fulltext/118983178/PDFSTART

Kane, R. A., Reinardy, J., Penrod, J. D., & Huck, S. (1999). After the hospitalization is over: A different perspective on family care of older people. *Journal of Gerontological Social Work, 31*, 119-141. doi:10.1300/J083v31n01_08

Kneeshaw M. F., Considine R. M., & Jennings, J. (1999). Mutuality and preparedness of family caregivers for elderly women after bypass surgery. *Applied Nursing Research, 12*, 128-135. doi:10.1016/S0897-1897(99)80034-2

Lazarus, R. S., & Folkman, S. (1984). *Stress, appraisal, and coping.* New York: Springer.

Li, H. J., & Shyu, Y. I. (2007). Coping processes of Taiwanese families during the postdischarge period for an elderly family member with hip fracture. *Nursing Science Quarterly, 20*, 273-279. doi:10.1177/0894318407303128

Lin, P. C., Hung, S. H., Liao, M. H., Sheen, S. Y., & Jong, S. Y. (2006). Care needs and level of care difficulty related to hip fractures in geriatric populations during the post-discharge transition period. *Journal of Nursing Research, 14,* 251-259. doi:10.1097/01.JNR.0000387584.89468.30

Lofland, J., Snow, D., Anderson, L., & Lofland, L. H. (2006). *Analyzing social settings: A guide to qualitative observation and analysis.* Florence, KY: Wadsworth.

Meleis, A. I., Sawyer, L. M., Im, E. O., Hilfinger Messias, D. K., & Schumacher, K. (2000). Experiencing transitions: An emerging middle-range theory. *Advances in Nursing Science, 23,* 12-28. Retrieved from http://journals.lww.com/advancesin nursingscience/Abstract/2000/09000/Experiencing_Transi tions__An_Emerging_Middle_Range.6.aspx

Morse, J. M. (2009). Exploring transitions. *Qualitative Health Research, 19,* 431.doi:10.1177/1049732308328547

Morse, J. M., & Field, P. A. (1995). *Qualitative research methods for health professionals.* Thousand Oaks, CA: Sage.

Navon, L., & Weinblatt, N. (1996). The show must go on—Behind the scenes of elderly spousal caregiving. *Journal of Aging Studies, 10,* 329-342. doi:10.1016/S0890-4065(96)90005-5

Naylor, M. D. (2000). A decade of transitional care research with vulnerable elders. *Journal of Cardiovascular Nursing, 14*(3), 1-14. Retrieved from http://ovidsp.tx.ovid.com/sp-3.2/ovid-web.cgi?&S=HLANFPLFEGDDDKLCNCDLDCGCECH NAA00&Link+Set=S.sh.15.17.22.27%7c4%7csl_10

Naylor, M. D. (2002). Transitional care of older adults. *Annual Review of Nursing Research, 20,* 127-147. Retrieved from http://www.ingentaconnect.com/content/springer/arnr/2002/00000020/00000001/art00007

Naylor, M. D., Brooten, D. A., Campbell, R. L., Maislin, G., McCauley, K. M., & Schwartz, J. S. (2004). Transitional care of older adults hospitalized with heart failure: A randomized, controlled trial. *Journal of the American Geriatrics Society, 52,* 675-684. doi:10.1111/j.1532-5415.2004.52202.x

Naylor, M. D., Hirschman, K. B., Bowles, K. H., Bixby, M. B., Konick-McMahan, J., & Stephens, C. (2007). Care coordination for cognitively impaired older adults and their caregivers. *Home Health Care Services Quarterly, 26*(4), 57-78. doi:10.1300/J027v26n04_05

Naylor, M. D., Stephens, C., Bowles, K. H., & Bixby, M. B. (2005). Cognitively impaired older adults: From hospital to home. *American Journal of Nursing, 105,* 52-61. Retrieved from http://journals.lww.com/ajnonline/Citation/2005/02000/Cognitively_Impaired_Older_Adults__From_Hos pital.28.aspx

Nolan, M. R., Lundh, U., Grant, G., & Keady, J. (Eds.). (2003). *Partnerships in family care: Understanding the caregiving career.* Maidenhead, UK: Open University Press.

Ory, M. G., Hoffman, R. R., Yee, J. L., Tennstedt, S., & Schulz, R. (1999). Prevalence and impact of caregiving: A detailed comparison between dementia and nondementia caregivers. *Gerontologist, 39,* 177-185. doi:10.1093/geront/39.2.177

Parry, C., Coleman, E. A., Smith, J. D., Frank, J., & Kramer, A. M. (2003). The care transitions intervention: A patient-centered approach to ensuring effective transfers between sites of geriatric care. *Home Health Care Services Quarterly, 22*(3), 1-17. doi:10.1300/J027v22n03_01

Parry, C., Kramer, H. M., & Coleman, E. A. (2006). A qualitative exploration of a patient-centered coaching intervention to improve care transitions in chronically ill older adults. *Home Health Care Services Quarterly, 25*(3-4), 39-53. doi:10.1300/J027v25n03_03

Pearlin, L. I., Mullan, J. T., Semple, S. J., & Skaff, M. M. (1990). Caregiving and the stress process: An overview of concepts and their measures. *Gerontologist, 30,* 583-594. doi:10.1093/geront/30.5.583

Pruchno, R. A., & Resch, N. (1989). Husbands and wives as caregivers: Antecedents of depression and burden. *Gerontologist, 29,* 159-165. doi:10.1093/geront/29.2.159

Redfern, S. J., & Norman, I. J. (1994). Validity through triangulation. *Nurse Researcher, 2,* 41-56.

Reuss, G. F., Dupuis, S. L., & Whitfield, K. (2005). Understanding the experience of moving a loved one to a long-term care facility: Family members' perspectives. *Journal of Gerontological Social Work, 46,* 17-46. doi:10.1300/J083v46n01_03

Sandelowksi, M. (1993). Rigor or rigor mortis—The problem of rigor in qualitative research revisited. *Advances in Nursing Science, 16*(2), 1-8.

Schumacher, K. L. (1995). Family caregiver role acquisition: Role-making through situated interaction. *Scholarly Inquiry for Nursing Practice, 9,* 211-226.

Schumacher, K. L., Jones, P. S., & Meleis, A. (1999). Helping elderly persons in transition: A framework for research and practice. In E. Swanson & T. Tripp-Reimer (Eds.), *Life transitions in the older adult: Issues for nurses and other health professionals* (pp. 1-26). New York: Springer.

Showalter, A., Burger, S., & Salyer, J. (2000). Patients' and their spouses' needs after total joint arthroplasty: A pilot study. *Orthopaedic Nursing, 19,* 49-62.

Shyu, Y. I. (2000a). The needs of family caregivers of frail elders during the transition from hospital to home: A Taiwanese sample. *Journal of Advanced Nursing, 32,* 619-625. Retrieved from http://www3.interscience.wiley.com/cgi-bin/fulltext/119010648/PDFSTART

Shyu, Y. I. (2000b). Role tuning between caregiver and care receiver during discharge transition: An illustration of role function mode in Roy's adaptation theory. *Nursing Science Quarterly, 13,* 323-331.doi:10.1177/08943180022107870

Shyu, Y. I. (2000c). Patterns of caregiving when family caregivers face competing needs. *Journal of Advanced Nursing, 31,* 35-43. Retrieved from http://www3.interscience.wiley.com/journal/121440743/abstract

Shyu, Y. L., Chen, M., Chen, S., Wang, H., & Shao, J. (2008). A family caregiver-oriented discharge planning program for older stroke patients and their family caregivers. *Journal of Clinical Nursing, 17,* 2497-2508. Retrieved from http://www3.inter science.wiley.com/cgi-bin/fulltext/121377510/PDFSTART

Skaff, M. M., Pearlin, L. I., & Mullan, J. T. (1996). Transitions in the caregiving career: Effects on sense of mastery. *Psychology and Aging, 11,* 247-257.

Wells, J. L., Seabrook, J. A., Stolee, P., Borrie, M. J., & Knoefel, F. (2003). State of the art in geriatric rehabilitation. Part II: Clinical challenges. *Archives in Physical Medicine and Rehabilitation, 84,* 898-903. doi:10.1016/S0003-9993(02) 04930-4

Wright, D. L., & Aquilino, W. S. (1998). Influence of emotional support exchange in marriage on caregiving wives' burden and marital satisfaction. *Family Relations, 47,* 195-204. Retrieved from http://www.jstor.org/stable/585624?cookieSet=1

Bios

Kerry Byrne, PhD, is a postdoctoral fellow in the Department of Sociology at the University of British Columbia, Vancouver, British Columbia, Canada.

Joseph B. Orange, PhD, is an associate professor in and the director of the School of Communication Sciences and Disorders in the Faculty of Health Sciences at the University of Western Ontario at London, Ontario, Canada.

Catherine Ward-Griffin, RN, PhD, is a professor and acting chair of graduate programs in the Arthur Labatt Family School of Nursing, the University of Western Ontario, London, Ontario, Canada.

APPENDIX

F

Nursing Research • November/December 2011 • Vol 60, No 6, 386–392

Sharing a Traumatic Event

The Experience of the Listener and the Storyteller Within the Dyad

Jeanne Cummings

▶ **Background:** Individuals who have experienced traumatic events often share their experiences in story form. This sharing has consequences for both storytellers and listeners. Understanding the experience of both members of the listener–storyteller dyad is of value to nurses who are often the listener within the nurse–patient dyad.

▶ **Objective:** The aim of this study was to illuminate the experiences of the listener and the storyteller when a traumatic event is shared within the dyad.

▶ **Methods:** The phenomenon was explored using an interpretive phenomenological approach. Participants consisted of 12 dyads, each with a storyteller and a listener. The storytellers were individuals who had been involved in U.S. Airways Flight 1549 when it crash-landed in the Hudson River in January 2009. Each storyteller identified a listener who had listened to them share their story of this event, dubbed *The Miracle on the Hudson*. In-depth interviews were conducted with each storyteller and each listener.

▶ **Results:** Five essential themes emerged from the data: Theme 1, The Story Has a Purpose; Theme 2, The Story as a Whole May Continue to Change as Different Parts Are Revealed; Theme 3, The Story Is Experienced Physically, Mentally, Emotionally, and Spiritually; Theme 4, Imagining the "What" as well as the "What If"; and Theme 5, The Nature of the Relationship Colors the Experience of the Listener and the Storyteller. Roy's Adaptation Model of Nursing was found to be applicable to the findings of this study.

▶ **Discussion:** For the participants in this study, the experience of sharing a traumatic event involved facts, feelings, and images. The story evolved as it was remembered, told, and listened to in a nonlinear, multifaceted way. The listener and the storyteller collaborated, adapted, and responded physically, mentally, emotionally, and spiritually.

▶ **Key Words:** dyad · Flight 1549 · listening · Miracle on the Hudson · nursing · storytelling · trauma

Trauma is any distressing event or psychological shock from experiencing a disastrous event (Webster's Dictionary, 2001, p. 760). The surgeon general has recognized trauma as a major public health risk (Courtois & Gold, 2009). Individuals can directly experience a trauma or can be indirectly traumatized through witnessing or other forms of

secondhand exposure (Courtois, 2002). In a national survey of the general population, 60% of men and 51% of women reported having experienced at least one traumatic event in their lifetime (Kessler, Sonnega, Bromet, Hughes, & Nelson, 1995).

People who have experienced traumatic events may tell trauma stories that are fragmented and disjointed, and understanding these stories can be complicated and challenging (Leydesdorff, Dawson, Burchardt, & Ashplant, 2009). Trauma is experienced subjectively; its meaning is very personal (BenEzer, 2009): "for a trauma survivor, putting the story and its imagery into words is the goal of recovery" (Herman, 1992, p. 177). Being asked to share traumatic experiences lets storytellers know that listeners recognize them and their suffering (Rosenthal, 2003). The absence of an invitation to share may convey the message that these experiences are unspeakable or unbearable to listen to; in addition, delayed disclosure and negative reactions to disclosure have been associated with poor adjustment (Ullman, 2007). When people avoid talking about a traumatic event with a victim, the victim may interpret it as a lack of concern and support (Guay, Billette, & Marchand, 2006). Esposito (2005) found that women who had been raped failed to disclose the rape during many subsequent encounters with healthcare providers because no one ever asked them about it. In a study of veterans, it was reported that when healthcare providers asked them about previous trauma, 71% disclosed a history of trauma; nearly 45% remembered receiving a negative response to their disclosure and 30% felt they had not been believed (Leibowitz, Jeffreys, Copeland, & Noel, 2008). Symonds (1980), who worked with crime victims, described *the second wound*, which he defined as "the victim's perceived rejection by and lack of expected support from the community, agencies, family, friends, and society in general" (p. 37). Nurses and other healthcare professionals risk creating a second wound if they do not acknowledge trauma, fail to invite the patient to share, or respond in a way that does not feel meaningful to the patient.

For nurses, listening is one way of responding and adapting to patients within the nurse-patient relationship. The essence of nursing through the ages has been rooted in the relationship between nurse and patient (Roy, 1988).

Jeanne Cummings, DNS, RN, NP, CS, BC, is Visiting Professor, The Graduate Center, City University of New York.
DOI: 10.1097/NNR.0b013e3182348823

In Roy's Adaptation Model of Nursing, the person is conceptualized as an adaptive system functioning toward a purpose (Roy, 1988). In Roy's theory, it is proposed that, as adaptive systems, humans respond to stimuli to initiate a coping process, which has an effect on behavior that leads to responses that are either adaptive or ineffective (Perrett, 2007).

Nurses who bear witness to trauma survivors should keep in mind that "just talking without being listened to is not enough; the one that talks must find someone who will listen" (Vajda, 2007, p. 90). In addition, as Bunkers (2010) observed, there is more to listening than hearing the words of another person. When nurses are listeners for storytelling patients, a dyad is formed. In a dyad, each person must relate directly to the other; thoughts and feelings are engaged (Moreland, 2010). The act of listening enables humans to be present and to bear witness to one another (Kagan, 2008). By remaining present, listeners can create a space for storytellers to reveal themselves, the experience, and the story. "Stories are told with, not only to, listeners" (Frank, 2000, p. 354). Pasupathi and Rich (2005) found that storytellers told shorter stories and experienced negative emotions when listeners were distracted. They also found that, when listeners did not respond to the meaning in the story, storytellers had problems completing the story.

Listening to the patient's story is part of the emotional labor of healthcare (Barrett et al., 2005). Repeatedly listening to trauma stories is not without effect on listeners. Exposure to accumulated stress and secondary trauma can result in compassion fatigue; individuals can become fatigued, depressed, and withdrawn and can lose interest. They can experience recurrent thoughts and images, somatic symptoms, and anger (Showalter, 2010). Shortt and Pennebaker (1992) found that, as dyads of listeners and storytellers shared a story of the Holocaust, the listeners' heart rate increased and the storytellers' heart rate decreased. Nurses and social workers were reported to have strong physical sensations when doing traumatic clinical work (Raingruber & Kent, 2003). Baird and Kracen (2006) documented secondary stress reactions and posttraumatic stress disorder symptoms in trauma therapists. These reactions may affect the treatment process as well as the therapist's own experience (Canfield, 2005). Listening to trauma stories may affect the listener; the storyteller may sense this and adapt by changing the way they share.

Nurse practitioners have described listening as the most valuable skill they have (Parrish, Peden, & Staten, 2008). Hearing the patient's story helps in understanding the patient as a person (Barrett et al., 2005). In spite of the emphasis in nursing education on the importance of listening to the patient, "there is a paucity of nursing literature on listening" (Kagan, 2008, p. 109). Little information is available on what listening to stories of traumatic events is like for nurses, how they may be affected by such stories, and how the patient experiences the nurse as listener. This study sought to illuminate the experience of the listener and the storyteller when a traumatic event is shared within the dyad by interviewing individuals who told their story of being

> *Sharing a traumatic event has consequences for both listener and storyteller.*

▼▼▼

involved in the crash-landing of a plane and the people who listened to them. The knowledge gained from this study has implications for individuals who share stories of traumatic events and the nurses and other healthcare professionals who listen to them.

Methods

Design

An interpretive phenomenological research approach, as outlined by van Manen (1997), guided this study. Van Manen believed that lived experience was the starting and ending point of phenomenological research (van Manen, 1997). This approach was chosen as a way to gain a deeper understanding of the lived experience of individual participants. The personal experiences that were part of the public traumatic event may not have been known by others. This study was done to illuminate the experience of the listener and the storyteller when a traumatic event was shared within the dyad.

Setting and Sample

The context was the crash-landing of a plane, which was the traumatic event. On January 15, 2009, U.S. Airlines Flight 1549, bound for Charlotte, North Carolina, took off from a New York airport carrying 150 passengers and 5 crew members. The plane lost engine thrust shortly after takeoff when a flock of Canadian geese flew into the engines. It crash-landed in the Hudson River in New York City, and all those on board survived. The good news of this event, which the media dubbed *Miracle on the Hudson*, spread throughout the country. Despite its outwardly happy ending, the event would be considered traumatic for the individuals involved.

Data Collection

A purposive sample was obtained in that individuals were sampled in order to purposefully inform an understanding of the phenomenon under study (Creswell, 2007). As primary investigator (PI), I obtained institutional review board approval from my academic setting. I then sent an invitation to participate to potential participants. It was sent via e-mail to 20 potential storyteller participants by an individual who had contact with those involved in Flight 1549. The invitation contained an overall description of the study, including the purpose, and the PI's name, background, and contact information. The 12 storyteller participants who responded and agreed to be in the study then asked someone who had listened to them tell their story previously if he or she would be interested in participating in the study as the listener member of the storyteller–listener dyad. If the listener agreed, he or she responded via e-mail. Listeners were then sent the original e-mail invitation.

The purposive sample consisted of 24 participants forming 12 dyads, each with a storyteller and a listener. These spouse, friend, sibling, and parent dyads included 9 men and 15 women, with ages ranging from 29 to 74 years. Signed consent, including permission to be audiotaped, was obtained from all participants who were made aware that their participation was voluntary and that they had the right to stop participation or withdraw from the study at any time without penalty. Information regarding the availability of mental health counseling was also provided to participants.

In-depth interviews were done face to face with 21 participants; the remaining three interviews were conducted on the telephone because of participant availability. Each storyteller and each listener were asked to speak about what their experience was like when the traumatic event was shared within the dyad. Each storyteller was asked, "Tell me what it was like to tell your story to [name of listener]." Each listener was asked, "Tell me what it was like listening to [name of storyteller] tell you [his or her] story." The interviewer encouraged participants to share their experiences by asking nonleading questions such as "Tell me more about your experience" until participants felt they had no more to say on the topic. The interviews were audiotaped, assigned pseudonym titles, and downloaded individually to a secure server. Each audiotape was transcribed verbatim by a transcriptionist who had completed the Human Subjects Research in Social and Behavioral Sciences module as well as the Research Integrity module. Names were removed during transcription. After the transcription was completed, each transcript was reviewed for completeness and to ensure that all identifying information was removed.

Data Analysis

Data analysis was carried out according to the process described by van Manen (1997). The following steps were taken to achieve rigor; preconceived notions and beliefs were put aside about the phenomenon under study. A holistic reading was done of each transcript to get a sense of it as a whole and then read again to see what statements or phrases seemed to best represent the experience of the participants. During these readings, notes were made in the margins, using different color highlighters for what appeared to be different categories of statements. Each of the statements or phrases was listed in categories that seemed to be related. After repeatedly reviewing and dwelling with the data, five essential themes were identified, after determining that the phenomenon would lose its meaning without the inclusion of these themes.

As a way to further maintain rigor, the PI collaborated with two professional colleagues and expert qualitative researchers who reviewed transcripts and findings; each had more than 20 years of experience in qualitative research. A journal was kept to record additional observations and personal reflections. Findings were presented and clarified with participants to assess whether the transcripts were accurate and whether the identified themes resonated with them. According to Lincoln and Guba (1985), "The criterion for objectivity is intersubjective agreement; if multiple observers agree on a phenomenon, then their collective judgment can be said to be objective" (p. 292). Saturation, as described by Lincoln and Guba (1985), was achieved upon interviewing nine dyads, as there was no new or different information emerging; however, a total of 12 dyads were interviewed to confirm redundancy and maintain rigor. There was intersubjective agreement on themes between the PI, participants, and expert qualitative researchers. Five essential themes were supported in the form of narrative excerpts from participants.

Results

The five essential themes and the data to support them are discussed in the sections that follow.

Essential Theme 1: The Story Has a Purpose for the Listener and the Storyteller

Purposes identified included sharing the facts and the special story, giving inspiration, and providing a benefit to the storyteller and the listener. Personal experience often differed from public media presentation. One storyteller noted, "I guess there's almost this compulsion to set the record straight and say, 'It's still a wonderful story, and we are so fortunate, and it could have been so much worse, but let me tell you, it wasn't as easy as you think.'"

Storytellers wanted to inspire: "I've seen the really, really strong inspirational impact it had on certain people. That's the kind of impact I want to have when I tell it because that's the most rewarding for me." In turn, many listeners described experiencing a feeling of awe while listening. Storytellers and listeners spoke of feeling that the story was special. A listener smiled and whispered, "I love the story." A storyteller described the story, "It's a little bit, maybe, too big of a word—sacred—but just special, very special." Many felt that an incomplete version was disrespectful. One storyteller felt that "the worst thing that can happen when you are telling somebody about something like this, it's either dismissiveness or indifference."

It was revealed repeatedly that the storytellers did not mind telling their story and felt that telling was helpful to them. One storyteller said, "I could probably go on a ramble about it as long as anybody would listen." She went on to say, "It was very therapeutic, saying it over and over; it helped me remember things." Another storyteller explained, "Talking about it was actually a way for me to release, not to keep it in, because I think I know myself enough: I keep it in, and it will just burn a hole." In some dyads, the listeners had the impression that the storyteller preferred to avoid telling the story. A listener shared her belief, "I know she did not want to tell it all the time." Another commented, "I did not have a sense that he needed to share or get support." These statements revealed that listeners sometimes had a different perception of the storyteller's desire to tell the story and were unaware of the benefit of doing so.

Another benefit of telling the story was reflected in the fact that, as time went on, listeners and storytellers noticed that the more they shared, the easier it got. They felt less emotionally and physically reactive. A storyteller explained, "Over time, I feel less bad about it. The trauma of the actual event has subsided some." A listener found that her responses had changed as well: "You know, I still get the chills on occasion, but it's not as emotional as it was for the first few months." A storyteller explained, "Going through it over and over and over again, it got easier and easier. I don't think I could have healed without—and I really feel that I healed from it." All participants spoke about learning and gaining a sense of understanding as they shared. A listener recalled, "Each time we'd share, we'd learn a little something." A storyteller recalled that, "Telling it, it helped me process it to a certain extent."

Essential Theme 2: The Story That Is Known as a Whole May Continue to Change as Different Parts of It Are Revealed

Participants talked about how the story was remembered, told, and listened to in bits and pieces—that there was a "worst part" to the story and that the story evolved as information was gathered. All participants were drawn to fill in the holes of the story or elaborate on specific parts. A storyteller explained, "So in the beginning, it was probably a lot of—I was probably—definitely more scattered. So I maybe couldn't have told it in a linear fashion." She remembered things as she shared: "So it was a progression to where my story is today, and I—it may change; I don't know that it's complete. I suspect there will be continued learnings, there will be the evolution." Listeners also were aware of the evolution of the story: "Listening in those respects over the next 4 or 5 months when bits and pieces would come in, it would be more of an unveiling of something." The listener and the storyteller often collaborated to piece the story together, accepting what they knew in the present moment to be the story while being open to the possibility of change in the future.

Even though parts of the story changed as information was gathered, the part of the story that was identified as the worst part never changed. A listener revealed the worst part for her: "He thought he was going to die. But the most painful was the next day, when I got to process it more." There is no way to know what the worst part was for each individual without asking them. A storyteller recounted what was the worst part for him: "We're going down, and he's already told us to brace for impact, and I start thinking about what I was thinking then…. That would get me choked up every time."

Essential Theme 3: The Story Is Often Experienced Physically, Mentally, Emotionally, and Spiritually

Both members of the dyad were aware of physical manifestations of emotion reflected in the body, the face, and the eyes of the other as the story was shared. Simultaneous listener–storyteller nonverbal communication added to the collaborative nature of the experience within the dyad. The observation, perception, and interpretation of these nonverbal cues affected the creation, cessation, and modification of dialogue as well as the images, emotions, and physical sensations experienced. For example, the responses of the listener often validated the storyteller: "Just to see the reaction on other people's faces makes you realize exactly how traumatic the experience was." This storyteller described her awareness of the listener as she spoke: "I do notice if I feel like they're actually interested in listening to what I'm saying or not. I notice it in people's faces." She found herself responding to these nonverbal cues: "I'm very big on mannerisms and stuff like that. If I felt like they were losing interest, then I probably would just quit talking about it."

Participants also had physical reactions to the experience. One listener remembered "that nonstop crying and the throwing up." A storyteller noted, "I can get varying degrees of physical response, tightening, tensing up, or I found myself fidgeting and stuff like that; the heart rate starts to go up a little bit." The listener in this dyad remembered she would "get goose bumps at a certain point when he would talk about it."

Listeners and storytellers experienced the story mentally through images. This occurred spontaneously at times, and at other times, the participant actively tried to picture things. In one dyad, the storyteller recalled, "So when I started telling about it was—it was the pictures playing over and over in my head." In the same dyad, the listener revealed, "I could almost tell you what she looked like; I could picture her there." Another listener talked about "seeing" the storyteller's experience as she escaped the cabin of the plane. "You know, getting out on that wing, I almost—it's almost like, you know, I can almost—I can see the light." He imagined being there: "I'll be thinking about it, and maybe listening to her, and at the same time maybe trying to imagine what it's like being right alongside of her." Participants often described a sense of derealization as they shared the story of the traumatic event. A storyteller felt as though he was "dreaming." A listener recalled thinking, "This is surreal."

While telling or listening, participants experienced the story emotionally. A storyteller elaborated: "When I talk about it and remind her how much she means, it definitely gets her emotional, I know it does. And I, in turn, get emotional." The listener in this dyad was clear about the emotional impact that listening had on her: "I was, like, traumatized by this, you know, by listening to it." She called her experience an "emotional roller coaster." Both listeners and storytellers reported feeling as though they were reliving the experience as it was shared. A storyteller recalled, "When I'm going through the narrative, it's like in a lesser degree as time has gone on—but it's kind of happening again, and instead of just talking about the emotional part, it's more like you're feeling the emotional part." A listener felt that things came alive as she listened: "And so as he speaks, and I'm listening, then I am, if you will, reprocessing. I'm reliving, I'm recounting. I'm—it's real."

Participants also had spiritual experiences. As one listener put it, "God was providing me a moment by moment peace" as the storyteller shared bits of what had happened early on. Another listener felt a presence. She had a "feeling wash over her" and felt as if "someone was trying to comfort me—like maybe it was the Holy Ghost."

Essential Theme 4: Imagining the "What" as Well as the "What If" Is Done by Both Listener and Storyteller

Many participants found themselves imagining what happened as well as what could have happened. When a storyteller imagined the what if, he thought about "the things I was going to miss out on, I wouldn't—all those missed-out-on things that haven't happened yet. And every time I'd think about that, and how lucky I am to do some of those things, I just get choked up." One storyteller imagined what it would be like to lose his wife, the listener, and, at the same time, what it would have been like for her to lose him: "I always try to reflect in other people's shoes, and if I lost my wife, it would be devastating. It would have been very painful for her [to lose me]. Still painful for her [to contemplate], I'm sure, but it didn't work out that way."

Many listeners imagined what had happened and what it was like for the storytellers by putting themselves in their shoes. A listener revealed, "Every time she was telling it, I would think—I would picture myself in her situation. I see me doing it. I wasn't listening as much as I was picturing myself in it." One listener imagined two aspects of walking in the other's shoes. First, she imagined how the storyteller had experienced the event: "It was amazing to listen and then try to put myself in his shoes to really try and comprehend the thought processes that he was describing." Second, she imagined experiencing the event herself: "Once I get a feel for things I step into a role, but I'm going to—so as he tells the story, then I try and put myself in his shoes, and how would I have reacted?"

Some participants, in contrast, felt that they could never imagine putting themselves in the shoes of the other: "There is no way you can understand; there's no way, even if you'd had a similar experience, that you can put yourself in their shoes." They may have understood the facts but have been unable to achieve a deeper understanding of the lived experience.

Essential Theme 5: The Nature of the Relationship Colors the Experience of the Listener and the Storyteller When a Traumatic Event Is Shared Within the Dyad

The listener, the context, the type of relationship, and the amount of time the dyad spent together affected the experience of sharing. A storyteller observed, "A lot of that storytelling has to do with the listener, too." He said that he "tells the story differently depending on who he is talking to." Sometimes storytellers altered the story to protect the listener. One storyteller told me, "I didn't want to burden her. I didn't want to—I just didn't want to upset *her*." The listener in this dyad explained, "She doesn't want me to really know how it really was…and she was worried about me." Other listeners felt that they had listened so often they knew the story by heart: "It's become very familiar, and I could almost, you know, recite at least parts of it."

Storytellers always made decisions about whom to share their story with: "It's almost like because it's such a personal and deep experience, you sort of don't want to waste it on people…. It's precious, like a piece of gold." They considered the reactions of listeners: "When somebody acknowledges your feelings—and not just acknowledges; somebody says, 'Oh, this must have been this and that'—it makes you more willing to discuss your feelings that maybe you were a little more reserved about before."

That some listeners felt they had had enough of listening and wanted to move on was evident in the study findings. A listener explained, "It's not so therapeutic for me to keep reliving that, I guess." Another listener described being "sick of hearing the story" and expressed a desire to "move on, some normalcy." As a way to cope, another listener revealed an attempt to actively try not to listen: "I just think I knew I'd heard it, and I didn't want to have to get it in my mind again." Another listener became "exhausted, definitely exhausted" after fully listening for a very long time. However, she was one of several listeners who said they would continue to listen if the storyteller needed them to: "I mean, I was there to support, as I still am, and that's just what you do." Adding, "I wouldn't have done anything differently."

> **Sharing stories of traumatic events is one way of responding and adapting to the stimulus of trauma.**

Continuing to listen for the sake of the other despite feeling as though they had had enough of listening may affect listeners as well as storytellers. Storytellers had some awareness of listener saturation and desire to move on. One storyteller believed that, after initially hearing the entire story, the listener had met her capacity for listening and had become saturated; he said, "She doesn't really want to hear it." Another storyteller worried about the effect on the listener: "I would not want to bore people…I don't want to wear somebody out with it."

All storytellers noted that when they were with other people who had shared the traumatic experience, they felt understood: "That's the best-case scenario because they really understand what's going on…because they understand what I went through." One storyteller added, "Unless you've lived it, there's no comparison."

Integrated Essential Essence

The meaning of phenomenological description lies in its interpretation, its aim to transform lived experience by breathing meaning into a textual expression of its essence (van Manen, 1997). A textual interpretative statement was formulated from essential themes as a summary of the experience. An integrated essential essence was created to capture the essence of the experience of the listener and the storyteller when a traumatic event is shared within the dyad. The Integrated Essential Essence is as follows. The traumatic event is lived by an individual who, in an attempt to understand his or her own experience and to eventually have it understood by another, forms a story about the event and his or her experience and shares it with a listener, forming a unique dyad. Seeking physical, psychic, and spiritual integrity, the listener and the storyteller collaborate, sharing the story of the traumatic event and the experience in a complex, nonlinear multifaceted way, continuously adapting while attempting to create a sense of meaning through the experience.

Discussion

Implications for Nursing

For nurses, inviting an individual to share his or her experience of a traumatic event is a way to say, "I see *you*; come, share your story with me, and I will listen." Initial assessments are not complete without this invitation. This study revealed a collaborative, adaptive process between listener and storyteller, consistent with Roy's Adaptation Model. It was revealed that the listener and the storyteller acted as interdependent parts, collaborating as they shared the story of the traumatic event within the dyad. Participant's individual patterns of adaptation and individual attempts at coping were illuminated, providing a deeper understanding of the lived experiences of these individuals.

Sharing stories of traumatic events is one way of responding and adapting to the stimulus of trauma. In this study, the results showed that despite feeling as though they had had enough of listening and wanted to move on, some listeners adapted by continuing to try to listen. Nurses may do the same. Just as some athletes develop stress injuries, some nurses who listen repeatedly to stories of traumatic events may develop stress injuries. This pattern may carry a risk for both nurse and patient. Nurses may continue to listen for the sake of their patients; however, they may experience compassion fatigue and, as a result, may tire, withdraw, and lose interest. Patients may sense this and adapt by altering their trauma story or by not sharing it at all. Focusing more intensively on listening within nursing curricula may be of value. Preventing stress injury, exploring ways to promoting resilience, and illuminating ways for nurses to be with patients so they are able to share their stories of traumatic events are of value to nursing.

Implications for Future Research
Nursing education includes the topic of therapeutic communication. However, few studies have explored how the patient experiences the nurse during this communication and what it is like for nurses to be fully present while listening. Further dyadic studies exploring the experience of sharing a traumatic event within the nurse–patient dyad may reveal patterns related to listening, being heard, presencing, resilience, and burnout or compassion fatigue.

Future studies exploring the experience of sharing a traumatic event in specific relationship dyads may reveal different patterns. For example, veterans are returning from war having experienced traumatic events. Exploring what it is like for these individuals and their significant others to share these events may add to the understanding of their experience.

Also highlighted in the results of this study was the sense of understanding that often exists among individuals who have shared similar experiences. Nurses who have experienced traumatic events and work-related stress injuries may benefit from sharing these with other nurses who have had similar experiences. This sense of mutual understanding may be a protective factor in recovery from work-related stress, burnout, and compassion fatigue.

Strengths and Limitations
A strength of this dyadic study was that it enabled the perspective of both listener and the storyteller to be illuminated. The findings may be of value to the nurse–patient dyad, because the nurse is often the listener to the patient storyteller when a traumatic event is shared. The fact that three participants were interviewed on the telephone may have changed what was shared; however, there did not seem to be any differences in the findings among these participants. A potential bias is that the PI's brother was a passenger on the plane. He was not a participant in the study.

Conclusions
This study illuminates the experience of the listener and the storyteller when a traumatic event is shared within the dyad. In this study, it was revealed that, when the traumatic event is shared, the story includes more than factual events; it is accompanied by feelings and images. The story evolved as it was remembered, told, and listened to in a nonlinear, multifaceted way. When the traumatic event is shared within the dyad, the listener and the storyteller collaborate, adapt, and respond physically, mentally, emotionally, and spiritually. ▼

Accepted for publication August 15, 2011.
The author thanks her brother (a passenger on Flight 1549) for his assistance in providing access to potential participants. The author also thanks the participants for generously sharing their experiences.
The author has no funding or conflicts of interest to disclose.
Corresponding author: Jeanne Cummings, DNS, RN, NP, CS, BC, The Graduate Center, City University of New York, Doctor of Nursing Science Program, 365 Fifth Avenue, New York, NY 10016-4309 (e-mail: JCummings225@gmail.com).

References
Baird, K., & Kracen, C. (2006). Vicarious traumatization and secondary traumatic stress: A research synthesis. *Counselling Psychology Quarterly, 19*, 181–188. doi: 10.1080/09515070600811899.
Barrett, C., Brothwick, A., Bugeja, S., Parker, A., Vis, R., & Hurworth, R. (2005). Emotional labour: Listening to the patient's story. *Practice Development in Health Care, 4*, 213–223. doi: 10.1002/pdh.17.
BenEzer, G. (2009). Trauma signals in life stories. In K. L. Rogers, S. Leydesdorff, & G. Dawson (Eds.). *Life stories of survivors of trauma* (pp. 29–44). New Brunswick, NJ: Transaction Publishers.
Bunkers, S. S. (2010). The power and possibility in listening. *Nursing Science Quarterly, 23*, 22–27. doi: 10.1117/0894318409353805.
Canfield, J. (2005). Secondary traumatization, burnout, and vicarious traumatization: A review of the literature as it relates to therapists who treat trauma. *Smith College Studies in Social Work, 75*, 81–101. doi: 10.1300/j497v75n02_06.
Courtois, C. A. (2002). Traumatic stress studies: The need for curricula inclusion. *Journal of Trauma Practice, 1*, 33–57. doi: 10.1300/J189v01n01_03.
Courtois, C. A., & Gold, S. (2009). The need for inclusion of psychological trauma in the professional curriculum: A call to action. *Psychological Trauma: Theory, Research, Practice, and Policy, 1*, 3–23. doi: 10.1037a0015224.
Cresswell, J. (2007). *Qualitative inquiry & research design, choosing among five approaches*. Lincoln, NE: Sage.
Esposito, N. (2005). Manifestations of enduring during interviews with sexual assault victims. *Qualitative Health Research, 15*, 912–927. doi: 10.117/1049732305279056.
Frank, A. W. (2000). The standpoint of the storyteller. *Qualitative Health Research, 10*, 354–365. doi: 10.1177/104973200129118499.
Guay, S., Billette, V., & Marchand, A. (2006). Exploring the links between posttraumatic stress disorder and social support: Processes and potential research avenues. *Journal of Traumatic Stress, 19*, 327–338. doi: 10.1002/jts.20124.
Herman, J. (1992). *Trauma and recovery*. New York, NY: Basic Books.
Kagan, P. N. (2008). Listening: Selected perspectives in theory and research. *Nursing Science Quarterly, 21*, 105–110. doi: 10.1177/0894318408315027.
Kessler, R. C., Sonnega, A., Bromet, E., Hughes, M., & Nelson, C. (1995). Posttraumatic stress disorder in the national comorbidity study. *Archives of General Psychiatry, 52*, 1048–1060.
Leibowitz, R. Q., Jeffreys, M. D., Copeland, L. A., & Noel, P. H. (2008). Veterans' disclosure of trauma to healthcare providers. *General Hospital Psychiatry, 30*, 100–103. doi: 10.1016/j.genhosppsych.2007.11.004.
Leydesdorff, S., Dawson, G., Burchardt, N., & Ashplant, T. G. (2009). Trauma and life stories. In K. L. Rogers, S. Leydesdorff, &

G. Dawson (Eds.), *Life stories of survivors of trauma* (pp. 1–26). New Brunswick, NJ: Transaction Publishers.

Lincoln, Y., & Guba, E. (1985). *Naturalistic inquiry*. Newbury Park, CA: Sage.

Moreland, R. (2010). Are dyads really groups? *Small Group Research, 41,* 251–267. doi: 10.1177/1046496409358618.

Parrish, E., Peden, A., & Staten, R. (2008). Strategies used by advanced practice psychiatric nurses in treating adults with depression. *Perspectives in Psychiatric Care, 44,* 232–240. doi: 10.1111/j.1744-6163.2008.00182.x.

Pasupathi, M., & Rich, B. (2005). Inattentive listening undermines self verification in personal storytelling. *Journal of Personality, 73,* 1051–1086. doi: 10.1111/j.1467-6494.2005.00338.x.

Perrett, S. E. (2007). Review of Roy Adaption Model-based qualitative research. *Nursing Science Quarterly, 20,* 349–356. doi: 10.1177/0894318407306538.

Raingruber, B., & Kent, M. (2003). Attending to embodied responses: A way to identify practice-based and human meanings associated with secondary trauma. *Qualitative Health Research, 13,* 449–468. doi: 10.1177/1049732302250722.

Rosenthal, G. (2003). The healing effects of storytelling on the conditions of curative storytelling in the context of research and counseling. *Qualitative Inquiry, 9,* 915–933. doi: 10.1177/1077800403254888.

Roy, C. Sr. (1988). An explication of the philosophical assumptions of the Roy Adaptation Model. *Nursing Science Quarterly, 1,* 26–34. doi: 10.1177/089431848800100108.

Shortt, J., & Pennebaker, J. (1992). Talking versus hearing about Holocaust experiences. *Basic and Applied Psychology, 13,* 165–179. doi: 10.1207/s15324834basp1302_2.

Showalter, S. (2010). Compassion fatigue: What is it? Why does it matter? Recognizing the symptoms, acknowledging the impact, developing the tools to prevent compassion fatigue and strengthen the professional already suffering from the effects. *American Journal of Hospice and Palliative Medicine, 27*(4), 239–242. doi: 10.1177/1049909109354096.

Symonds, M. (1980). The second injury to victims. *Evaluation and Change, 4,* 36–38.

Ullman, S. E. (2007). Relationship to perpetrator, disclosure, social reactions, and PTSD symptoms in child sexual abuse survivors. *Journal of Child Sexual Abuse, 16,* 19–36. doi: 10.1300/j070v16n01-02.

Vajda, J. (2007). Two survivor cases: Therapeutic effect as side product of the biographical narrative interview. *Journal of Social Work Practice, 21,* 89–102. doi: 10.1080/02650530601173664.

van Manen, M. (1997). *Researching lived experience* (2nd ed.). Winnipeg, Manitoba, Canada: Althouse Press.

Webster's dictionary. (4th ed.). (2001). New York, NY: Ballentine Books.

Journal of Cardiovascular Nursing
Vol. 00, No. 0, pp 00–00 | Copyright © 2011 Wolters Kluwer Health | Lippincott Williams & Wilkins

Effect of Culturally Tailored Diabetes Education in Ethnic Minorities With Type 2 Diabetes
A Meta-analysis

Soohyun Nam, PhD, RN, NP; Susan L. Janson, DNSc, RN, FAAN; Nancy A. Stotts, EdD, RN, FAAN; Catherine Chesla, DNSc, RN, FAAN; Lisa Kroon, PharmD, CDE

Background: Diabetes is a major cause of cardiovascular morbidity and mortality. Ethnic minorities experience a disproportionate burden of diabetes; however, few studies have critically analyzed the effectiveness of a culturally tailored diabetes intervention for these minorities. **Objective:** The aim of this study was to evaluate the effectiveness of a culturally tailored diabetes educational intervention (CTDEI) on glycemic control in ethnic minorities with type 2 diabetes. **Method:** We searched databases within PubMed, Cumulative Index to Nursing and Allied Health Literature (CINAHL), Education Resources Information Center (ERIC), PsycINFO, and ProQuest for randomized controlled trials (RCTs). We performed a meta-analysis for the effect of diabetes educational intervention on glycemic control using glycosylated hemoglobin (HbA_{1c}) value in ethnic minority groups with type 2 diabetes. We calculated the effect size (ES) with HbA_{1c} change from baseline to follow-up between control and treatment groups. **Results:** The 12 studies yielded 1495 participants with a mean age of 63.6 years and a mean of 68% female participants. Most studies (84%) used either group education sessions or a combination of group sessions and individual patient counseling. The duration of interventions ranged from 1 session to 12 months. The pooled ES of glycemic control in RCTs with CTDEI was −0.29 (95% confidence interval, −0.46 to −0.13) at last follow-up, indicating that ethnic minorities benefit more from CTDEI when compared with the usual care. The effect of intervention was greatest and significant when HbA_{1c} level was measured at 6 months (ES, −0.41; 95% confidence interval, −0.61 to −0.21). The ES also differed by each participant's baseline HbA_{1c} level, with lower baseline levels associated with higher ESs. **Conclusions:** Based on this meta-analysis, CTDEI is effective for improving glycemic control among ethnic minorities. The magnitude of effect varies based on the settings of intervention, baseline HbA_{1c} level, and time of HbA_{1c} measurement. More rigorous RCTs that examine tailored diabetes education, ethnically matched educators, and more diverse ethnic minority groups are needed to reduce health disparities in diabetes care.

KEY WORDS: culturally tailored intervention, diabetes mellitus, ethnic minority, meta-analysis, type 2

Diabetes is a major cause of cardiovascular morbidity and mortality in the United States. The prevalence rates of diabetes have continued to increase for the past decade, with racial/ethnic minority populations having disproportionate burden of disease.[1] The Centers for Disease Control and Prevention reported

Soohyun Nam, PhD, RN, NP
Postdoctoral Fellow, School of Nursing, Department of Health Systems and Outcomes, Johns Hopkins University, Baltimore, Maryland.

Susan L. Janson, DNSc, RN, FAAN
Professor, Department of Community Health, School of Nursing, University of California, San Francisco.

Nancy A. Stotts, EdD, RN, FAAN
Professor, Department of Physiological Nursing, School of Nursing, University of California, San Francisco.

Catherine Chesla, DNSc, RN, FAAN
Professor, Department of Family Health Care Nursing, School of Nursing, University of California, San Francisco.

Lisa Kroon, PharmD, CDE
Professor, Department of Clinical Pharmacy, School of Pharmacy, University of California, San Francisco.

Support for this study was received from the California Endowment and American Association of Colleges of Nursing, University of California, San Francisco–Graduate Student Research Award, and the Sigma Theta Tau National Honor Society of Nursing, Alpha Eta Chapter. Editorial support provided by the Johns Hopkins University School of Nursing Center for Collaborative Intervention Research. Funding for the Center is provided by the National Institute of Nursing Research (P30 NRO 8995).

The content is solely the responsibility of the authors and does not necessarily represent the official views of the National Institute of Nursing Research or the National Institutes of Health.

Correspondence
Soohyun Nam, PhD, RN, NP, The Johns Hopkins University School of Nursing, 525 North Wolfe St, Baltimore, MD 21205-2110 (soohnam@gmail.com).

DOI: 10.1097/JCN.0b013e31822375a5

183

that the prevalence rate of diabetes is 8.7% among non-Hispanic whites, 9.5% among Hispanics, and 13.3% among African Americans.[2] In addition, African Americans, Hispanic/Latino Americans, American Indians, and some Asian Americans and Native Hawaiians or other Pacific Islanders are at particularly high risk for type 2 diabetes and its complications. African Americans have 2 to 4 times the rate of renal disease, blindness, amputations, and amputation-related mortality of that of non-Hispanic whites.[3,4] Similarly, Latinos have higher rates of renal disease and retinopathy.[3,4] Although the reasons for the disparities in diabetes prevalence and health outcomes are multifactorial—genetic, environmental, and cultural[5–7]—there is little evidence that ethnic minority groups benefit from traditional diabetes educational programs. The likely reason for this lack of evidence is that ethnic minorities are often not included as a subgroup in most large trials and the attrition rate of the ethnic minorities is higher than for non-Hispanic whites. Data from the Third National Health and Nutrition Examination Survey indicate that glycemic control is poorer for ethnic minority groups compared with whites and show that participation rates of ethnic minorities in educational programs are low and attrition is high.[8,9]

Possible barriers to participation in diabetes education may be language, socioeconomic factors, cultural/lifestyle factors, and health beliefs. Furthermore, some studies show that traditional risk reduction approaches have not been effective for certain ethnic groups. Less success has frequently been reported with dietary self-management, lifestyle change, weight loss, and adherence to treatment regimens among African Americans compared with whites.[10–12] Therefore, ethnic minority groups have often been labeled "noncompliant" and have worse health outcomes than do individuals of other cultures.[13,14] The failure of traditional educational approaches for ethnic minorities may be due to a lack of cultural competency on the part of providers and failure to address issues of relevance to the population.[10]

In an effort to reduce significant health care disparities and improve access to care for various ethnic and racial groups, designing and evaluating culturally tailored interventions have become an important priority of the public health system. For our meta-analysis, culturally tailored diabetes interventions refer to incorporating the following factors into the interventions: cultural beliefs, family participation, values, customs, food patterns, language, low literacy, culturally specific educational materials, and health practices.

Previous meta-analyses have demonstrated the effect of various educational interventions on glycemic control, quality of life, and other psychosocial factors[15–17]; however, these studies have not focused specifically on ethnic minorities with type 2 diabetes, nor have cul-

turally tailored interventions been addressed. Identifying an effective diabetes educational strategy for ethnic minorities is crucial for reducing the health disparity gap. Therefore, the purpose of this meta-analysis was to bridge this gap by evaluating the effect of culturally tailored diabetes education (CTDE) on glycemic control in ethnic minorities with type 2 diabetes.

Method

Search Process and Selection of Studies

We searched PubMed, CINAHL, ERIC, and PsycINFO for published studies and ProQuest database for dissertations and theses using the following key words: *type 2 diabetes, diabetes mellitus, health education, diabetes education, counseling, minority, ethnic minority, race,* and *behavioral intervention.* The following medical subject heading terms were also used in the search: *patient education, diabetes mellitus, type 2, non-insulin-dependent, minority group, ethnic group, intervention,* and *program.* We limited our search to English-language, both published and unpublished studies between 1980 and 2009. We also used the Cochrane Collaboration database, a manual review of *Diabetes Care* and *Diabetes Educator* (1990–2009), previous meta-analyses, and review articles as sources for identifying articles.

Randomized controlled trials (RCTs) that had diabetes educational interventions (no drug intervention) performed only in ethnic minority groups with type 2 diabetes and that reported both preintervention and postintervention glycosylated hemoglobin (HbA_{1c}) values were included. Quasi-experimental studies (ie, studies with lack of comparison group) were excluded.

Quality Assessment

Study quality was assessed using 4 items from relevant literature.[18,19] This method assigns 1 point for each ordered criterion: descriptions of appropriate randomization procedures, information about the number of withdrawals/dropouts and reasons, description of culturally tailored interventions, and description of inclusion and exclusion criteria. The highest possible study score was 8; each item had a possible score of 0 to 2 (0 = absent, 1 = partially described, 2 = clearly described). For purposes of this analysis, studies with scores of 0 to 5 were considered to be low quality and those with scores of 6 to 8 were considered to be high quality.

Data Extraction and Calculation of Effect Size

To compare studies, we used a data collection sheet and described the year of publication, study design, study sample, setting, type of intervention, type of intervention provider (eg, nurse, dietitian, certified diabetes educator, other professionals), country, intensity/duration of intervention, and time to outcome measure (months).

To generate a summary estimate, we conducted a meta-analysis on the results comparing intervention to control groups. The effect size (ES), defined as the difference in the change of a measurement from baseline to follow-up between control and treatment groups, was calculated for HbA_{1c}.

Analysis

We performed a meta-analysis for the effect of diabetes educational intervention on glycemic control only in ethnic minority groups with type 2 diabetes, using HbA_{1c} level as the outcome measure. We used a random effects model to calculate pooled weighted mean differences with 95% confidence intervals (CIs). The random effects model assumes that each study is estimating different effects, which varies according to different methods, outcomes, and participants studied.[20]

Although the main aim of a meta-analysis is to produce an estimate of the average effect seen in trials comparing therapeutic strategies, we cannot assume that the effect of a given treatment is identical across different groups of patients. Therefore, we planned 3 specific subgroup analyses a priori based on key design issues and conducted the analysis. The first subgroup analysis was conducted by baseline HbA_{1c} level; the second, by intervention setting; and the third, by intervention duration (ie, 3, 6, and 12 months). Sensitivity analyses were performed to determine whether the results varied by potentially influential studies (ie, extreme ES, large sample size). The sensitivity analysis was also conducted to compare high- and low-quality studies with the overall ES.

The test for heterogeneity assesses the degree of variability in the summary measures among the included studies. Statistically significant heterogeneity means that the results of the studies are not consistent. The presence of heterogeneity often indicates that there are methodological differences in the mechanism of randomization, patient sample, interventions, length of follow-up, and the extent of withdrawals between included studies.[21] Heterogeneity should not necessarily always be viewed as a negative aspect of a systematic review. It may simply alert the investigators to different aspects of the intervention or study designs that have the potential to affect the results.[22]

The method for identifying heterogeneity in the studies was planned through (1) observation of the forest plot to examine how well the CIs overlay; (2) performance of χ^2 test with a P value of >0.1, and (3) by quantifying the effect of heterogeneity using I^2, where I^2 values of 25%, 50%, and 75% represent low,

moderate, and high levels of heterogeneity, respectively.[23] A small P value ($P < .1$) from the χ^2 test was used to indicate evidence of heterogeneity. When heterogeneity was visually or statistically present, we explored the source of heterogeneity using subgroup and sensitivity analysis. We also used a random effects model when heterogeneity was present; this approach provides a more conservative estimate of the pooled estimate and CIs.

We explored publication bias using a funnel plot, in which symmetry about the line of no effect suggests little influence of publication bias.[24] We also used an adjusted rank correlation model proposed by Begg and Mazumdar[25] and Egger's linear regression model.[26] We used StataSE version 10 for this meta-analysis.

Results

Extensive searching identified 12 RCTs for inclusion.[27–38] Papers were commonly excluded because the study lacked an intervention, HbA_{1c} levels, or ethnicity-specific data. Studies with quasi-experimental "before and after" designs (no comparison group) were also excluded. Studies that included type 1 diabetes or gestational diabetes or that did not report the results by type of diabetes or ethnicity were excluded (Figure 1). Unpublished studies were sought by using ProQuest and Clinical Trial registries, but none of them was eligible for the review because of study design (lack of intervention and comparison group), population of interest (no ethnic specific data), or no HbA_{1c} results.

Participant Demographics Across Studies

A total of 1,495 participants were included in the 12 studies, with a mean age of 63.6 years and a mean of 68% female participants. Among the 12 studies, 4 studies included African Americans, 3 studies included Hispanic Americans, 4 studies included Asians, and 1 study included others (eg, Canadian-Portuguese). The mean baseline HbA_{1c} level was 8.6% (SD, 1.4%; median, 8.5%).

Study Characteristics

The characteristics of the 12 studies are described in Table 1. Eight (67%) studies were conducted within the United States. The mean sample size of the 12 studies was 124 (SD, 100; median, 88).

Intervention and Intervention Provider

Most studies (84%) used either group education sessions or a combination of group sessions and individual patient counseling; 16% of the studies used only individual sessions as a mode of instruction. Fifty percent of studies reported usual care as the control group

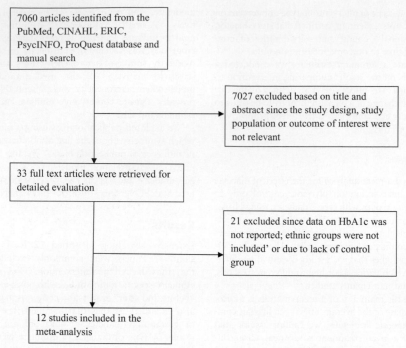

FIGURE 1. *Flowchart of selection of studies for inclusion in the meta-analysis. Abbreviation: HbA$_{1c}$, glycosylated hemoglobin.*

condition; the other 50% reported some type of minimal intervention as the control. The following intervention providers were reported: nurses (36%), dieticians (36%), certified diabetes educators (5%), other professionals (eg, pharmacists, physiotherapists, psychologists, and social workers: 9%), and nonprofessional staff (14%).

Duration, Frequency, and Settings

The duration of intervention ranged from 1 session to 12 months (median, 3 months), with a frequency of 1 session to 25 weekly or biweekly sessions. Three studies provided the diabetes educational intervention for 1 month or less; 8 studies provided the educational intervention for 1 to 3 months; and 1 study provided the educational intervention for 12 months. The number of contact hours of the intervention ranged from 1 session to more than 30 hours, but most studies did not describe the number of contact hours in 1 session in the intervention and control groups. Therefore, it was difficult to analyze the relationship between the effect of the intervention and the intensity/dose of the intervention. The settings of interventions were hospital-based outpatient clinics or hospital diabetes education centers (58%) and community-based settings (42%).

Educational Interventions

All studies included interventions focused on CTDE. To ensure the cultural appropriateness of the intervention, bilingual/bicultural professional educators or nonprofessional workers provided the education. The components of culturally tailored intervention included the following: teaching/counseling about dietary change by modifying ethnic foods and recipes; teaching/counseling of activity change using culturally appropriate activities (eg, dancing and walking); delivery of intervention in the preferred language, including all materials (ie, non-English materials); attendance by family member to elicit home-based support; and use of visual aids to tailor to low-literacy needs.

The main subject of most interventions was diabetes knowledge (eg, symptoms of hypoglycemia/hyperglycemia, complications of diabetes, and medications) and diabetes self-management including diet, physical activity, and blood glucose monitoring. Other topics included psychosocial strategies (eg, coping skill, stress management, problem solving) and risk management of cardiovascular diseases. Approximately two-thirds of the studies encouraged patients to bring support persons (family or friends) to the educational sessions to foster family participation in managing diabetes.

TABLE 1   Overview of Reviewed Studies

Anderson et al, 2005 (n = 239)	Aims	To evaluate the impact of a problem-based empowerment patient education program specially tailored for urban African Americans with type 2 diabetes
	Country	United States
	Methods	RCT
	Participants	96% African American with type 2 diabetes in urban area in Detroit
		Inclusion criteria: not stated
		Exclusion criteria: not stated
	Intervention	Intervention: 2-h weekly group sessions for 6 wk
		Control group: wait-listed
		Setting: convenient community-based location
		Duration of intervention: 6 wk
		Duration of follow-up: 6 wk as RCT; thereafter, non-RCT at 12 wk, 6 mo, and 1 y
		Provider: certified diabetes educator
	Outcome	HbA$_{1c}$, lipid, BP, weight, DCP questionnaire, DES-SF, subscale of the Diabetes Attitude scales
	Quality	4
Anderson-Loftin et al, 2005 (n = 97)	Aims	To test the effects of a culturally competent, dietary self-management intervention on physiological outcomes and dietary behaviors for African Americans with type 2 diabetes
	Country	United States
	Methods	RCT
	Participants	Inclusion criteria
		1. African American
		2. Medical diagnosis of type 2 diabetes
		3. Aged ≥18 y
		4. At least 1 of the following indicators of diabetes complications defined as high risk and modifiable by diet: (a) HbA$_{1c}$ >8%, (b) cholesterol >200 mg/dL, (c) triglycerides >200 mg/dL, (d) LDL cholesterol >100 mg/dL, (e) BMI >25 kg/m^2, and (f) high-fat dietary patterns (score on the FHQ >2.5).
		Exclusion criteria: 1. Mental or physical limitations that would preclude participation in group activities and discussion
	Intervention	Intervention: 4 weekly classes in low-fat dietary strategies, 5 monthly peer-professional group discussions, and weekly telephone follow-up
		Control group: referral to a local 8-h traditional diabetes class
		Setting: diabetes education center in a rural South Carolina county
		Duration of intervention: 4 wk
		Duration of follow-up: 6 mo
		Provider: nurse case manager and registered dietician
	Outcome	HbA$_{1c}$, lipids, BMI, dietary behaviors, FHQ
	Quality	8
Agurs-Collins et al, 1997 (n = 64)	Aims	To evaluate a weight loss and exercise program designed to improve diabetes management in older African Americans
	Country	United States
	Methods	RCT
	Participants	African American
		Inclusion criteria
		1. Obese African American with type 2 diabetes
		2. ≥55 y of age
		3. ≥120% weight standard
		4. HbA$_{1c}$ >8%
		Exclusion criteria: contraindication for exercise
	Intervention	Intervention: weekly nutrition sessions (60 min) with exercise training (30 min) for 3 mo, then 3 mo on biweekly problem-solving (90 min) sessions and 1 individual diet counseling
		Control: 1 class on glycemic control at 3 wk from start; 2 letters with written information on nutrition at 3 and 6 mo
		Setting: urban hospital clinics
		Duration of intervention: 6 mo
		Duration of follow-up: at 3 and 6 mo
		Provider: dietician and exercise physiotherapist with experience in working with African Americans
	Outcome	HbA$_{1c}$, weight, BMI, waist-hip ratio, BP, lipid profile, physical activity, nutrition knowledge, dietary component, dietary components
	Quality	6

(continues)

TABLE 1	Overview of Reviewed Studies, continued

Brown et al, 2002 (n = 252)		
	Aims	To determine the effect of a culturally competent diabetes self-management intervention in Mexican Americans with type 2 diabetes
	Country	United States
	Methods	RCT
	Participants	256 Mexican Americans with type 2 diabetes
		Inclusion criteria
		1. Not having participated in a previous intervention
		2. 35–70 y of age
		3. Having type 2 diabetes from 35 y of age
		4. 2 verifiable FBG test results ≥140 mg/dL or taking or have taken insulin or oral hypoglycemic agents for ≥1 y in the past
		Exclusion criteria
		1. Pregnancy
		2. Medical conditions preventing changes in diet and exercise
	Intervention	Intervention: 2-h weekly group educational sessions for 3 mo, 6 mo biweekly support sessions, and thereafter 2-h monthly support groups sessions for 3 mo
		Control: 1-y wait-listed group. Usual care from their private physicians or at local clinics
		Setting: community- based sites (schools, churches, county agricultural extension offices, adult day care center, and health care clinics)
		Duration of intervention: 12 mo
		Duration of follow-up: 12 mo
		Provider: bilingual Mexican American dietician, nurse, and community health worker
	Outcome	HbA$_{1c}$, FBG, diabetes knowledge and diabetes-related health beliefs, BMI, lipids
	Quality	7
Gucciardi et al, 2007 (n = 61)	Aims	To examine the impact of 2 culturally competent diabetes education methods, individual counseling, and individual counseling in conjunction with group education on nutrition adherence and glycemic control
	Country	Canada
	Methods	RCT
	Participants	Canadian-Portuguese with type 2 diabetes in Toronto urban area in Canada
		Inclusion criteria
		1. Type 2 diabetes
		2. Speaking Portuguese
		Exclusion criteria
		1. Renal dialysis
		2. Prior attendance at a similar education program
		3. Diagnosis of mental illness
	Intervention	Intervention: individual counseling of 1 initial assessment and following appointment are scheduled on a need basis per person + group education classes (15 h) over 3 consecutive weekdays
		Control: Group education classes (15 h) over 3 consecutive weekdays
		Setting: hospital-based diabetes education center
		Duration of intervention: 3 group meetings of 6.5 h each and individual meetings scheduled on a need basis per participants. Duration of the period was not stated
		Duration of follow-up: 3 mo
		Provider: Portuguese-speaking dietician, nurse, pharmacist, and registered physiotherapist, psychologist and social worker
	Outcome	1. TPB scale—attitude, subjective norms, perceived behavior control, and intentions toward nutrition adherence
		2. Self-reported nutrition adherence (Summary of Diabetes Self-care Activities Questionnaire)
		3. HbA$_{1c}$
	Quality	8
Hawthorne et al, 1997 (n = 201)	Aims	To design and evaluate a structured pictorial teaching program for Pakistani Moslem patients in Manchester with type 2 diabetes
	Country	United Kingdom
	Methods	RCT
	Participants	British Pakistani with type 2 diabetes
		Inclusion criteria
		1. Pakistani origin with type 2 diabetes
		Exclusion criteria
		1. Previous diabetes education
		2. Spouse receiving or received diabetes education in the past
		3. Planning to go abroad
		4. Not in good health

	TABLE 1 **Overview of Reviewed Studies, continued**	
	Intervention	Intervention group: 1 session of one-to-one pictorial flash-card education (purpose of glucose monitoring, how to control blood sugar, diabetic complications, and the purpose of regular screening) with a trained link worker Control: not stated Setting: primary and secondary clinics Duration of intervention: 1 session Duration of follow-up: 6 mo Provider: trained link worker
	Outcome	Diabetes knowledge, attitudes and self- care behaviors assessed with questionnaire, HbA_{1c}, cholesterol level
	Quality	4
Kim et al, 2009 (n = 79)	Aims	To test the efficacy of culturally tailored diabetes intervention on HbA_{1c}, QoL, diabetes knowledge, self-efficacy, and self-care behaviors
	Country	United States
	Methods	RCT

	Participants	KAIs with type 2 diabetes
		Inclusion criteria
		  1. Self-identification as KAIs
		  2. Aged ≥30 y
		  3. Self-identification as having diabetes with an uncontrolled glucose level >7.5% within the past 6 mo
		  4. Resident of Baltimore-Washington
		Exclusion criteria: not stated

	Intervention	Intervention: 2-h weekly diabetes group education for 6 wk and monthly telephone counseling with a bilingual nurse for 24 wk Control: delayed intervention that joined the intervention group after 30 wk Setting: community-based location Duration of intervention: 30 wk Duration of follow-up: 30 wk for the RCT component Provider: bilingual Korean American nurses and dietician
	Outcome	HbA_{1c}, cholesterol, QoL, diabetes knowledge, self-efficacy, and self-care behaviors
	Quality	6
Middelkoop et al, 2001 (n = 113)	Aims	To examine if culturally specific diabetes intervention led to a decrease HbA_{1c} level, improvement in lipid profile, or a decrease in BMI
	Country	The Netherlands
	Methods	RCT

	Participants	South Asians in the Netherlands
		Inclusion criteria
		  1. South Asian origin
		  2. Type 2 diabetes
		Exclusion criteria: comorbidity (ie, recent myocardial infarction or dementia)

	Intervention	Intervention: approximately 4-7 intensive guidance visits for the first 3 mo, with less frequent subsequent visits Control: wait-list group that joined the intervention group after 6 mo Setting: general practices and outpatient clinic Duration of intervention: 6 mo Duration of follow-up: 6 mo for the RCT component Provider: specialist nurse and dietician trained in South Asian culture
	Outcome	HbA_{1c}
	Quality	4
O'Hare et al, 2004 (n = 325)	Aims	To test the hypothesis that enhanced diabetes care tailored to the needs of the South Asian community with type 2 diabetes would improve risk factor for diabetic vascular complications and ultimately reduce morbidity and mortality
	Country	United Kingdom
	Methods	RCT

	Participants	South Asians with type 2 diabetes
		Inclusion criteria
		  1. South Asian origin
		  2. Type 2 diabetes
		  3. At least 1 of the following risk factor: high BP, HbA_{1c} >7%, total cholesterol >5.0 mmol/L
		Exclusion criteria: not stated

(continues)

TABLE 1	Overview of Reviewed Studies, continued	
	Intervention	Intervention: extra weekly diabetes clinic at the primary care centers
		Control: usual care, no further resources were provided
		Setting: primary care center
		Duration of intervention: 1 y
		Duration of follow-up: 1 y
		Provider: diabetes nurse specialist, practice nurse, and dietician, all aided by a link worker
	Outcome	BP, HbA_{1c}, total cholesterol
	Quality	5
Rosal et al, 2005 (n = 25)	Aims	To assess the feasibility of a self-management education in low-income, Spanish-speaking individuals and, second, to have preliminary data of intervention effect
	Country	United States
	Methods	RCT
	Participants	Spanish-speaking individual with type 2 diabetes, >18 y of age
		Inclusion criteria
		1. Having a health care provider
		2. Having a physician-confirmed diagnosis of type 2 diabetes
		3. >18 y of age
		4. Doctor's approval to participate in the PA of the intervention
		5. Home telephone
		6. Able to provide informed consent in English or Spanish
		Exclusion criteria
		1. History of diabetes ketoacidosis
		2. Current gestational diabetes
		3. Planning to move out of the area during the study period
		4. Steroid use during the previous year
		5. Having had a cardiovascular event in the previous 6 mo
	Intervention	Intervention: 1 h of initial individual sessions, followed by 2–3 h of weekly group sessions for 10 wk and two 15-min individual sessions during the 10-wk period. Primary care physicians received copies of laboratory results at each assessment point
		Control: usual care and primary care physician received copies of laboratory results as intervention group did
		Setting: community room
		Duration of intervention: 10 wk
		Duration of follow-up: 6 mo
		Provider: bilingual nutritionist, diabetes nurse, and assistant
	Outcome	1. Feasibility (rate of attendance, recruitment, and assessment completion)
		2. HbA_{1c}
		3. Lipid profile
		4. BP
		5. Height
		6. Weight
		7. Hip-waist ratio
		8. Behavioral: 2 unannounced 24-h dietary recall, modified version of the Community Healthy Activities Model Program for Seniors PA questionnaire, 24-h SMBG recall
		9. Audit of diabetes knowledge
		10. Audit of diabetes-dependent QoL
		11. Insulin Management Self-efficacy Scale
		12. Center for Epidemiological Studies–Depression scale
	Quality	5
Skelly et al, 2005 (n = 39)	Aims	To test the effectiveness of an in-home, nurse-delivered symptom-focused teaching/counseling intervention with older rural African American women with type 2 diabetes
	Country	United States
	Methods	RCT
	Participants	Older African American women in rural in North Carolina
		Inclusion criteria
		1. Aged 50–85 y
		2. Women with type 2 diabetes
		3. No cognitive, affective, or functional dysfunction
		Exclusion criteria
		1. BDI-II score of 29
		2. Short Portable Mental Status Questionnaire, error 8-109 (depression or intellectual impairment)

TABLE 1	Overview of Reviewed Studies, continued

	Intervention	Intervention: individual biweekly visits to individual's home lasting <1 h, with 4 Diabetes Symptom–Focused Management intervention modules and 2 preintervention visits. Total time spent with participants was 6 h
		Control: received the 2 preintervention visits during which demographic data were collected and the study instruments were administered. Controls also received a telephone call at a midpoint between baseline and final evaluation details. Total time spent was 3 h and a telephone call
		Setting: community setting
		Duration of intervention: 12 wk
		Duration of follow-up: 12 wk
		Provider: nurse
	Outcome	Symptom distress and its effects on QoL, diabetes knowledge, HbA₁c, QoL, diabetes self-care practice, and patient satisfaction with the intervention as assessed using structured in-depth interviews
	Quality	5
Vincent et al, 2007 (n = 17)	Aims	To test the feasibility and examine the effects of a culturally tailored intervention for Mexican Americans with type 2 diabetes on outcomes of self-management
	Country	United States
	Methods	RCT
	Participants	Mexican Americans in Tucson, Arizona
		Inclusion criteria
		1. Self-identification as Mexican American
		2. 18–75 y of age
		3. Fluency in Spanish
		4. Ability to walk without assistance
		Exclusion criteria
		1. Pregnancy
		2. Medical condition (heart failure)
		3. Cognitive impairment
		4. Participated a diabetes self-management program within the previous 12 mo
	Intervention	Intervention: 2-h weekly group sessions for 8 wk
		Control: usual care consisted of a 10- to 15-min encounter with a physician or nurse practitioner 2 to 4 times per year
		Setting: community health clinic
		Duration of intervention: 8 wk
		Duration of follow-up : 12 wk
		Provider: not stated
	Outcome	Feasibility and acceptability (assessed by examining ease of recruitment and retention rate), BP, HbA₁c, blood glucose, weight, BMI, diabetes knowledge, self-efficacy, self-management activity
	Quality	6

Abbreviations: BDI-II, Beck Depression Inventory Short Form; BMI, body mass index; BP, blood pressure; DCP, Diabetes Care Profile; DES-SF, Diabetes Empowerment Scale Short Form; FBG, fasting blood glucose; FHQ, Food Habits Questionnaire; HbA₁c, glycosylated hemoglobin; KAIs, Korean American Immigrants; LDL, low-density lipoprotein; PA, physical activity; QoL, quality of life; RCT, randomized controlled trial; SMBG, Self-monitoring Blood Glucose; TPB, Theory of Planned Behavior.

Follow-up

The duration of follow-up ranged from 12 weeks to 1 year (mean [SD], 6.4 [3.2] months). Median follow-up duration for the reviewed studies was 6 months. Follow-up for conducting outcome assessments was made by telephone interviews or by home or clinic visits.

Outcomes

Results from this meta-analysis are reported for the primary outcome of HbA₁c as a reflection of glycemic control. The main results are reported as overall effects of CTDE on glycemic control compared with the control group. We reported the subgroups based on baseline HbA₁c levels, settings of intervention, and reported

time of HbA₁c measurement. All results are based on random effects models.

Effect sizes (mean difference) for HbA₁c are depicted in Table 2. Most interventions produced a decline in HbA₁c levels compared with controls. Because the main aim of our meta-analysis was to evaluate the effect of culturally tailored intervention on glycemic control among ethnic minorities, we analyzed RCTs with only culturally tailored interventions. The pooled ES of the 12 RCTs with culturally tailored intervention was −0.29 when measured at the last follow-up (Figure 2); the result was statistically significant (95% CI, −0.46 to −0.13). This indicates that the intervention was effective in improving HbA₁c among ethnic minorities with type 2 diabetes. We computed the ES

TABLE 2 Estimated Effect Size With 95% CIs			
Element	Category	No. of Studies	Effect Size (95% CI)
Overall		12	−0.29 (−0.46 to −0.13)
Settings of intervention	Clinic or hospital based	7	−0.26 (−0.44 to −0.09)
	Community based	5	−0.34 (−0.69 to 0.01)
Time of HbA$_{1c}$ measurement	3 mo	8	−0.21 (−0.47 to 0.05)
	6 mo	5	−0.41 (−0.61 to −0.21)
	12 mo	2	−0.14 (−0.39 to 0.11)
Baseline HbA$_{1c}$	≤8.5%	7	−0.31 (−0.52 to −0.09)
	>8.5%	5	−0.29 (−0.58 to 0.01)
Quality	Low quality (0–5)	6	−0.17 (−0.39 to 0.05)
	High quality (≥6)	6	−0.41 (−0.59 to −0.24)

Abbreviations: CI, confidence interval; HbA$_{1c}$, glycosylated hemoglobin.

using a random effects model to account for significant heterogeneity among interventions across studies (χ^2 = 22.07, df = 11, P = .024).

The following subgroup analyses were performed for pooled ES of glycemic change based on key design issues: settings of intervention, time of HbA$_{1c}$ measurement, and baseline HbA$_{1c}$ level (Table 2). For participants who attended clinic- or hospital-based diabetes education centers, HbA$_{1c}$ values in those who attended CTDE was significantly improved compared with the control group (ES, −0.26; 95% CI, −0.44 to −0.09), with nonsignificant heterogeneity (χ^2 = 8.32, df = 6, P = .215). Although the ES for the studies with community-based CTDE was greater than for the study for clinic settings, the result was not statistically significant (ES, −0.34; 95% CI, −0.69 to 0.01).

Larger declines in HbA$_{1c}$ levels compared with controls were seen at 6 months (ES, −0.41; 95% CI, −0.61 to −0.21); the result demonstrated that at 6 months, the average person in the intervention group was better off than 66% of the control group. However, the results of HbA$_{1c}$ change in 3 months (ES, −0.21; 95% CI, −0.47 to 0.05) and 12 months (ES, −0.14; 95% CI, −0.39 to 0.05) showed not only smaller changes compared with 6 months but also nonsignificant results.

The pooled ES differed by baseline HbA$_{1c}$ level; therefore, we divided the studies into 2 groups by the median HbA$_{1c}$ value, 8.5%. The ES was −0.31 (95% CI, −0.52 to −0.09) for studies with a baseline HbA$_{1c}$ level of 8.5% or lower and −0.29 (95% CI, −0.58 to 0.01) for studies with a baseline HbA$_{1c}$ level greater

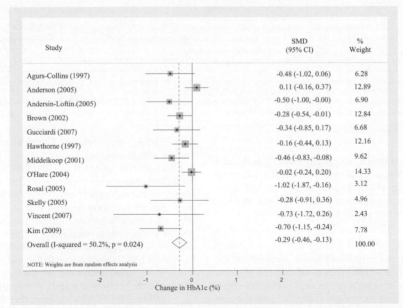

FIGURE 2. *The effect of culturally tailored intervention on glycosylated hemoglobin (HbA$_{1c}$). Abbreviations: CI, confidence interval; SMD, standard mean difference.*

than 8.5%, showing that a lower baseline HbA_{1c} level was associated with a larger ES.

We performed sensitivity analyses by excluding outlier studies one at a time (ie, extreme ES or large sample size) and based on quality rating (quality rating: <6 vs ≥6). When the Rosal et al[35] study was removed, the ES for the remaining studies was −0.26 (95% CI, −0.42 to −0.10). Removing the O'Hare et al[34] study resulted in an ES of −0.39 (95% CI, −0.51 to −0.16) for the remaining studies. Without the Vincent et al[37] study, the ES for the other 11 studies was −0.28 (95% CI, −0.45 to −0.12). Pooled ESs differed by study quality. The ES for the low-quality studies (quality rating: <6, n = 6) was −0.17 (95% CI, −0.39 to 0.05), whereas the high-quality studies (quality rating: ≥6, n = 6) had the largest ES of −0.41 (95% CI, −0.59 to −0.24), with nonsignificant heterogeneity (χ^2 = 3.20, df = 5, P = .67).

Assessment of Publication Bias

We conducted funnel plots, Egger's test, and Begg's test to assess publication bias. If publication bias does not exist, the plot should reveal that the largest studies cluster around the midpoint or top of the funnel; an equal number of smaller studies should be present on both sides of the funnel. The funnel plot for this meta-analysis seemed slightly asymmetrical. The hole in the lower right-hand corner indicates that smaller studies showing no effect are absent. Egger's test and Begg's test showed a small P value, which indicates evidence of publication bias.

Discussion

This meta-analysis provides evidence of the benefit of CTDE on glycemic control for ethnic minorities with type 2 diabetes. The HbA_{1c} improves with CTDE, with a pooled ES of −0.29 when measured at the last follow-up. In our analysis, the summary ES of −0.29 suggests that the average person in the intervention group is better off than 61% of the control group. We cannot directly compare our results with those of other meta-analyses because no previous meta-analyses focused specifically on CTDE intervention for various ethnic minorities. Compared with the previous meta-analyses that did not include a substantial number of ethnic minorities, the ES for HbA_{1c} from our meta-analysis is slightly smaller (pooled ES ranged from −0.36 to −0.43).[15,16] A possible explanation for the small effect is that care delivered to the control groups varied greatly and the control groups also received frequent attention from health care providers during the study periods. Because our main effect, net glycemic change, is the difference between the amount of improvement in the intervention group and that in the

control group, the true effect of the intervention may be underestimated because of the Hawthorne effect in the control groups, that is, the tendency for control subjects to improve when enrolled in research studies. Most studies included for this meta-analysis provided some minimal interventions to the control group; thus, the improvement occurred in both intervention and control groups. Conducting an RCT with ethnic minorities who often have very limited resources (ie, no health insurance, no opportunity for health education in their native language) is likely to put researchers in ethical and logistical dilemmas. That is, it may not be feasible to take something away from this vulnerable population without giving any direct benefit through the research participation. Future efforts should be made in considering alternative methods and design of research to meet both the needs of ethnic minority communities and the scientific rigor of the research.

In analyzing ES by the time of HbA_{1c} measurement, the ES at 6 months was the largest and significant compared with the ES at 3 and 12 months. The effect peaked at 6 months, with a decline to earlier levels after 6 months. The analysis shows that at least 6 months is needed to see a decrease in HbA_{1c} level in ethnic minority groups. This result is generally consistent with the studies of Norris et al[17] and Brown,[39] which found that the benefit of diabetes education declines from 1-3 months[17] to 1-6 months[39] after the intervention ceases. Taken together, these findings suggest the need for maintenance programs for people with type 2 diabetes.

Unlike previous studies, we found that baseline HbA_{1c} level affected the HbA_{1c} outcome. The culturally tailored intervention was more effective for those with baseline HbA_{1c} level equal to or less than 8.5% than for those who had HbA_{1c} level greater than 8.5%. This is a new finding, not previously reported, and suggests that ethnic minorities with a higher HbA_{1c} level may need additional intervention and that further investigation about hard-to-change subgroups is warranted.

A previous meta-analysis[39] found that HbA_{1c} level decreased more when the intervention was delivered in clinic- or hospital-based diabetes educational center settings than in community settings. In our analyses, the ES was −0.34 (95% CI, −0.69 to 0.01) for the studies with community-based CTDE and −0.26 (95% CI, −0.44 to −0.09) for the studies with clinic settings, which was statistically significant. However, our results need to be interpreted with caution because the number of studies included in our subgroup analysis was small and because of its small ES difference. The nonsignificant result of community-based CTDE might have been attributable to the small number of studies available for our subgroup analyses (community-based intervention: n = 5). Future meta-analysis is needed as more studies with community-based interventions for ethnic minorities become available.

When results were stratified by quality score, the ES was −0.41 (CI, −0.59 to −0.24) and −0.17 (CI, −0.39 to 0.05) for studies with high and low quality scores, respectively. Larger declines in HbA_{1c} levels were shown in the studies with more rigorous intervention and design (quality score ≥6).

There are several limitations to our analysis. Our meta-analysis was confined to English-language articles, which could introduce selection bias. However, the ethnic minority group in this analysis is considered in relation to the dominant ethnic group. Therefore, the population in a study reported by a language other than English, with participants who live in their own country, would not be considered as an ethnic minority for this review. In addition, Moher et al[40] found that excluding non-English studies had little impact on overall estimates and that language-restricted meta-analyses overestimated treatment effect by only 2%, on average, compared with language-inclusive meta-analyses.

We included only published data after searching the unpublished literature and excluding studies that did not meet the inclusion criteria. Therefore, our result may be affected by the possibility of publication bias; that is, unpublished studies not identified in our search may have influenced our results. Many of the studies included in this analysis had methodological limitations common in undertaking research of ethnic minorities. For example, none of the studies were long-term (>12 months), and so clinically important, long-term outcomes could not be analyzed. In addition, high attrition, moderate attendance, and complex, multifaceted interventions made subgroup comparisons difficult to interpret with confidence.

It was difficult to analyze the data by type of interventionist because most of the studies used a combination of different providers (eg, "nurse and dietician" or "diabetes educator and community worker") rather than only 1 type of provider. We also chose to look only at the outcome of glycemic control because of potential

problems with pooling ES from studies where outcomes were not measured uniformly (eg, knowledge, attitude, treatment satisfaction, or adherence). None of the included studies reported blinding, although it would have been difficult to mask both intervention and control groups, given the nature of the behavioral interventions.

The results of our meta-analysis are likely generalizable to African American or Hispanic women in the United States because participants in a majority of the studies were women, and of 12 studies, 7 included either African Americans or Hispanic Americans. More research is needed in various ethnic minorities other than African Americans and Latinos. For example, there were no published studies of CTDE among Native Americans.

Despite the limitations, findings from this study suggest important directions for future research and current clinical practice. Ethnic minorities with type 2 diabetes may benefit from linguistically and culturally matched providers for their diabetes care. The duration of intervention, baseline HbA_{1c} level, and settings of interventions should be carefully considered in designing culturally tailored diabetes interventions to maximize the effect.

Cardiovascular diseases, specifically macrovascular events (eg, stroke and myocardial infarction) are the major source of mortality in individuals with type 2 diabetes. One of the most important goals in diabetes management is to reduce cardiovascular morbidity and mortality by effectively delivering diabetes education.

More research with ethnic minorities, including various settings and focusing on participants' characteristics, is warranted to guide culturally competent clinical practice for better diabetes care among ethnic minorities and, in turn, to reduce the burden of cardiovascular diseases.

Conclusions

Ethnic minority populations continue to grow in the United States and experience a disproportionate burden of disease from diabetes. Our analysis supports the short-term effect of CTDE on glycemic control over usual care among ethnic minorities. The effect varies depending on baseline HbA_{1c} level and settings; however, findings from the subgroup analyses should be considered as preliminary evidence of the effect of CTDE based on the small number of included studies. For more definitive estimates of the effect of CTDE, additional analyses should be conducted when more studies with CTDE become available.

Further research is also needed to better understand how interventions improve glycemic control and to pinpoint what the critical component of intervention is for ethnic minorities with type 2 diabetes. There is a need for long-term, multicenter RCTs that compare different ethnic minorities and different types of providers and settings. More important, future research should provide adequate information regarding detailed description of the interventions, duration and frequency of sessions, and allocation concealment if randomization is performed to widely disseminate effective diabetes educational programs for reducing health disparities in diabetes care.

REFERENCES

1. McBean AM, Li S, Gilbertson DT, Collins AJ. Differences in diabetes prevalence, incidence, and mortality among the elderly of four racial/ethnic groups: whites, blacks, Hispanics, and Asians. *Diabetes Care.* 2004;27(10): 2317–2324.
2. Diabetes Public Health Resource. 2005 National diabetes fact sheet. Atlanta, GA: Centers for Disease Control and Prevention; March 12, 2010. http://www.cdc.gov/diabetes/pubs/estimates05.htm#prev3. Accessed August 2, 2010.
3. Carter JS, Pugh JA, Monterrosa A. Non-insulin dependent diabetes mellitus in minorities in the United States. *Ann Intern Med.* 1996;125(3):221–232.
4. Lanting LC, Joung IM, Mackenbach JP, Lamberts SW, Bootsma AH. Ethnic differences in mortality, end-stage complications, and quality of care among diabetic patients: a review. *Diabetes Care.* 2005;28(9):2280–2288.
5. Walsh ME, Katz MA, Sechrest L. Unpacking cultural factors in adaptation to type 2 diabetes mellitus. *Med Care.* 2002;40(1 suppl):I129–I139.
6. Yamada Y, Matsuo H, Segawa T, et al. Assessment of genetic factors for type 2 diabetes mellitus. *Int J Mol Med.* 2006;18(20):299–308.
7. Li S, Zhao JH, Luan J, et al. Genetic predisposition to obesity leads to increase risk of type 2 diabetes [published online ahead of print January 26, 2011]. *Diabetologia.* http://www.springerlink.com.ezproxy.welch.jhmi.edu/content/565265v1642255n0/. Accessed January 28, 2011.
8. Harris MI, Eastman RC, Cowie CC, Flegal KM, Eberhardt MS. Racial and ethnic differences in glycemic control of adults with type 2 diabetes. *Diabetes Care.* 1999;22(3): 403–408.
9. Thackeray R, Merrill RM, Neiger BL. Disparities in diabetes management practice between racial and ethnic groups in the United States. *Diabetes Educ.* 2004;30(4): 665–675.
10. Kumanyika SK, Ewart CK. Theoretical and baseline considerations for diet and weight control of diabetes among Blacks. *Diabetes Care.* 1990;13(11):1154–1162.
11. Kumanyika SK, Herbert PR, Cutler JA, et al. Feasibility and efficacy of sodium reduction in the Trials of Hypertension Prevention, phase I. Trials of Hypertension Collaborative Research Group. *Hypertension.* 1993;22(4): 502–512.
12. Wing RR, Anglin K. Effectiveness of a behavioral weight control program for blacks and whites with NIDDM. *Diabetes Care.* 1996;19(5):409–413.
13. Delamater AM, Jacobson AM, Anderson BJ, et al. Psychosocial therapies in diabetes: report of the Psychosocial Therapies Working Group. *Diabetes Care.* 2001;24(7): 1286–1292.
14. Karter AJ, Ferrara A, Darbinian JA, Ackerson LM, Selby JV. Self-monitoring of blood glucose: language and financial barriers in a managed care population with diabetes. *Diabetes Care.* 2000;23(4):477–483.

15. Gary TL, Genkinger JM, Guallar E, Peyrot M, Brancati FL. Meta-analysis of randomized educational and behavioral interventions in type 2 diabetes. *Diabetes Educator.* 2003; 29(3):488–501.
16. Ismail K, Winkley K, Rabe-Hesketh S. Systemic review and meta-analysis of randomized controlled trials of psychological interventions to improve glycemic control in patients with type 2 diabetes. *Lancet.* 2004;363(9421): 1589–1597.
17. Norris SL, Lau J, Smith S, Schmid C, Engelgau M. Self-management education for adults with type 2 diabetes: a meta-analysis of the effect on glycemic control. *Diabetes Care.* 2002;25(7):1159–1171.
18. Hayden JA, Côté P, Bombardier C. Evaluation of the quality of prognosis studies in systematic reviews. *Ann Intern Med.* 2006;144(6):427–437.
19. Jadad AR, Moore RA, Carroll D, et al. Assessing the quality of reports of randomized clinical trials: is blinding necessary? *Control Clin Trials.* 1996;17(1):1–12.
20. Lipsey MW, Wilson DB. *Practical Meta-analysis: Applied Social Research Methods Series.* Thousand Oaks, CA: Sage; 2000.
21. Thompson SG. *Systematic Reviews in Health Care: Meta-analysis in Context.* 2nd ed. London, England: BMJ; 2001.
22. Bent S, Shojania KG, Saint S. The use of systematic reviews and meta-analyses in infection control and hospital epidemiology. *Am J Infect Control.* 2004;32(4):246–254.
23. Higgins JT, Thompson SG, Deeks JJ, Altman DG. Measuring inconsistency in meta-analysis. *BMJ.* 2003;32:557–560.
24. Ferrer RL. Graphical methods for detecting bias in meta-analysis. *Fam Med.* 1998;30(8):579–583.
25. Begg CB, Mazumdar M. Operating characteristics of a rank correlation test for publication bias. *Biometrics.* 1994;50(4): 1088–1101.
26. Egger M, Smith GD, Schneider M, Minder C. Bias in meta-analysis detected by a simple, graphical test. *BMJ.* 1997; 315(7109):629–634.
27. Anderson-Loftin W, Barnett S, Sullivan P, Hussey J, Tavakoli A. Soul food light: culturally competent diabetes education. *Diabetes Educ.* 2005;31(4):555–563.
28. Agurs-Collins TD, Kumanyika SK, Ten Have TR, Adams-Campbell LL. A randomized controlled trial of weight reduction and exercise for diabetes management in older African-American subjects. *Diabetes Care.* 1997;20(10): 1503–1511.
29. Anderson RM, Funnell MM, Nwankwo R, Gillard ML, Oh M, Fitzgerald T. Evaluating a problem-based empowerment program for African Americans with diabetes: results of randomized controlled trial. *Ethn Dis.* 2005;15(4): 671–678.
30. Brown SA, Garcia AA, Kouzekanani K, Hanis CL. Culturally competent diabetes self-management education for Mexican Americans. *Diabetes Care.* 2002;25(2): 259–268.
31. Gucciardi E, DeMelo M, Lee RN, Grace SL. Assessment of two culturally competent diabetes education methods: individual versus individual plus group education in Canadian Portuguese adults with type 2 diabetes. *Ethn Health.* 2007;12(2):163–187.
32. Hawthorne K, Tomlinson S. One-to-one teaching with pictures-flashcard health education for British Asians with diabetes. *Br J Gen Pract.* 1997;47(418):301–304.
33. Middelkoop BC, Geelhoed-Duijvestijn P, van der Wal G. Effectiveness of culture-specific diabetes care for Surinam South Asian patients in the Hague. *Diabetes Care.* 2001; 24(11):1997–1998.

34. O'Hare JP, Raymond NT, Mughal S, et al. UKADS Study Group. Evaluation of delivery of enhanced diabetes care to patients of South Asian ethnicity: the United Kingdom Asian Diabetes Study (UKADS). *Diabet Med*. 2004;21(12): 1357–1365.

35. Rosal M, Olendzki B, Reed GW, Gumieniak O, Scavron J, Ockene I. Diabetes self-management among low-income Spanish-speaking patients: a pilot study. *Ann Behav Med*. 2005;29(3):225–235.

36. Skelly AH, Carlson JR, Leeman J, Holditch-Davis D, Soward A. Symptoms-focused management for African American women with type 2 diabetes: a pilot study. *Appl Nurs Res*. 2005;18(4):213–220.

37. Vincent D, Pasvogel A, Barrera L. A feasibility study of a culturally tailored diabetes intervention for Mexican Americans. *Biol Res Nurs*. 2007;9(2):130–141.

38. Kim MT, Han H, Song H, et al. A community-based, culturally tailored behavioral intervention for Korean Americans with type 2 diabetes. *Diabetes Educ*. 2009;35(6): 986–994.

39. Brown S. Meta-analysis of diabetes patient education research: variations in intervention effects across studies. *Res Nurs Health*. 1992;15(6):409–419.

40. Moher D, Pham B, Klassen TP, et al. What contributions do languages other than English make on the results of meta-analyses? *J Clin Epidemiol*. 2000;53(9):964–972.

Lead Article

A Metaethnography of Traumatic Childbirth and its Aftermath: Amplifying Causal Looping

Qualitative Health Research
21(3) 301–311
© The Author(s) 2011
Reprints and permission:
sagepub.com/journalsPermissions.nav
DOI: 10.1177/1049732310390698
http://qhr.sagepub.com
$\circledS$SAGE

Cheryl Tatano Beck[1]

Abstract

Integrating results from multiple analytic approaches used in a research program by the same researcher is a type of metasynthesis that has not often been reported in the literature. In this article the findings of one type of qualitative synthesis approach, a metaethnography, of six qualitative studies on birth trauma and its resulting posttraumatic stress disorder from my program of research are presented. This metaethnography provides a wide-angle lens to view and interpret the far-reaching, stinging tentacles of this often invisible phenomenon that new mothers experience. I used Noblit and Hare's seven-step approach for synthesizing the findings of qualitative studies. The original trigger of traumatic childbirth resulted in six amplifying feedback loops, four of which were reinforcing (positive direction), and two which were balancing (negative direction). Leverage points that identify where pressure in the amplifying causal loop can break the feedback loop where necessary are discussed.

Keywords

childbirth; metaethnography; metasynthesis; qualitative analysis; trauma

As Lisa recalled, "I am amazed that three and a half hours in the labor and delivery room could cause such utter destruction in my life. It truly was like being a victim of a violent crime of rape" (Beck, 2004a, p. 32). What happened to this mother that turned her birthing dream into a rape scene? The purpose of this article is to present the results of a metaethnography which focused not only on answering this question, but also on the repercussions of traumatic childbirth for women. By synthesizing the results of six qualitative studies on birth trauma and its resulting posttraumatic stress disorder (PTSD) from my research program, I used a wide-angle lens to view and interpret the far-reaching, stinging tentacles of this often invisible phenomenon. In two of the qualitative studies I examined the experience of a traumatic childbirth (Beck, 2004a, 2006b). My focus in the remaining four studies was the aftermath of birth trauma (Beck, 2004b; 2006a; Beck & Watson, 2008; Beck & Watson, 2010).

Metasynthesis

Metasynthesis is "an interpretive integration of qualitative findings that are themselves interpretive syntheses of data, including the phenomenologies, ethnographies, grounded theories, and other integrative and coherent descriptions or explanations of phenomena, events, or cases that are the hallmarks of qualitative research" (Sandelowski & Barroso, 2007, p. 151). The aim of a metasynthesis is not to focus on the similarities of the results of the qualitative studies included in the metasynthesis, but instead to delve further into these findings to unearth new information to increase our understanding of the phenomenon (Paterson, Thorne, Canam, & Jillings, 2001). Sandelowski and Barroso differentiated between qualitative metasynthesis and qualitative metasummary. Qualitative metasummary is "a quantitative oriented aggregation of qualitative findings that are themselves topical or thematic summaries or surveys of data" (p. 151). Qualitative metasyntheses are more than just summaries. Their end product is a new interpretation of the findings.

Metasyntheses help to prevent what Glaser and Strauss (1971, p. 181) warned as qualitative research studies' results remaining as "respected little islands of knowledge separated from others and not helping to build a cumulative

[1]University of Connecticut, Storrs, Connecticut, USA

Corresponding Author:
Cheryl Tatano Beck, University of Connecticut School of Nursing, 231 Glenbrook Road, Storrs, CT 06269-2026, USA
Email: cheryl.beck@uconn.edu

197

body of knowledge in a substantive area." With more and more focus on metasynthesis, qualitative scholars are now delving further into its implications and applications (Thorne, Jensen, Kearney, Noblit & Sandelowski, 2004). Examples of recent metasyntheses span topics such as withdrawing life-sustaining treatments (Meeker & Jezewski, 2009), mothers' confidence in breastfeeding (Larsen, Hall, & Aagaard, 2008), diabetes in nine South Asian communities (Fleming & Gillibrand, 2009), healing from sexual violence (Draucker et al., 2009), and the hope experience of family caregivers of chronically ill persons (Duggleby et al., 2010).

Three types of metasyntheses are available to researchers (Sandelowski, Docherty, & Emden, 1997). The most frequently used type involves synthesizing results across studies on the same topic conducted by different researchers. A second type consists of using quantitative approaches to synthesize qualitative results from cases across different studies. Integrating results from multiple analytic approaches used in a research program by the same researcher is the third type. An example of this third kind of qualitative metasynthesis is a synthesis of the transition to parenthood of infertile couples (Sandelowski, 1995). This is the only metasynthesis located to date in which a series of qualitative research studies on a phenomenon conducted by the same researcher were synthesized.

Kearney (2001) described current approaches to the synthesis of findings of qualitative research studies into a new integrated whole as the meta family. Included in this meta family are such approaches as metastudy, metainterpretation, metaethnography, and grounded formal theory. Kearney placed these different synthesis approaches on an interpreting–theorizing continuum. On the theorizing end is formal grounded theory (Glaser, 2007), and on the interpretive end is metaethnography (Noblit & Hare, 1988).

Research Design

This metaethnography of birth trauma and its resulting PTSD resulting from childbirth was generated from the findings of six studies I conducted which were published between 2004 and 2010 (Beck 2004a, 2004b, 2006a, 2006b; Beck & Watson, 2008, 2010). Metaethnography is the synthesis of interpretive research. It involves a rigorous approach for constructing substantive interpretations about a group of qualitative studies. A metaethnographer compares and analyzes texts to create new interpretations by translating studies into one another. Noblit and Hare (1988) proposed that translating studies involves making analogies between the studies and also among the studies. An interpretive form of knowledge synthesis is achieved inductively. The aims of metaethnography are to enable:

1. More interpretive literature reviews
2. Critical examination of multiple accounts of an event, situation, and so forth
3. Systematic comparison of case studies to draw cross-case conclusions
4. A way of talking about our work and comparing it to the works of others
5. Synthesis of ethnographic studies (Noblit & Hare, 1988, p. 12)

Sample

These six studies are profiled in Tables 1 and 2. In the first study, "Birth Trauma: In the Eye of the Beholder," I focused on the experience of traumatic childbirth (Beck, 2004a). In the second study I examined PTSD following birth trauma (Beck, 2004b). In the third study I examined the anniversary of birth trauma (Beck, 2006a). These first three studies were phenomenological studies. The fourth study was a narrative analysis of birth trauma stories (Beck, 2006b). The fifth and sixth studies in my program of research were phenomenological studies looking at the impact of birth trauma on breastfeeding (Beck & Watson, 2008), and on the experience of subsequent childbirth after a previous traumatic birth (Beck & Watson, 2010). The total number of participants in these six studies was 175 mothers. Thirty-eight of the 40 mothers who participated in the first study on birth trauma (Beck, 2004a) also participated in the PTSD-following-childbirth study (Beck, 2004b). I achieved data saturation in each study. All the studies adhered to ethical standards. I received institutional review board approval for each study and informed consent was obtained from all participants.

Qualitative studies on traumatic childbirth have been conducted by researchers other than me, including Ayers (2007) and Nicholls and Ayers (2007). The studies conducted by these authors were not pertinent to the current metaethnography and thus were not included in it, because this metaethnography was a synthesis of results used in a program of research by the same researcher, that being myself.

Data Analysis

I used Noblit and Hare's (1988) seven-step approach for synthesizing the findings of qualitative studies. These steps overlapped and repeated as the synthesis was conducted, and included:

1. Choosing a phenomenon to be studied
2. Identifying which qualitative studies were pertinent
3. Reading the qualitative studies to be included in the synthesis

Table 1. Demographic Characteristics of Participants in the Individual Studies Included in the Metaethnography

Study	Sample Size	Country (N)	Age Range	Parity (N)	Marital Status (N)	Delivery Type (N)
Beck (2004a)	40	New Zealand (23) United States (8) Australia (6) United Kingdom (3)	25-40	Multiparas (24) Primiparas (16)	Married (34) Divorced (3) Single (3)	Vaginal (22) Cesarean (18)
Beck (2004b)	38	New Zealand (22) United States (7) Australia (6) United Kingdom (3)	25-44	Multiparas (26) Primiparas (12)	Married (34) Divorced (2) Single (2)	Vaginal (21) Cesarean (17)
Beck (2006a)	11	United States (6) New Zealand (3) Australia (1) United Kingdom (1)	26-38	Multiparas (8) Primiparas (3)	Married (11)	Vaginal (7) Cesarean (3) Both (1)
Beck (2006b)	37	United States (20) New Zealand (8) Australia (4) United Kingdom (4) Canada (1)	24-54	Multiparas (14) Primiparas (19) Missing (4)	Married (31) Divorced (1) Single (1) Missing (4)	Vaginal (18) Cesarean (13) Both (6)
Beck & Watson (2008)	52	New Zealand (28) United States (11) Australia (6) United Kingdom (4) Canada (3)		Multiparas (21) Primiparas (31)	Married (46) Living with partner (5) Separated (1)	Vaginal (26) Cesarean (25) Both (1)
Beck & Watson (2010)	35	United States (15) United Kingdom (8) New Zealand (6) Australia (5) Canada (1)	27-51	Multiparas (52)	Married (34) Divorced (1)	Vaginal (25) Cesarean (10)

4. Deciding how the studies were related to one another. Here the researcher lists the key metaphors in each study and how they are related to each other. Noblit and Hare use the term *metaphor* to refer to concepts, themes, or phrases when synthesizing studies. Three differing assumptions can be made regarding how studies are related: "(a) the accounts are directly comparable as 'reciprocal' translations; (b) the accounts stand in relative opposition to each other and are essentially 'refutational'; or (c) the studies taken together present a 'line of argument' rather than a reciprocal or refutational translation" (p. 36). In this metaethnography, the assumption was one of reciprocal translations.

5. Translating each study's metaphors into the metaphors of the others, and vice versa. Noblit and Hare described these translations as "especially unique syntheses because they protect the particular, respect holism, and enable comparison" (p. 28).

6. Synthesizing the translations, wherein a whole is created which is something more than the individual parts imply.

7. Expressing the synthesis, most often through the written word; however, plays, art, videos, or music are other options.

Care must be taken during the data analysis phase of a qualitative synthesis, as Sandelowski et al. warned:

Qualitative metasynthesis is not a trivial pursuit, but rather a complex exercise in interpretation: Carefully peeling away the surface layers of studies to find their hearts and souls in a way that does the least damage to them. Synthesists must analyze studies in sufficient detail to preserve the integrity of each study and yet not become so immersed in detail that no useable synthesis is produced. (1997, p. 370)

Table 2. Methodological Characteristics of the Qualitative Studies Included in the Metaethnography

Author	Year	Qualitative Research Design	Data Analysis
Beck	2004a	Phenomenology	Colaizzi
Beck	2004b	Phenomenology	Colaizzi
Beck	2006a	Narrative Analysis	Burke
Beck	2006b	Phenomenology	Colaizzi
Beck & Watson	2008	Phenomenology	Colaizzi
Beck & Watson	2010	Phenomenology	Colaizzi

Note. All studies had methodological characteristics of convenience sampling and Internet data collection.

Results

I constructed a detailed table of key metaphors from each of the six studies to facilitate the reciprocal translations (Table 3). These individual study metaphors were clustered into three overarching themes: stripped of protective layers, invisible wounds, and insidious repercussions. Under the theme of stripped of protective layers were the key metaphors that revealed that in birth trauma women perceived they were systematically stripped of essential protective layers, leaving them exposed and feeling very vulnerable. The overarching theme of invisible wounds addressed both the short- and long-term distressing emotions women struggled to cope with after experiencing a traumatic birth, such as fear, terror, grief, and feeling like a rape victim. Included under insidious repercussions were the often invisible detrimental effects of birth trauma on mothers' interactions with their infants.

Two of the six studies (Beck, 2004a; Beck, 2006b) included in the metaethnography uncovered the essence of what constituted traumatic childbirth for the women. The key metaphors in these two studies started the devastating domino effects that permeated mothers' lives as their dreams of motherhood were shattered. In my phenomenological study of traumatic childbirth (Beck, 2004a), a resounding characteristic of this phenomenon was that, just like beauty, birth trauma was in the eye of the beholder. What women perceived as a traumatic birth clinicians might have been viewed as a routine, normal delivery. Women felt abandoned, stripped of their dignity, and not cared for as an individual who deserved to be treated with respect. Obstetric staff neglected to communicate with mothers. Women often felt invisible, as Nicole explained:

After an hour trying to deliver the baby with a vacuum extractor, the obstetrician said it was too late for an emergency cesarean. The baby was truly stuck. By now the doctors are acting like I'm not there. The attending physician was saying, "We

may have lost this bloody baby." The hospital staff discussed my baby's possible death in front of me, and argued in front of me just as if I weren't there. (Beck, 2004a, pp. 32-33)

Some women felt their trust in their respective obstetric care provider was betrayed, because they perceived that they received unsafe care but were powerless to rectify the dangerous situation. Mothers' traumatic experiences were pushed into the background as family and clinicians celebrated the birth of a live, healthy infant.

I later examined traumatic childbirth using a different qualitative research design, that being narrative analysis (Beck, 2006b). Using Burke's (1969) dramatistic pentad as the structure for viewing mothers' narratives, his ratio imbalance of act:agency appeared prominently in the narratives. Center stage in a woman's birth trauma narrative was how acts were performed during the birthing process. The manner in which obstetrical staff provided care to women during childbirth demonstrated a glaring absence of caring. The following is an excerpt from Michelle's narrative of the uncaring manner (agency) of the nurse who was present as the mother gave birth to her stillborn preterm infant:

My husband went to get the nurse. The nurse said, you have only just had the gel, you couldn't be having IT yet. I said, yes. She is about to be born. The nurse checked and the head was visible. She looked shocked and said wait. I'll have to get a dish and returned with a green kidney shaped dish. The way she held the dish and the look on her face, I knew she did not want to be in the room. My husband held the dish for her. I then gave a little push and my daughter (still in her little sack) slipped quietly in the dish. The nurse took the dish from my husband and covered my daughter with a sheet. She then walked off without saying a word about where she was going. I called to her. Where are you taking her??? (I had not even seen her properly as she was still in her sack). The nurse said, I have to take IT to the doctor. She wants to see IT. Also the nurse continued to refer to me by my last name, not my first name. I said but I want to see my daughter. She said, Why? IT's dead. She then said I have to get someone to wash IT so IT can be examined. (Beck, 2006b, p. 461)

As the metaethnography progressed and more of the key metaphors were translated into each other, I had an "Aha!" moment. Operating in the aftermath of birth trauma—with its domino effects on various aspects of motherhood—was amplifying causal looping. In amplifying causal looping, "as consequences become continually causes and causes

Table 3. Individual Study Metaphors as Related to the Overarching Themes

Study	Stripped of Protective Layers	Invisible Wounds	Insidious Repercussions
Beck (2004a) Birth trauma: In the eye of the beholder	To care for me: Was that too much to ask? To communicate with me: Why was this neglected? To provide safe care: You betrayed my trust and I felt powerless	Fear Horror Terror Felt like a rape victim	The end justifies the means: At whose expense? At what price?
Beck (2004b) PTSD due to childbirth: The aftermath	Seeking to have questions answered and wanting to talk, talk, talk Isolation from world of motherhood	Going to the movies: Please don't make me go A shadow of myself: Too numb to try and change Dangerous trio of anger, anxiety, and depression: Spiraling downward	World of motherhood: Dreams shattered
Beck (2006a) Anniversary of birth trauma: Failure to rescue	Failure to rescue Lack of caring Lack of communication	The prologue: An agonizing time The actual day: A celebration of a birthday or torment of an anniversary	The epilogue: A fragile state Subsequent anniversaries: For better or worse Emotional bonding with infant missing
Beck (2006b) Pentadic cartography: Mapping birth trauma narratives	Act: agency ratio imbalance Powerless	Terrified Shock Loss Grief Flashbacks Like being raped	Suicidal thoughts
Beck & Watson (2008) Impact of birth trauma on breastfeeding		Proving oneself as a mother: Sheer determination Making up for an awful arrival: Atonement to the baby Just one more thing to be violated: Mother's breasts Intruding flashbacks: Stealing anticipated joy	Disturbing detachment: An empty affair
Beck & Watson (2010) Subsequent childbirth after a previous traumatic birth	Frighteningly alone	Riding the turbulent wave of panic during pregnancy Fear Anxiety Dread Terror Denial	Numbness to fetus Still elusive: The longed-for healing experience Grieving for what could have been Past can never be changed

continually consequences one sees either worsening or improving progressions or escalating severity" (Glaser, 2005, p. 9). Causal loops involve feedback behavior in which the effects of a change serve to intensify or oppose the original change. Feedback is an important concept to consider. A change in one factor can impact another factor, which then can affect the first factor. When feedback decreases the impact of a change, it is sometimes referred to as a balancing loop. In contrast, a reinforcing loop occurs when feedback increases the impact of a change. This causal looping can amplify in either a positive or negative direction. The term *positive* does not necessarily

mean that the changes are good; it only means that the changes are reinforced. *Negative* only indicates that changes are resisted; it does not necessarily mean the effects or changes are bad.

The amplifying feedback loops that emerged from this metaethnography of the five phenomenological studies and one narrative analysis on traumatic childbirth are illustrated in Figure 1. A successive series of amplifying feedback loops occurred. The original trigger of traumatic childbirth resulted in six amplifying feedback loops, four of which were reinforcing (positive direction), and two of which were balancing (negative direction).

Reinforcing Loop #1

The first reinforcing feedback loop focused on the detrimental effects that the posttraumatic stress symptoms resulting from childbirth can have on mothers' breastfeeding experiences. When attempting to breastfeed, some women suffered with uncontrollable flashbacks to their traumatic birth. As Molly revealed:

> I had flashbacks to the birth every time I would feed him. When he was put on me in the hospital, he wasn't breathing and he was blue. I kept picturing this; and could still feel what it was like. Breastfeeding him was a similar position as to the way he was put on me. (Beck & Watson, 2008, p. 234)

For some mothers, these intruding flashbacks were so distressing that they made a decision to stop breastfeeding. Angie admitted that, "The flashbacks to the birth were terrible. I wanted to forget about it and the pain, so stopping breastfeeding would get me a bit closer to my 'normal' self again" (Beck & Watson, 2008, p. 234).

Avoidance of triggers to the recollection of the original trauma, in this case traumatic birth, permeated mothers' lives. Their infants were constant reminders of their birth trauma. For some mothers, feeling detached from their babies and distancing themselves from this trigger hindered their breastfeeding. Rachael shared,

> Breastfeeding my son in the first few months, certainly the first 6 but possibly as much as 9 months, was an empty affair. I felt nothing at all. Breastfeeding was just one of the many things I did while remaining totally detached from my baby. (Beck & Watson, 2008, p. 234)

Nancy, who had an emergency cesarean birth under general anesthesia, revealed, "I didn't feel like a real mother, as I was unable to give my daughter a normal birth. I felt very disconnected from this baby as I breastfed her" (Beck & Watson, 2008. p. 235).

Women traumatized during childbirth often felt like victims of rape: violated and stripped of their dignity. Hypervigilance is one of the clusters of symptoms of posttraumatic stress. Some women became vigilant about protecting their bodies from being violated yet again. This hypervigilance focused on their breasts and hindered their breastfeeding. Jeanne, whose labor had been induced and who had a failed vacuum extraction followed by a cesarean birth, shared the following:

> When I breastfed my baby, I felt like it was one more invasion up on my body and I couldn't handle

that after the labor I had suffered. Whenever I put her to breast, I wanted to scream and vomit at the same time. (Beck & Watson, 2008, p. 233)

In the following comment Leslie was referring to the staff in the neonatal intensive care unit who were trying to help her breastfeed her preterm infant: "I was sick of everyone grabbing my breasts like they didn't belong to me. My breasts were just another thing to be taken away and violated" (Beck & Watson, 2008, p. 233).

In this first amplifying causal loop the posttraumatic stress symptoms of birth trauma had a positive (reinforcing) effect on breastfeeding experiences, which in turn intensified women's distress and posttraumatic stress symptoms, creating a vicious cycle of trauma and distress.

Balancing Loop #1

The first balancing loop, like the first reinforcing loop, involved the feedback between posttraumatic stress and breastfeeding. In this causal loop, some factors related to breastfeeding opposed the original effects of posttraumatic stress from birth trauma and helped to diminish these distressing symptoms. One of the themes in my phenomenological study with Watson (2008) on the impact of birth trauma on breastfeeding was "Helping to heal mentally: Time out from the pain in one's head." For some women, breastfeeding helped to heal them. *Soothing* was a term used by some mothers to describe breastfeeding. Karen, who had experienced a terrifying postpartum hemorrhage, explained:

> Breastfeeding was a timeout from the pain in my head. It was a "current reality"—a way to cling onto some "real life," whereas all the trauma that continued to live on in my head belonged to the past, even though I couldn't seem to keep it there. (Beck & Watson, 2008, p. 233)

Reinforcing Loop #2

This second reinforcing causal loop involved the feedback between posttraumatic stress following childbirth and mother–infant interaction. This positive amplifying loop was operating in all the studies included in this metaethnography. In my study on PTSD resulting from childbirth (Beck, 2004b), a disturbing theme revealed that posttraumatic stress choked off lifelines to the world of motherhood. Women's dreams of how motherhood would be were shattered. With PTSD, some women distanced themselves from their infants. Their infants were triggers to intensifying their posttraumatic stress symptoms, such as flashbacks and nightmares. As Linda described,

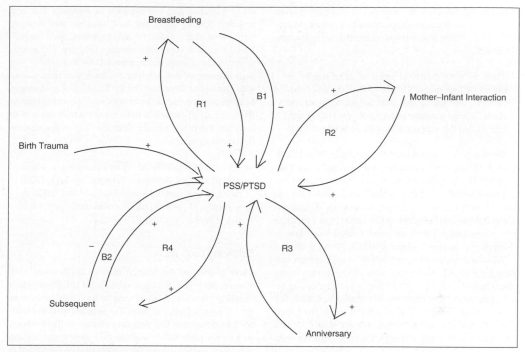

Figure 1. Amplifying causal loop diagram illustrating traumatic childbirth and its aftermath
R = reinforcing loop; B = balancing loop; PSS/PTSD = posttraumatic stress symptoms/posttraumatic stress disorder.

At night I tried to connect/acknowledge in my heart that this was my son, and I cried. I knew that there were great layers of trauma around my heart. I wanted to feel motherhood. I wanted to experience and embrace it. Why was I chained up in the viselike grip of this pain? (Beck, 2004b, p. 222)

The disturbing detachment from their infants of mothers suffering with posttraumatic stress symptoms was confirmed in the breastfeeding study (Beck & Watson, 2008).

In the anniversary-of-birth-trauma study (Beck, 2006a), some mothers revealed that the traumatic effects of birth left them feeling like they were not real mothers, and that an emotional bond with their infants was missing. Debbie recalled the following about her child's first birthday:

I wanted to die. I felt nothing for her and found it hard to celebrate the joy of this child that meant so little to me. I took excellent care of her, but it was as if I was babysitting; the emotional bond just wasn't there. (Beck, 2006a, p. 386)

From the subsequent childbirth-after-previous-traumatic-birth study results (Beck & Watson, 2010), we now are privy to the reinforcing effect—this time the effect on mother–fetus bonding. During their pregnancies women experienced terror, panic, and fear as they waited for 9 months for the dreaded labor and delivery. Some women turned to denial of their pregnancy to "survive" this period. Laurie shared that, throughout her pregnancy, she "felt numb to my baby" (p. 245).

Reinforcing Loop #3

The third reinforcing feedback loop in this metaethnography concerned the anniversary-of-birth trauma (Beck, 2006a). Feedback from the yearly anniversary increased the impact of the posttraumatic stress symptoms and amplified distress in mothers. It was not just the actual day of the anniversary that amplified this distress, but also the prologue of weeks and sometimes months leading up to the anniversary of traumatic birth. Fear, grief, anxiety, dread, depression, and guilt were just some of the distressing emotions women struggled with as the anniversary approached. The calendar, seasons, and clock times were all triggers to flareups of posttraumatic stress symptoms. Anna, whose birth trauma occurred near Halloween, explained:

> There is also a distinct smell of dead leaves in the air that screams, "October!" Hearing the word, October, and seeing the word in writing gives me chills. When I would see decorations for Halloween, fear rushed through my body. (Beck, 2006a, p. 385)

Women also struggled with the actual day: Was it a celebration of their child's birthday, or the torment of an anniversary? The birthday of Shannon's child triggered the following flashback of this mother's emergency cesarean birth: "I can't stop seeing images of a woman drugged and strapped down and being gutted like a fish. I can't get those or my own images out of my mind. I didn't know how to celebrate my daughter's birthday" (Beck, 2006a, p. 386).

Women often paid a heavy toll as a result of their surviving the actual anniversary. One of the themes in my phenomenological study (2006a) was "The epilogue: A fragile state." Mothers vividly shared how they felt at anniversary time, as the invisible wounds from their traumatic births were reopened. Women needed time to heal their raw wounds. Christine described this reinforcing effect:

> As hard as I try to move away from the trauma, at birthday anniversary time I am pulled straight back as if on a giant rubber band into the midst of it all and spend MONTHS AFTER trying to pull myself away from it again. (Beck, 2006a, p. 387)

Reinforcing Loop #4

Results of the phenomenological study of subsequent childbirth after a previous traumatic birth (Beck & Watson, 2010) provided data upon which the fourth reinforcing causal loop was based. During pregnancy, women rode a turbulent wave of panic and other distressing emotions as their posttraumatic stress symptoms increased in intensity. Nicole revealed the following about the entire period of her pregnancy: "My 9 months of pregnancy were an anxiety filled abyss which was completely marred as an experience due to the terror that was continually in my mind from my experience 8 years earlier" (Beck & Watson, 2010, p. 245).

Women employed numerous strategies during pregnancy to break the reinforcing cycle of one traumatic birth followed by another traumatic birth. Examples of various strategies include exercise, yoga, relaxation techniques, keeping a journal, hypobirthing (a method of natural childbirth

using relaxation and self-hypnosis to eliminate fear and tension), reading about the birth process, and creating birth-oriented art. Sadly, for some women, their longed-for healing birth experience remained elusive. The amplifying feedback loop was reinforced. An example of one such instance of this positive feedback was from Carol, who had opted for a homebirth. Because of postpartum hemorrhage she had to be transported by ambulance to the hospital, all the while terrified she would not live to raise her baby. She vividly described her experience on the operating table:

> With my legs held in the air by two strangers while a third mopped the blood between my legs, I felt raped all over again. I wanted to die. I had failed as a woman. My privacy had been invaded again. I felt sick. (Beck & Watson, 2010, p. 247)

Balancing Loop #2

Three fourths of the women in my (2010) study with Watson described that their subsequent childbirth was a "healing experience," or at least "a lot better" than their prior traumatic birth had been. The second balancing feedback loop captures this opposing change to the feedback loop. A reverence was brought to their subsequent birthing processes, and the women felt empowered. What helped to initiate this balancing feedback loop? Some reasons mothers gave included (a) being treated with respect, dignity, and compassion; (b) having pain relief taken seriously; (c) improved communication with labor and delivery staff; and (d) not feeling rushed to deliver. Kathryn described this negative (balancing) feedback loop:

> It was as healing and empowering as I had always hoped for. I did not want any high tech management. My homebirth was the proudest day of my life and the victory was sweeter because I overcame so very much to come to it. (Beck & Watson, 2010, p. 247)

Discussion

Leverage points identify where pressure in the amplifying causal loop can produce desired outcomes, namely breaking the feedback loop where necessary (Newell, Proust, Dyball, & McManus, 2007). Obviously, with birth trauma, the ideal intervention is to prevent it, to treat each woman during the birthing process as if she were a survivor of previous trauma (Crompton, 2003). Highley and Mercer (1978) expressed it best, as they reminded clinicians of the reverence that needs to be provided to women in labor:

Being able to assist a woman in one of the greatest tasks of her life—giving birth to and mothering a baby—is a privilege and challenge that touches every nurse who assists in her care. The challenge extends not only to the concrete physical help that the mother needs, but to the subtle consideration and attention which help her maintain her self-control and thus her self-respect. (p. 41)

The panoramic view provided by this metaethnography (see Figure 1) clearly illustrates the multiple, repetitive, reinforcing, amplifying causal loops that permeate mothers' lives as they struggle with the long-term aftermath of traumatic childbirth. Four of the six amplifying loops are reinforcing, thus intensifying posttraumatic stress symptoms in mothers. Leverage points abound for interrupting these positive amplifying causal loops. Clinicians fail to rescue women with birth trauma time and time again: during breastfeeding, during their interactions with their infants, during yearly anniversaries, and in subsequent childbirth. Many precious opportunities to balance these causal loops are lost. Obstetric care providers need to ensure that women are surrounded with protective layers during the birthing process. These protective layers include feeling cared for, being communicated with, being treated with respect and dignity, allowing some control when appropriate, supporting women, and providing assurance.

To help prevent the four reinforcing causal loops from coming into play, clinicians need to be vigilant in observing women for any symptoms indicating that they might have experienced a traumatic birth. Instruments are available to screen women in the postpartum period for posttraumatic stress symptoms. One such instrument is the Post-Traumatic Stress Symptoms Scale (Foa, Riggs, Dancu & Rothbaum, 1993). If women screen positive for elevated symptom levels, referrals to mental health professionals can be made. Treatment options, such as eye movement desensitization reprocessing, have been shown to be effective in women with posttraumatic stress symptoms resulting from traumatic childbirth (Sandstrom, Wiberg, Wikman, Willman, & Hogberg, 2008).

Regarding Reinforcing Loop #1, an example of one leverage point is providing intensive one-on-one support for traumatized women as they initiate breastfeeding. For the second reinforcing loop, periodic routine assessment of mother–infant interactions during the postpartum period can be one leverage point. These assessments can provide an opportunity to identify women struggling with posttraumatic stress symptoms.

Yearly physical exams for children provide a golden opportunity for clinicians to try and interrupt Reinforcing Loop #3. At these well-child checkups, mothers should also be the focus of health care providers. Women need to be asked if they are struggling around the yearly anniversary of their children's birth.

Leverage points to address Reinforcing Loop #4 can and should occur throughout the 9 months of pregnancy. If a woman is a multipara, an essential component of her initial prenatal visit should be a discussion of the mother's perception of her previous births. Were any of those births perceived as traumatic births? England and Horowitz (1998) urged clinicians to encourage wounded mothers to grieve their prior traumatic births so as to lift the burden of their invisible pain. To try and prevent another traumatic birth, clinicians can share with women the strategies other mothers used (Beck & Watson, 2010).

Some of the amplifying causal loops discovered in this metaethnography confirmed results reported in qualitative studies conducted by other researchers. For example, Reinforcing Loop #2, mother–infant interactions, supported findings from Nicholls and Ayers' (2007) study of PTSD in six couples. The women commented on poor bonding with their infants, "putting on an act" with their babies because they did not have any positive feelings toward their babies. Overprotective/anxious bonding and avoidant/rejecting bonding were reported by these mothers.

The essence of what constituted traumatic childbirth identified in this metaethnography confirmed results of previous qualitative studies. For example, in Ayers' (2007) study with 25 mothers with posttraumatic stress symptoms, women used adjectives like *panicky*, *alarmed*, *scared*, and *helpless* to describe their traumatic births. Some mothers shared that they dissociated and had thoughts of death during labor.

Ideas for further research can be gleaned from this metaethnography. Some of the "domino effects" of traumatic childbirth are apparent from this synthesis, but more qualitative research can be conducted to discover what other insidious effects of birth trauma permeate women's lives. For example, are mothers' interactions with their older children also affected? Additional research to identify more balancing feedback loops is also warranted. Since all six studies included in this metaethnography were conducted via the Internet, replication of these qualitative studies with non-Internet samples is needed.

The reinforcing amplifying feedback loops discovered in this metaethnography provide compelling evidence to help bring visibility to this mostly invisible phenomenon. A mother in one of my studies (Beck, 2004b) said it best when describing her PTSD following childbirth: "It's like an invisible wall around the sufferer" (p. 221). In the recent United States national survey, Listening to Mothers II, 9% of new mothers screened positive for meeting the *DSM-IV* (American Psychiatric Association, 2000) criteria for a diagnosis of PTSD following childbirth

(Declercq, Sakala, Corry, & Applebaum, 2008). The qualitative results of this metaethnography of traumatic childbirth "put the flesh on the bones" of this sobering quantitative statistic of the state of new mothers in the United States (Patton, 1990).

Declaration of Conflicting Interests

The author declared no conflicts of interest with respect to the authorship and/or publication of this article.

Funding

The author received no financial support for the research and/or authorship of this article.

References

American Psychiatric Association. (2000). *Diagnostic and statistical manual of mental disorders* (4th ed.). Washington, DC: Author.

Ayers, S. (2007). Thoughts and emotions during traumatic birth: A qualitative study. *Birth, 34,* 253-263. doi:10.1111/j.1523-536x2007.0018.x

Beck, C. T. (2004a). Birth trauma: In the eye of the beholder. *Nursing Research, 53,* 28-35. doi:10.1097/00006199-20040 1000-00005

Beck, C. T. (2004b). Post-traumatic stress disorder due to childbirth: The aftermath. *Nursing Research, 53,* 216-224. doi:10.1097/00006199-200407000-00004

Beck, C. T. (2006a). The anniversary of birth trauma: Failure to rescue. *Nursing Research, 55,* 381-390. doi:10.1097/0000 6199-200611000-00002

Beck, C. T. (2006b). Pentadic cartography: Mapping birth trauma narratives. *Qualitative Health Research, 16,* 453-466. doi:10. 1177/1049732305285968

Beck, C. T, & Watson, S. (2008). Impact of birth trauma on breastfeeding: A tale of two pathways. *Nursing Research, 57,* 228-236. doi:10.1097/01.nnr.0000313494.87282.90

Beck, C. T, & Watson, S. (2010). Subsequent childbirth after a previous traumatic birth. *Nursing Research, 59,* 241-249. doi:10.1097/nnr.06013e3181e501fd

Burke, K. (1969). *A grammar of motives.* Berkley, CA: University of California Press.

Crompton, J. (2003, summer). Post-traumatic stress disorder and childbirth. *Childbirth Educators New Zealand Education Effects,* 25-31.

Declercq, E. R., Salaka, C., Corry, M. P., & Applebaum, B. O. (2008). *New mothers speak out: National survey results highlight women's postpartum experiences.* New York: Childbirth Connection. Retrieved from Childbirth Connection Web site at http://www.childbirthconnection.org/listeningtomothers/

Draucker, C. B., Martsolf, D. S., Ross, R., Cook, C. B., Stidham, A. W., & Mweemba, P. (2009). The essence of healing from sexual violence: A qualitative metasynthesis. *Research in Nursing & Health, 32,* 366-378. doi:10.1002/nur.20333

Duggleby, W., Holtslander, L., Kylma, J., Duncan, V., Hammond, C., & Williams, A. (2010). Metasynthesis of the hope experience of family caregivers of persons with chronic illness. *Qualitative Health Research, 20,* 148-158. doi:10.1177/1049732309358329

England, P., & Horowitz, R. (1998). *Birthing from within.* Albuquerque, NM: Partera Press.

Fleming, E., & Gillibrand, W. (2009). An exploration of culture, diabetes, and nursing in the South Asian community. *Journal of Transcultural Nursing, 20,* 146-155. doi:10.1177/1043659608330058

Foa, E. B., Riggs, D. S., Dancu, C. V., & Rothbaum, B. O. (1993). Reliability and validity of a brief instrument for assessing posttraumatic stress disorder (PSS-SR). *Journal of Traumatic Stress, 6,* 459-473. doi:10.1002/jts.2490060405

Glaser, B. G. (2005). *The grounded theory perspective III: Theoretical coding*: Mill Valley, CA: Sociology Press.

Glaser, B. G. (2007). *Doing formal grounded theory: A proposal.* Mill Valley, CA: Sociology Press.

Glaser, B. G., & Strauss, A. L. (1971). *Status passage.* Chicago: Aldine-Atherton.

Highley, B., & Mercer, R. T. (1978). Safeguarding the laboring woman's sense of control. *MCN: The American Journal of Maternal Child Nursing, 4,* 39-41. doi:10.1097/00005721-197801000-00013

Kearney, M. H. (2001). New directions in grounded formal theory (pp. 227-246). In R. S. Schreiber & P. N. Stern (Eds.), *Using grounded theory in nursing.* New York: Springer.

Larsen, J. S., Hall, E. O. C., & Aagaard, H. (2008). Shattered expectations: When mothers' confidence in breastfeeding is undermined—A metasynthesis. *Scandinavian Journal of Caring Science, 22,* 653-661. doi:10.1111/j.1471-6712 .2007.00572.x

Meeker, M. A., & Jezewski, M. A. (2009). Metasynthesis: Withdrawing life-sustaining treatments. The experience of family decision-makers. *Journal of Clinical Nursing, 18,* 163-173. doi:10.111/j.1365-2702.2008.02465.x

Newell, B., Proust, K., Dyball, R., & McManus, P. (2007). Seeing obesity as a systems problem. *NSW Public Health Bulletin, 18,* 214-218. doi:10.1071/nb07028

Nicholls, K., & Ayers, S. (2007). Childbirth-related post-traumatic stress disorder in couples: A qualitative study. *British Journal of Health Psychology, 12,* 491-509. doi:10.1348/135910706x120627

Noblit, G. W., & Hare, R. D. (1988). *Meta-ethnography: Synthesizing qualitative studies.* Newbury Park, CA: Sage.

Paterson, B. L., Thorne, S. E., Canam, C., & Jillings, C. (2001). *Meta-study of qualitative health research.* Thousand Oaks, CA: Sage.

Patton, M. Q. (1990). *Qualitative evaluation and research methods.* Newbury Park, CA: Sage.

Sandelowski, M. (1995). A theory of the transition to parenthood of infertile couples. *Research in Nursing & Health, 18,* 123-132. doi:10:1002/nur.4770180206

Sandelowski, M., & Barroso, J. (2007). *Handbook for synthesizing qualitative research*. New York: Springer.

Sandelowski, M., Docherty, S., & Emden, C. (1997). Qualitative metasynthesis: Issues and techniques. *Research in Nursing & Health, 20*, 365-371. doi:10.1002/(sici)1098-240x(199708)

Sandstrom, M., Wiberg, B., Wikman, M., Willman, A. K., & Hogberg, U. (2008). A pilot study of eye movement desensitization and reprocessing treatment (EMDR) for post-traumatic stress after childbirth. *Midwifery, 24*, 62-73. doi:10-1016/j.midw.2006.07.008

Thorne, S., Jensen, L., Kearney, M. H., Noblit, G., & Sandelowski, M. (2004). Qualitative metasynthesis: Reflections on methodological orientation and ideological agenda. *Qualitative Health Research, 14*, 1342-1365. doi:10.1177/1049732304269888

Bio

Cheryl Tatano Beck, DNSc, CNM, FAAN, is a distinguished professor at the University of Connecticut School of Nursing in Storrs, Connecticut, USA.

Answers to Selected Study Guide Exercises

CHAPTER 1

A. FILL IN THE BLANKS

1. paradigm
2. constructivism
3. Positivism
4. applied
5. clubs
6. clinical
7. generalizability
8. cause
9. assumption
10. Empirical
11. determinism
12. Replication
13. methods
14. qualitative
15. biases
16. Quantitative

B. MATCHING EXERCISES

1. a	2. b	3. d	4. b	5. a
6. b	7. d	8. b	9. c	10. a

D. APPLICATION EXERCISES

Exercise D.1: Questions of Fact (Appendix A)

a. Yes, this was a systematic study that tested the efficacy of an intervention designed to improve the psychosocial health of chronically ill rural women.
b. It was a quantitative study. The researchers systematically measured several psychosocial outcomes (e.g., self-esteem, stress) using scales that yielded quantitative information.

c. The underlying paradigm was positivism/postpositivism.
d. Yes, the study involved the collection of information through the senses (i.e., through scrutiny of study participants' responses to series of questions).
e. This study was applied research—there was a practical problem that the researchers wanted to solve (i.e., a problem relating to the psychosocial health of chronically ill rural women).
f. Yes, this study was concerned with evaluating whether the intervention *caused* improvements to the psychosocial health of the women in the study. In this and most studies, there is an underlying assumption that phenomena are multiply determined. Thus, women's scores on the various psychosocial scales are *caused* by a number of factors, and this study tested whether one of the causes is the women's participation in a special intervention.
g. The purposes of the study could be described as prediction and control—the investigators examined possible methods of controlling (improving) psychosocial outcomes. The purpose could also be called explanatory—the researchers designed their intervention on a conceptualization of the problem that purported to explain how women adapt to a chronic illness.
h. Yes, this study directly addressed a question relevant to the *treatment* of patients—a therapy question. The results of this study, together with those from other similar studies, could provide guidance about evidence-based treatment decisions.

209

Exercise D.2: Questions of Fact (Appendix B)

a. Yes, this was a systematic study of breast-feeding promotion in a neonatal intensive care unit (NICU).

b. It was a qualitative study. The researcher used loosely structured methods to capture in an in-depth fashion the experiences of nurses and mothers with high-risk infants in the NICU, relative to the promotion of breast-feeding.

c. The underlying paradigm is constructivism (naturalism).

d. Yes, the study involved the collection of information through the senses (e.g., through conversations with nurses, through direct observation of practices in the NICU, and through scrutiny of documents in the NICU).

e. This study is best described as basic—to gain a better understanding of the structure and processes of the culture in a particular NICU. Interventions could, however, be designed that are based on the study findings.

f. No, this study is not cause probing per se. Qualitative studies seldom focus on causes and effects, although in-depth scrutiny of phenomena can sometimes suggest causal linkages.

g. The purpose of the study can be described as exploration into the everyday world of NICU processes and transactions, with emphasis on actions and interactions relating to breast-feeding.

h. This study addresses the evidence-based practice (EBP) question described in the textbook as "Meaning and Processes," i.e., developing an in-depth understanding of the NICU environment and processes.

CHAPTER 2

A. FILL IN THE BLANKS

1. guideline
2. Systematic
3. pilot
4. Cochrane
5. outcome
6. population
7. Therapy
8. AGREE
9. PICO
10. Meta-analysis
11. comparison
12. evidence hierarchy
13. intervention
14. meta-synthesis
15. Evidence-based practice (EBP)

B. MATCHING EXERCISES

1. c   2. b   3. c   4. b   5. d
6. a   7. a   8. b

C. STUDY QUESTIONS

C.1   a. I   b. P   c. C   d. I   e. O
       f. P   g. I   h. O   i. C   j. O

D. APPLICATION EXERCISES

Exercise C.1: Questions of Fact (Appendix C)

a. The purpose of the evidence-based project was to develop, implement, and evaluate the effectiveness of a standardized nursing procedure to increase the identification of depression in family members of active duty soldiers.

b. The setting for the project was a military family practice clinic located on a U.S. Army infantry post in Hawaii.

c. The project was guided by the Iowa Model of Evidence-Based Practice to Promote Quality Care.

d. The authors described the project as having *both* a problem-focused trigger and a knowledge-focused trigger. With regard to the former, the introduction indicated that "The absence in this clinic of a systematic method to screen family members of deployed soldiers for depression and the inability to estimate rates of depression in this clinical population were the problem-focused triggers for this project." The authors cited national standards and guidelines calling for the screening of all adults for depression in primary care settings as the knowledge-focused triggers.

e. There were 3 authors for this report, and presumably they were major team members on this project. Two authors were masters-prepared officers in the U.S. Army Nurse Corps, and the third was an instructor at the University of Hawaii. The article also indicates that a "multidisciplinary panel of stakeholders", which included advance practice registered nurses (APRNs), physicians, certified nurse assistants, RNs, a psychologist, and clinic administrators, formed the EBP team. It is not unusual for EBP project teams to comprise research and clinical staff and to be multidisciplinary.

f. The report did not discuss implementation at length, but it did state that the project team was led by a change champion (an APRN) and an opinion leader (a physician), who were persuasive and influential in the clinic. The article stated that "The EBP project received enthusiastic support throughout the organization and at the highest levels of nursing leadership".

g. Yes, the report described the study that was undertaken as a pilot study.

h. Yes, one of the purposes of this pilot study was to evaluate the effectiveness of the newly developed practice guideline for screening for depression.

Exercise C.2: Questions of Fact (Appendix G)

a. Yes, the article by Nam and colleagues described a systematic review undertaken to summarize evidence on culturally tailored educational interventions to promote improved glycemic control among ethnic minorities with Type 2 diabetes. Systematic reviews are an especially important type of preappraised evidence. The particular type of systematic review in this example was a meta-analysis.

b. The meta-analysis in this study integrated information from several studies, including randomized controlled trials (RCTs), and so evidence from this study would be at the top rung of the evidence hierarchy portrayed in Figure 2.1.

c. The researchers stated that "The aim of this study was to evaluate the

effectiveness of a culturally tailored diabetes educational intervention (CTDEI) on glycemic control in ethnic minorities with type 2 diabetes".

CHAPTER 3

A. FILL IN THE BLANKS

1. dependent
2. gain
3. data
4. sample
5. operational
6. theory
7. statistical
8. literature
9. emergent
10. experimental
11. trial
12. phenomenology
13. ethnography
14. saturation
15. Population
16. grounded
17. construct
18. effect
19. design
20. causal
21. themes
22. variable
23. participant
24. variable
25. independent
26. relationship
27. observational

B. MATCHING EXERCISES

B.1. 1. a 2. c 3. b 4. a 5. b
6. c 7. c 8. c 9. b 10. c

B.2. 1. b 2. c 3. a 4. c 5. c
6. b 7. d 8. d

B.3. 1. a 2. b 3. a 4. c 5. b
6. c 7. d 8. c 9. b 10. a

B.4. 1. c 2. b 3. a 4. a 5. b
6. d 7. e 8. b 9. c 10. d

C. STUDY QUESTIONS

C.2

a. Independent variable (IV) = participation versus nonparticipation in assertiveness training; dependent or outcome variable (DV) = psychiatric nurses' effectiveness

b. IV = patients' postural positioning; DV = respiratory function

c. IV= amount of touch by nursing staff; DV = patients' psychological well-being

d. IV = frequency of turning patients; DV = incidence of decubitus

e. IV = history of parents' abuse during their childhood; DV = parental abuse of their own children

f. IV = patients' age and gender; DV = tolerance for pain

g. IV= pregnant women's number of prenatal visits; DV = labor and delivery outcomes

h. IV = children's experience (vs. nonexperience) of a sibling death; DV = levels of depression

i. IV = gender; DV = compliance with a medical regimen

j. IV = participation versus nonparticipation in a support group among family caregivers of AIDS patients; DV = coping

k. IV = time of day; DV = elders' hearing acuity

l. IV = location of giving birth—home versus hospital; DV = parents' satisfaction with the childbirth experience

m. IV = type of diet in the outpatient setting among patients undergoing chemotherapy; DV = incidence of positive blood cultures

C.5.

a. An ethnographic study would not be experimental—no intervention would be introduced.

b. The independent variable is relaxation therapy (the intervention), and the dependent variable or outcome variable is pain.

c. Grounded theory studies are not clinical trials, which involve an intervention.

d. Study participants would not be exposed to an intervention in phenomenological studies.

e. In experimental studies, decisions about data collection would be made well before going out into the field to implement the intervention.

C.6.

a. Ethnographic
b. Phenomenological
c. Grounded theory

D. APPLICATION EXERCISES

Exercise D.1: Questions of Fact (Appendix D)

a. All four researchers were nurses, and three of them (Jurgens, Hoke, and Reigel) were doctorally prepared. The research team included a mix of nurses with primarily clinical responsibilities (Hoke) and academic jobs (e.g., Reigel). All four researchers worked in the northeast region of the United States (New York and Pennsylvania).

b. The study participants were elders with heart failure.

c. Participants were recruited from tertiary care hospitals in Philadelphia and New York. The data were collected in the patients' rooms at the hospitals.

d. It is not particularly easy to identify the independent variables in this study—and there are several of them. In the abstract, the researchers state that the purpose of the study was to examine "contextual factors related to symptom recognition and response," and it is a complex array of contextual factors that are independent variables—that is, the factors presumed to influence symptom recognition and delayed response. Later in the paper (just before the section labeled "Methods"), the authors indicated that a study purpose was to "determine the influence of sociodemographic, clinical, cognitive, emotional, and social contextual factors"—all of which can be considered independent variables—on symptom duration. A few specific examples include gender (sociodemographic), year of heart failure diagnosis (clinical), somatic perceptions (cognitive appraisal), anxiety (emotional), and marital status (social contextual). None of these variables are *inherently* independent variables.

e. The dependent variable in this study was duration of heart failure symptoms. This variable is not *inherently* a dependent variable—one could readily imagine studies that seek to ascertain what effect duration of symptoms has on other variables (e.g., length of stay in hospital, mortality and morbidity, etc.).

f. The report did not use the terms "independent variable" or "dependent variable" in describing the purpose of their research. However, in a paragraph in the Data Analysis subsection that is rather technical and that concerns potential problems with the data analysis, the authors did refer to the set of variables being assessed for their influence on symptom duration as independent variables.

g. Symptom duration was operationalized as duration of several specific symptoms, such as dyspnea, dyspnea on exertion, fatigue, edema, orthopnea, weight gain, and chest pain. These were measured as duration of symptom in *hours* "from the time a participant was first aware of symptoms until arrival at the hospital." (For the purpose of analysis and reporting, however, duration was measured in days rather than hours).

h. The data in this study were both quantitative and qualitative. The researchers administered a number of scales that yielded numeric information (e.g., somatic perceptions, anxiety) but also asked a number of broad questions in a conversational manner about factors involved in their decision to seek care.

i. Yes, the researchers investigated the relationship between the various "contextual factors" on the one hand and symptom duration on the other. In the context of this study, it is best to consider the relationships functional rather than causal—although it is certainly plausible that certain contextual factors *caused* delays in seeking care for the symptoms, and the authors' conceptual model suggests a causal pathway. One issue in this study is that the data were collected at a single point in time, and so it is not possible to sort out whether some of the contextual factors actually preceded symptom duration. Perhaps symptom duration affected anxiety rather than vice versa, for example.

j. This was a nonexperimental (observational) study.

k. There was no intervention in this study. The researchers captured characteristics of the study participants at one point in time without intervening in any way.

l. The study involved the statistical analysis of the quantitative data and qualitative analysis of the narrative data.

Exercise D.2: Questions of Fact (Appendix F)

a. There was only one researcher in this study—which is fairly rare in quantitative studies but more common in qualitative ones. Jeanne Cummings, a doctorally prepared nurse, was (at the time the article was published) a visiting professor in the City University of New York.

b. The study participants were 12 dyads of *storytellers* and *listeners*. The storytellers were people who had been involved in a widely publicized disaster—the crash landing of U.S. Airways Flight 1549 into the Hudson River in January, 2009. The listeners were people with whom the storytellers had shared the story of the traumatic event.

c. The context of the study was the crash landing of the airplane into the Hudson River. There was, however, no specific setting for the storytelling (which would have occurred in multiple, varied settings). Almost all study participants were interviewed in person (only three were interviewed over the telephone), but information about where the interviews took place was not provided.

d. The key concept was the storytelling aspect of a particular traumatic event.

e. No, there were no *independent variables* or *dependent variables* in this qualitative study.

f. The data for this study were qualitative.

g. Although this study did not explicitly focus on relationships, the analysis revealed that the nature of the relationship between the storyteller and the listener did "color" or affect the listener's and storyteller's experience during the telling of the story (Theme 5).

h. This study was described as an interpretive phenomenological study.

i. This study was nonexperimental.

j. There was no intervention in this study, as is usually the case in qualitative inquiries.

k. The study did not report any statistical information (e.g., the average age of the participants). The study involved the qualitative analysis of rich, narrative data.

CHAPTER 4

A. FILL IN THE BLANKS

1. Bias
2. title
3. reflexivity
4. level
5. trustworthy
6. significant
7. IMRAD
8. blinding (or masking)
9. abstract
10. confounding
11. journal
12. valid
13. inference
14. Reliability
15. control
16. Randomness
17. Transferability

B. MATCHING EXERCISES

1. c	2. d	3. b	4. a	5. c
6. e	7. d	8. b	9. c	10. e
11. b	12. d			

D. APPLICATION EXERCISES

Exercise D.1: Questions of Fact (Appendix A)

a. Yes, the structure of the Weinert and colleagues' article follows the IMRAD format. There is an Introduction that begins with the first words ("Chronic illness") and includes two subsections labeled "Background" and "Purpose." Then there are Methods, Results, and Discussion sections.

b. The abstract is a "new style" abstract with subheadings, as is now required for articles submitted to the journal *Nursing Research*, which published this paper.

c. Yes, the abstract includes all this information organized into sections called Background, Objective, Methods, Results, and Discussion.

d. The article is written in the passive voice. For example, the first sentence states that "The WTW study was approved and monitored by the University Institutional Review Board for the Protection of Human Subjects." In the active voice, this could be stated as follows: "The University's Institutional Review Board approved and monitored this research."

e. This study is experimental. The researchers intervened by offering a computer-based intervention to some chronically ill rural women who participated in the study but withholding it from others.

f. Yes, the abstract states that 309 middle-aged rural women who had chronic conditions were *randomized* into either the intervention group or a control group (in the paragraph on Methods).

Exercise D.2: Questions of Fact (Appendix E)

a. Yes, the report basically follows the IMRAD format. The first part of the article is the introduction, with a subsection labeled "Literature Review." The next section is called Methodology. The "Results" are labeled "Findings" in this paper, and the final section is the Discussion.

b. The abstract is a traditional narrative style abstract. The journal in which the article was published, *Qualitative Health Research,* requires an abstract of no more than 150 words with no subheadings. This abstract had 147 words.

c. The abstract indicates the study purpose in the first sentence ("to develop a theoretical framework about caregivers' experiences..."). Then there is a brief statement about methods (a grounded theory approach was used, and data were collected at three points in time with 18 caregivers). Key findings were then highlighted, and the last sentence notes that the findings have important implications for clinicians, researchers, educators, and decision makers.

d. The presentation is in both the active and the passive voice. As an example of the passive voice, the first sentence of the Methodology section states, "A constructivist grounded theory methodology *was used.*" The authors switched to the active voice in the first paragraph under the Data Collection subsection: "The first author conducted 45 face-to-face interviews..."

e. Yes, this study was a grounded theory study, which is appropriate for understanding social processes relating to a phenomenon. Here, the researchers were interested in understanding the processes in which spousal caregivers engaged during their spouses' transition from a geriatric rehabilitation unit to home.

CHAPTER 5

A. FILL IN THE BLANKS

1. codes
2. Anonymity
3. risk
4. Beneficence
5. Process consent
6. stipend

7. Belmont
8. misconduct
9. implied
10. assent
11. confidentiality
12. disclosure
13. institutional review board (IRB)
14. dilemma
15. vulnerable groups
16. Informed consent
17. Debriefing
18. minimal

B. MATCHING EXERCISES

1. d	2. b	3. c	4. b	5. a
6. d	7. b	8. a	9. c	10. a
11. b	12. d			

D. APPLICATION EXERCISES

Exercise D.1: Questions of Fact (Appendix D)

a. Yes, in the last paragraph of the "Sample" subsection, the researchers indicated that the study protocol was reviewed and approved by the IRBs of both Stony Brook University and the University of Pennsylvania.

b. No, the study participants were adults with a chronic illness and would not be considered "vulnerable."

c. There is no reason to suspect that participants were subjected to any physical harm or discomfort or psychological distress. Only people who were medically stable were eligible to participate in the study, as a precaution for avoiding undue stress. The content of the interview does not appear stressful, and the qualitative portion of the interview may have been mildly therapeutic because it gave participants a chance to share their thoughts and concerns.

d. It does not appear that participants were deceived in any way.

e. There is no reason to suspect any coercion was used to force unwilling people to participate in the study. Nineteen people who were recruited for the study declined to participate, suggesting that participation was truly voluntary.

f. The report indicated that written consent was obtained from all participants. It is not possible to determine the extent to which disclosure was "full," but there does not appear to be any reason to conceal information in this study.

g. The article did not indicate the steps the researchers took to protect the privacy and confidentiality of participants, but presumably adequate protections were in place, given that approval was given by two IRBs. Presumably, statements regarding privacy and confidentiality were made in the informed consent form.

Exercise D.2: Questions of Fact (Appendix B)

a. Yes, the report indicates that approval for the study was granted by the "Human Subjects' Committees," presumably the committee in the children's hospital where the study took place and perhaps also (because *Committees* is plural) the committee of Cricoo-Lizza's institutional affiliation at the time of the research.

b. The focus of the study was nurses in the NICU, not the mothers or their infants. The nurses would not be considered vulnerable.

c. Participants were not subjected to any physical harm or discomfort. Nurses were observed performing their normal duties. It is possible that there was a certain degree of self-consciousness when the study started, but it is likely that the nurses became accustomed to the presence of the researcher, who was probably considered a colleague.

d. Participants were probably not deceived. The article states that "information was provided to the nurses through the intranet, staff meetings, and individual encounters in the NICU." It might be noted, though, that observations were made "unobtrusively," meaning that nurses were not always aware that their

interactions with families were under direct scrutiny—and presumably families were not aware either. Notification about the observations undoubtedly would have affected the very interactions of interest, and behaviors would likely have been atypical, undermining the study purpose. The nurses under observation knew that Cricco-Lizza was a nurse researcher who was interested in learning about their perspectives on infant feeding.

e. It does not appear that any coercion was involved.

f. The report stated that the researcher obtained written informed consent from the 18 key informants who were formally interviewed. Informed consent was not obtained from the 114 nurses who were considered "general informants," nor from any family members.

g. Cricco-Lizza stated that the interviews with key informants took place in a private room near the NICU. She did not explicitly discuss who had access to the audiotaped interviews or the transcripts, but it seems safe to presume that they were safeguarded. No names were used in the article. When verbatim quotes were presented in the report, the researcher said things such as: "One nurse said" or "one key informant stated."

CHAPTER 6

A. FILL IN THE BLANKS

1. problem
2. statement of purpose
3. question
4. hypothesis
5. relation ship
6. test
7. independent
8. nondirectional
9. proof
10. two
11. simple
12. research
13. null

B. MATCHING EXERCISES

B.1. 1. b   2. c   3. a   4. b   5. a
        6. c   7. b   8. a

B.2. 1. a   2. c   3. d   4. a   5. b
        6. d   7. a   8. c   9. b   10. d
        11. b   12. c   13. b   14. a   15. c

C. STUDY QUESTIONS

C.4 Independent variable = I, dependent/outcome variable = O

2a. I = type of stimulation (tactile vs. verbal); O = physiological arousal

2b. I = infants' birthweight; O = hypoglycemia in term newborns

2c. I = use versus nonuse of isotonic sodium chloride solution; O = oxygen saturation

2d. I = patients' fluid balance; O = success in being weaned from mechanical ventilation

2e. I = patients' gender; O = amount of narcotic analgesics administered by nurses

3a. I = prior blood donation versus no prior donation; O = amount of anxiety

3b. I = amount of conversation initiated by nurses; O = patients' ratings of nursing effectiveness

3c. I = ratings of nurses' informativeness; O = amount of preoperative stress

3d. I = pregnancy status; O = incidence of peritoneal infection

3e. I = type of delivery (vaginal vs. cesarean) O = incidence of postpartum depression

D. APPLICATION EXERCISES

Exercise D.1: Questions of Fact (Appendix D)

a. The first two paragraphs of this report stated the essence of the problem—namely, that hospital readmissions for patients with heart failure (HF) are potentially preventable, and that patients delay responding to their HF symptoms.

b. The authors stated their purpose (their specific objectives) at the end of the introduction, in a subsection labeled "Conceptual Framework." Several purposes were stated, two of which were descriptive and involved use of the verb "describe": To *describe* the experience of and the cognitive and emotional responses to the symptoms of decompensated HF; and to *describe* self-care behaviors prior to seeking care for decompensated HF. These descriptive aims do not, in themselves, provide insight into whether a qualitative or quantitative approach would be used, and in fact these researchers gathered both qualitative and quantitative data. The third aim was to *determine* the influence of sociodemographic, clinical, cognitive, emotional, and social contextual factors on symptom duration. This aim is consistent with a quantitative study that examines relationships among variables, as was the case.

c. The article did not explicitly state research questions, although they could be inferred from the purpose statement. For example, the question corresponding to the first descriptive aim might be: What are the experiences of, and the cognitive and emotional responses to, the symptoms of decompensated HF?

d. No hypotheses were formally stated.

e. The aim concerning factors affecting symptom duration could be the basis for several hypotheses. For example, one of the factors being examined in relation to symptom duration was an emotional factor, anxiety. One directional hypothesis would be: Patients with HF who are less anxious will have longer duration of symptoms before seeking help than patients who are more anxious.

f. Yes, the researchers used hypothesis-testing statistical tests.

Exercise D.2: Questions of Fact (Appendix B)

a. The first paragraph indicated that the research focused on the problem of breast-feeding promotion in neonatal intensive care units (NICUs). The next two paragraphs elaborate on the problem, noting that maternity practices in the United States often impede breast-feeding and the uptake of evidence-based practice guidelines.

b. Cricco-Lizza stated the purpose in the abstract: "Purpose: This study explored the structure and process of breast-feeding promotion in the NICU." This statement is reiterated in the very first sentence of the report and again in the last sentence of the introduction.

c. Specific research questions were not articulated.

d. No hypotheses were stated—nor would one have been appropriate in this qualitative study.

e. No, no hypotheses were tested. Qualitative studies do not use statistical methods to test hypotheses.

CHAPTER 7

A. FILL IN THE BLANKS

1. primary
2. secondary
3. ancestry
4. bibliographic
5. keywords
6. CINAHL
7. MEDLINE®
8. Boolean
9. MeSH
10. PubMed
11. author

B. MATCHING EXERCISES

B.1. 1. d   2. b   3. c   4. b   5. a
         6. c   7. b   8. d

D. APPLICATION EXERCISES

Exercise D.1: Questions of Fact (Appendix G)

a. This review was a systematic review—a meta-analysis.

b. Yes, the introduction described a research problem that the researchers addressed. The problem might be stated as followed: diabetes is a major health problem in the United States and racial/ethnic minority population have a disproportionate burden of disease. There is little evidence that ethnic minority groups benefit from traditional diabetes education programs, perhaps because of providers' lack of cultural competency and their failure to address issues of relevance to these populations. Designing and evaluating culturally tailored programs have become priorities of the public health system, but findings about their effectiveness have not been systematically integrated.

c. Yes, there was a statement of purpose in the abstract and in the last sentence of the introduction: "The purpose of this meta-analysis was to bridge the gap by evaluating the effect of culturally tailored diabetes education (CTDE) on glycemic control in ethnic minorities with type 2 diabetes."

d. The researchers used six different electronic databases in their literature search (PubMed, CINAHL, ERIC, PsycInfo, ProQuest, and the Cochrane Collaboration database).

e. The key words were *type 2 diabetes, diabetes mellitus, health education, diabetes education, counseling, minority, ethnic minority, race,* and *behavioral intervention.* Additional subject heading terms were used (e.g., *patient education* and *intervention).* The terms concerned the population (ethnic minority, type 2 diabetes) and the independent variable (health education, diabetes education). It does not appear that the search included the dependent variable of concern, i.e., glycemic control.

f. Yes, the researchers restricted their search to English-language publications.

g. No, the researchers searched for both published and unpublished studies (e.g., dissertations).

h. Twelve studies were included in the meta-analysis

i. All studies included in the review were quantitative; meta-analyses integrate quantitative findings.

Exercise D.2: Questions of Fact (Appendix H)

a. Beck undertook a systematic review of qualitative studies relating to birth trauma—a type of metasynthesis that is called a metaethnography, as explained in more detail in Chapter 19. In this case, the metasynthesis involved synthesizing results from multiple analytic approaches in a research program by the same researcher (Beck).

b. The purpose of this metasynthesis was to integrate and amplify findings from qualitative studies on birth trauma and the resulting posttraumatic stress disorder. Beck indicated her purpose in the first paragraph.

c. This particular synthesis integrated information from qualitative studies on traumatic births that had previously been conducted by Beck herself in her extensive program of research on traumatic births.

d. Six of Beck's prior studies were included in this metasynthesis.

e. The six studies in the review included five phenomenological studies and one narrative analysis (see Chapter 14).

CHAPTER 8

A. FILL IN THE BLANKS

1. framework
2. conceptual
3. map
4. model
5. description
6. middle-range
7. human beings, environment, health, nursing
8. Pender

9. Parse
10. Rogers
11. Adaptation
12. self-efficacy

B. MATCHING EXERCISES

B.1. 1. c   2. e   3. d   4. e   5. d
          6. a   7. b   8. d

B.2. 1. c   2. d   3. g   4. a   5. f
          6. b   7. h   8. e

D. APPLICATION EXERCISES

Exercise D.1: Questions of Fact (Appendix D)

a. Jurgens and colleagues used as a conceptual framework the Self-Regulation Model of Illness. This model was developed by health psychologists, primarily Howard Leventhal. An overview of this model can be found on the Internet: http://media.wiley.com/product_data/excerpt/70/04700240/0470024070.pdf

b. The Self-Regulation model was not described in the textbook, but it is a model that has been used by other nurse researchers.

c. Yes, a schematic model of the Self-Regulation Model of Illness was included as Figure 1.

d. The key concepts in the model are (1) physical stimuli (e.g., symptoms); (2) cognitive representation of illness (e.g., perceived causes); (3) emotional representation of illness (e.g., anxiety); (4) coping; (5) appraisal of the situation; and (6) response to the physical stimuli (symptoms)—seeking care.

e. According to the model, the decision to seek care is *directly* affected by a person's *appraisal* of the health threat and efficacy of coping, which are developed along both cognitive and emotional pathways.

f. The decision to seek care is *indirectly* affected by all of the factors that lead to an appraisal of the health threat, including the physical symptoms themselves, the person's level of anxiety, perceptions of causes and consequences of the threat, and the person's coping skills.

g. The report did not articulate formal conceptual definitions of each construct in the model. For example, there is no conceptual definition of "coping" or "anxiety." Nevertheless, the overall model was fairly well explained in a section of the article labeled "Conceptual Framework."

h. No, the article did not present formal hypotheses deduced from the conceptual model. The researchers stated, "We propose that delay in seeking care is due to the difficulty that HF patients experience in discerning the quality and meaning of their symptoms." A formal hypothesis might be: "HF patients who are less well able to detect and interpret their symptoms are more likely to delay seeking care." The researchers also said that a goal was to "determine the influence of sociodemographic, clinical, cognitive, emotional, and social contextual factors on symptom duration during this time." They did not state a hypothesis predicting *which factors* might affect symptom duration, such as: "Symptom duration will be greater among those who are older and have higher levels of anxiety." Symptom duration, a major dependent variable in this study, is not the endpoint in the conceptual model.

Exercise D.2: Questions of Fact (Appendix E)

a. No, the authors did not describe any priori framework or theory that guided this research. For example, there was no mention of symbolic interactionism. Given space constraints in journals, however, this does not mean that the study lacked a conceptual framework.

b. Yes, the purpose of the study was to generate a theory that was grounded in the experiences of the study participants. The authors referred to their grounded theory as *Reconciling in response to fluctuating needs*.

c. Yes, Figure 1 of the report was a schematic model depicting the researchers' grounded theory. The figure was a good way to illustrate three overlapping phases of reconciling (*getting ready, getting into it,* and *getting on with it*), as well as three subprocesses of reconciliation: *navigating, safekeeping,* and *repositioning*.

d. Inasmuch as this was a grounded theory study, no hypotheses were tested. A grounded theory study sometimes results in the identification of hypotheses that can be tested in a future quantitative study.

CHAPTER 9

A. FILL IN THE BLANKS

1. validity
2. crossover
3. attrition
4. selection
5. random
6. blinding (or masking)
7. control
8. Mortality
9. prospective or cohort
10. statistical
11. internal
12. external
13. cross-sectional
14. counter factual
15. case–control
16. longitudinal
17. Matching
18. power
19. history threat
20. wait-listed
21. baseline
22. quasi-experiments
23. relationships
24. retrospective

B. MATCHING EXERCISES

B.1 1. b   2. b   3. a   4. d   5. b
       6. a   7. d   8. a   9. b   10. d

C. STUDY QUESTIONS

C.2   2.a. Both   2.b. Nonexperimental
        2.c. Both   2.d. Nonexperimental
                      2.e. Nonexperimental
                      3.a. Nonexperimental
        3.b. Both   3.c. Nonexperimental
                      3.d. Nonexperimental
                      3.e. Nonexperimental

D. APPLICATION EXERCISES

Exercise D.1: Questions of Fact (Appendix A)

a. Yes, the purpose of the study was to evaluate the effects of a computer-delivered intervention for chronically ill rural women.

b. The design for this study was experimental.

c. The manipulated independent variable was participation versus nonparticipation in the special intervention that was being evaluated for its efficacy. The dependent variables included several measures of psychosocial health, including social support, self-esteem, acceptance of illness, depression, stress, and loneliness.

d. Yes, randomization was used. Eligible participants were enrolled and then randomly assigned to either the computer intervention group or a control group, in 8 blocks of approximately 40 women (about 20 per group in each block).

e. The control group strategy in this study was the absence of a special intervention. The control group completed questionnaires but did not receive any special services, nor were control group members put on a waiting list to receive the intervention at a later point in time.

f. In this study, data were collected from experimental and control group members both before and after the intervention. Thus, we could call the design a pretest–posttest (before–after) experimental design. (Because there were two points of data collection after the intervention—immediately postintervention and then 6 months later—we could also refer to this design as a *repeated measures design*, a term not mentioned in the textbook.)

g. The article states (in the subsection labeled "Design") that "the research staff was not blinded to the participant groups, and certainly the participants themselves knew whether or not they were in the group receiving the intervention."

h. The data were collected three times (before the intervention, immediately after it [approximately 3 months after baseline], and then 6 months later). Because Weinert and colleagues assessed the long-term effects of the intervention, the study can be considered longitudinal.

i. Weinert and colleagues used three methods to control confounding variables, the most important of which was randomization to groups. The researchers also used statistical control, although this may not be easy for students to understand. In the subsection on analysis, the authors indicated that they used an analysis in which the participants' score on each outcome at baseline (e.g., baseline stress) was statistically controlled in the analysis of postintervention outcomes (e.g., postintervention stress). Finally, another method (although this method was not explicitly used as a control method) was homogeneity. All of the study participants were women (not men), lived in rural areas (not urban or suburban areas), and had a chronic (not acute) illness.

j. Through randomization, virtually all participant characteristics (e.g., age, income, marital status, type of chronic illness, etc.) would have been controlled. Through statistical control, initial levels of each outcome were controlled. Through homogeneity, gender, area of residence, and acute versus chronic illness were controlled (i.e., held constant).

k. Yes, there was attrition. As shown in Figure 1, only 118 out of 155 initial members of the experimental group (76%) completed the intervention and both intervention assessments. In the control group, 132 out of 154 initial members (86%) completed all assessments. Thus, the overall rate of attrition was 19% (59 ÷ 309).

l. In this study, it would have been difficult to achieve constancy of conditions. The intervention itself was delivered in a manner that made it possible for women in the treatment group to participate at any convenient time (or to *not* participate). Researchers had no control over such factors as privacy, comfort, time of day the intervention was used, etc. Data were collected via self-administered questionnaire, and again there would have been no opportunity to ensure that conditions were constant or even similar. On the other hand, by having a standardized Internet-based program, the researchers had control over some aspects that would be difficult to achieve if the intervention had been delivered "live" in various community settings.

m. As noted in the previous question, the researchers did not have much control over the intervention, except to offer it to those in the experimental group and withhold it from those in the control group. It would have been possible for those in the treatment group to get virtually no intervention, and it might have been possible for those in the control group to get alternative (and varying) forms of social support and health-related information. Given the decentralized nature of the intervention, this was not an aspect over which researchers had control.

Exercise D.2: Questions of Fact (Appendix D)

a. No, there was no intervention in this study.

b. The study design was nonexperimental.

c. As noted in our comments in Chapter 3, identifying the independent variables in this study is not straightforward. In essence, the independent variables are various factors hypothesized to influence the dependent variable (delayed response), such as year of heart failure diagnosis, cognitive appraisal, and so on.

d. No, the researchers could not have experimentally manipulated any of the contextual independent variables.

e. The researchers stated that their design was mixed methods, a design we discuss in Chapter 18. The quantitative portion of the study used a descriptive correlational design.

f. No, there was no randomization in this study. Matching was not used either. Homogeneity was used to a certain extent—for example, all study participants were elders who had been diagnosed with heart failure. The analysis section is likely too complex for most of you at this point, but we can point out that the researchers did use statistical methods to control a few of the participants' background characteristics, such as age and gender (although these were not really *controlled* because the researchers had a substantive interest in these variables).

g. No, there was no blinding in this study. Blinding is seldom used in nonexperimental studies, although it is possible (and sometimes advisable) to use blinding with the people collecting data in a nonexperimental study—that is, to not tell them the study hypotheses.

h. This study was cross-sectional. All data were collected at a single point in time.

i. Jurgens and colleagues were asking a Cause/Etiology question: What are the factors that can contribute to a delayed response in seeking help for heart failure symptoms?

CHAPTER 10

A. FILL IN THE BLANKS

1. Consecutive
2. eligibility
3. size
4. population
5. strata
6. quota
7. target
8. probability
9. representativeness
10. Convenience
11. random
12. bias
13. systematic
14. power analysis
15. self-report
16. closed-ended
17. open-ended
18. scale
19. interview
20. Likert
21. visual
22. set
23. social
24. observational
25. checklist
26. Time

B. MATCHING EXERCISES

B.1 1. c   2. a   3. d   4. b   5. d
6. b   7. c   8. d   9. a   10. b

B.2 1. a, c   2. a, b   3. b, c
4. b   5. b   6. a, b, c
7. a, b, c   8. a, b

B.3 1. b   2. a   3. c   4. d   5. a
6. b   7. c   8. b

C. STUDY QUESTIONS

C.1

a. Simple random
b. Convenience
c. Systematic
d. Quota
e. Purposive
f. Consecutive

C.2

The sampling interval is 20. After the first element (23) is selected, the next three would be 43, 63, and 83.

D. APPLICATION EXERCISES

Exercise D.1: Questions of Fact

a. None of the studies in the appendices used probability samples of participants. However, in the Yackel et al. study, one outcome (compliance with documentation) was measured by means of an audit of randomly sampled charts.

b. The quantitative studies in the Appendices A and E used convenience sampling.

c. It appears that the pilot test of the EBP project described in Appendix C used consecutive sampling—i.e., all eligible patients within a certain time frame.

Exercise D.2: Questions of Fact

a. All three studies in these appendices used structured self-reports as a method of data collection. Weinert and colleagues used mailed questionnaires, and these questionnaires incorporated several psychosocial scales. Yackel and colleagues gathered data on the satisfaction of providers and nursing staff with regard to the screening program using a self-report item, measured on a Likert scale (described in the "Results" section). Jurgens administered several psychosocial scales, presumably in a paper-and-pencil format, and also interviewed study participants. The dependent variable—length of time to respond to symptoms—was quantified based on information obtained in the interview.

b. In both the Weinert and the Yackel et al. studies, it appears that observational methods were used to monitor intervention fidelity, although these methods were not described in detail and the data were not used to capture independent or dependent variables.

c. None of the three studies involved the collection of biophysiologic data specifically to address the study questions.

d. Records were used extensively in the Yackel study. For example, the primary outcome was how many patients were screened positive for depression before and after the screening program was implemented, and these data were obtained from records. Nurse compliance in documentation was assessed by means of an audit of randomly selected charts. Time-and-motion data for the length of time it took to screen patients were also obtained through records. In the Jurgens et al. study, the researchers used medical records to derive a NYHA functional class.

Exercise D.3: Questions of Fact (Appendix D)

a. The target population was elders with heart failure (presumably those living in northeast regions of the United States). The accessible population was elders with heart failure (HF) who were hospitalized in one of two hospitals, one located in New York and the other in Philadelphia.

b. To be eligible for this study, people had to be 65 or older, cognitively intact, medically stable, fluent in English, willing to provide consent, with a confirmed diagnosis of HF but living independently in the community, and able to manage their illness.

c. The sampling method was the most widely used type of nonprobability sampling, convenience sampling.

d. The article does not provide much information about methods used to recruit participants. All participants were patients hospitalized in an emergency department or as inpatients, and presumably health care staff (or one of the researchers) approached potentially eligible patients and invited them to participate.

e. It appears that a total of 96 patients were invited to participate, 19 of whom declined, for a response rate

of 80% (Information about refusers is at the end of the subsection labeled "Study Sample.").

f. The sample size in this study was 77 patients with HF. Participants were enrolled over a 19-month period, from October 2004 to May 2006.

g. Yes, the article states that a power analysis was performed, but the details of this power analysis were not described. The researchers concluded that a sample size of 77 was adequate for an exploratory study. (However, later in the paper, in discussing the study's strengths and limitations, the authors acknowledged that the sample was "limited for quantitative analysis."

h. Yes, the section labeled "Study Sample" and Table 2 summarize some of the major demographic and clinical characteristics of the sample. The sample was about evenly split in terms of gender and married versus unmarried. The majority of patients were non-Hispanic whites with at least a high school diploma. Only a minority had a household income of $40,000 or greater. Functional capacity tended to be low, and the average amount of time since HF diagnosis was about 5 years.

i. The authors adapted several existing scales, making modifications that improved the scales' usefulness in this research. For example, they used a scale called the Heart Failure Somatic Perception Scale to assess perceived symptom severity. The original scale had 12 items, but the researchers developed 5 additional items and administered the full 17-item scale. Modifications were also made to the Responses to Symptoms Questionnaire. Some items were deleted, and a few items were reworded.

j. The article does not provide much information on who collected the data, nor on how they were trained. (In the section on "Limitations" at the end of the paper, the authors hint that the data were collected by research assistants).

CHAPTER 11

A. FILL IN THE BLANKS

1. ordinal
2. ratio
3. nominal
4. interval
5. rules
6. internal
7. psychometric
8. error
9. true
10. Reliability
11. test–retest
12. observer
13. alpha
14. validity
15. content
16. criterion
17. groups
18. sensitivity
19. specificity
20. cutoff

B. MATCHING EXERCISES

B.1
1. d	2. a	3. d	4. b	5. c
6. a	7. b	8. d	9. c	10. b
11. b	12. a			

B.2
1. a	2. c	3. d	4. c	5. b
6. b	7. a	8. c		

C. STUDY QUESTIONS

C.1

Two of these attributes—attitudes toward abortion and achievement motivation—are sufficiently enduring that they are unlikely to change markedly from one month to the next, unless there was an intervention specifically designed to modify them. Thus, the test–retest approach would be an appropriate method of assessing reliability for these two traits. Nursing effectiveness is likely to be fairly stable, but *might* be modified over a 1-month period, depending on the nurses' amount of experience and any intervening instruction or activities. The reliability of measures of stress and depression should not be assessed with a test–retest method (unless the time frames are quite short) because both these traits can fluctuate and be modified over time.

C.3

a. High reliability of an instrument is necessary for strong validity, but it does not guarantee it.
b. The internal consistency of an instrument does not address whether it yields stable measurements over time.
c. The low validity coefficient could reflect a problem with the criterion measure rather than with the scale. For example, if the criterion had low reliability, this would depress the validity coefficient.
d. A true score can never be known. A reliability coefficient provides information about how good an approximation a *set* of obtained scores will be, on average, in representing true scores, but an individual true score cannot be inferred.
e. Validation efforts lend evidence in support of an inference of construct validity, but no amount of evidence *proves* construct validity.
f. Expert opinions yield one type of evidence about the validity of a measure, but one person's opinion would never yield sufficient *assurance*.

C.4.

a. The 15-item scale would likely be more reliable; longer scales are usually more reliable than shorter ones.
b. Stress would likely be more uniformly high among patients just diagnosed with cancer; the higher similarity of these scores would tend to depress reliability because it would be harder to reliably discriminate among people with high levels of stress.

c. Nursing knowledge would probably be more varied among seniors (some of whom have mastered nursing content and others of whom have not) than among freshmen. Therefore, reliability would be expected to be higher among senior students.

D. APPLICATION EXERCISES

Exercise D.1: Questions of Fact

The levels of measurement of key variables in the two studies in Appendices A and D are shown in the following table:

Exercise D.2: Questions of Fact (Appendix A)

a. All of the scales used in the Weinert et al. study were assessed for internal consistency reliability using Cronbach alpha, both by previous researchers and by the study team itself. The reliability coefficients were all presented in Table 1, in column 4 as published in other reports ("Reported α") and then in column 5 for this study ("Study α"). As computed using study data, the values of alpha were as follows: The Personal Resource

Level of Measurement	Appendix A, Weinert et al.[a]	Appendix D, Jurgens et al.
Nominal	Receipt/nonreceipt of computer intervention; race; marital status; type of chronic illness; children in the home or not	Presence/absence of specific symptoms; gender; race/ethnicity; marital status; types of comorbid illnesses; having had a prior hospital admission for heart failure (HF)
Ordinal	Income category	Scores on individual items on the "Response to Symptoms Questionnaire;" functional performance class (1 to 4); comorbidity categories (low, medium, high); education; total household income category
Interval	Social support (scores on Personal Resource Questionnaire); self-esteem (scores on Rosenberg Self-Esteem Scale); acceptance of illness (scores on Acceptance of Illness Scale); stress (scores on Perceived Stress Scale); depression (scores on Center for Epidemiological Studies-Depression scale); loneliness (UCLA Loneliness Scale)	Perceived symptom distress (scores on Heart Failure Somatic Perception Scale and subscales)
Ratio	Age, education (years of schooling); number of hours of work per week; years since diagnosis of chronic health condition	Duration of various symptoms before hospitalization (in hours); time since HF diagnosis; age

[a]Table 2 lists a variable, "degree of difficulty with vision, hearing, mobility, pain, fatigue, and coordination;" this variable was not described but would have been measured on an ordinal or interval scale.

Questionnaire: .93; Self-Esteem Scale: .90; Acceptance of Illness scale: .82; Perceived Stress Scale: .90; CES-D Depression Scale: .92; and UCLA Loneliness Scale: .92. It is quite likely that several of these measures had also been assessed for test–retest reliability, but this information was not presented in the report.

b. The researchers selected instruments that have a strong reputation, and all had undergone some type of formal validity assessments. As shown in Table 1, the Acceptance of Illness scale had undergone content validation. All the others had been assessed for construct validity (convergent and divergent validation, not described in the textbook, are approaches to construct validation).

c. Weinert and colleagues reported reliability assessments from other researchers, but they also computed Cronbach alphas using data in their own study. There was no discussion of validation of the scales within this study, but the positive intervention effects observed in this study, which were consistent with the researchers' conceptual model, offer some further evidence of the instruments' validity.

d. No, there was no information about the specificity or sensitivity of any of the instruments used in this study. (The reference to sensitivity analyses in the Results section is unrelated to the characteristics of any measure; this analysis strategy is discussed in a later chapter).

CHAPTER 12

A. FILL IN THE BLANKS

1. Inferential
2. negative, positive

3. unimodal, bimodal
4. normal
5. symmetric
6. mean
7. mode
8. variability
9. standard
10. range
11. cross-tab (or contingency)
12. Odds ratio
13. standard error of the mean (SEM)
14. Alpha
15. nonparametric
16. Type I
17. Type II
18. beta, power
19. positive
20. N
21. level
22. t-test
23. confidence
24. analysis of variance (ANOVA)
25. effect
26. correlation
27. power
28. Pearson's r
29. chi-squared
30. regression
31. analysis of covariance
32. Cohen's d or the d statistic
33. Logistic

B. MATCHING EXERCISES

B.1   1. b   2. a   3. c   4. d   5. b
         6. b   7. a   8. a   9. c   10. a

C. STUDY QUESTIONS

C.1.
Unimodal, fairly symmetric

C.2.
Mean: 81.8; Median: 83; Mode: 84

C.3.

| | Gender | | | | Total | |
| | Girls | | Boys | | | |
Status	n	%	n	%	n	%
OBSERVED FREQUENCIES FOR CHILDREN WITH LACTOSE INTOLERANCE						
Lactose Intolerant	16	26.7	12	20.0	28	23.3
Not Lactose Intolerant	44	73.3	48	80.0	92	76.7
TOTAL	60	100.0	60	100.0	120	100.0

C.4. Absolute Risk, exposed group (AR_E) = .60; Absolute Risk, nonexposed group (AR_{NE}) =.90; Absolute Risk Reduction (ARR) = .30; Odds Ratio (OR) = .167

C.7.   a. Chi-squared   b. *t*-test
   c. Pearson's *r*   d. ANOVA

C.8.   a. Logistic regression   b. ANCOVA
   c. MANOVA   d. Multiple regression

D. APPLICATION EXERCISES

Exercise D.1: Questions of Fact

a. All three of the studies reported some percentages. Weinert et al., for example, reported many demographic characteristics of their sample as percentages in Table 2 (e.g., percent Caucasian, 93% in the intervention group, and 89% in the control group). Yackel et al. reported satisfaction with the screening program in percentages (e.g., 95% of nurses strongly agreed that screening enhanced quality of care 1 year after program implementation). Jurgens et al. reported some background characteristics (Table 2) and symptom prevalence (Table 3) as percentages (e.g., 88% of participants reported dyspnea).

b. All three studies reported means. Weinert et al. reported several means and standard deviations (SDs)—for example, for age (for the intervention group, M = 56.1, SD = 7.7) and years of schooling (for the intervention group, M = 14.8, SD = 2.4). Yackel and colleagues reported some means but not standard deviations; for example, they reported that the mean time added per patient encounter after the screening program was introduced was 2 minutes, 53 seconds. Jurgens et al. also reported means and SDs. For example, Table 4 presents this information for six scores on scales measuring physical, cognitive, and emotional response (e.g., for symptom anxiety, M = 2.84, SD = 1.28).

c. Yackel et al. did not report medians, but the other two research teams did. Weinert et al. reported the median age of participants (56 years) in the text, and some medians are also shown in Table 2 (e.g., the median number of years since the onset of symptoms was 13 in the intervention group). In the Jurgens et al. study, Table 3 presents the median duration of various symptoms, in days, before hospital admission. Jurgens et al. noted that median duration rather than means was reported because there were extreme values (outliers) for duration that skewed the distribution.

d. Consistent with the fact that modes tend to be unstable indexes of central tendency and not used frequently, only one article reported a mode. Weinert and colleagues noted that the modal age of study participants was 60 years, suggesting a negative skew to the age distribution.

Exercise D.2: Questions of Fact (Appendix A)

a. The baseline characteristics of the two groups were presented in Table 2. The researchers did perform statistical tests to assess the comparability of the two groups with regard to the six outcome variables, but the results were not reported in a straightforward fashion (they are shown in Figure 3, as will be discussed in question d). If statistical tests were performed to compare the baseline demographic characteristics of the two groups, these were not presented in the report. Perusing Table 2, it appears that the two groups were fairly comparable in most respects at baseline (although only a statistical test would be conclusive). For example, the two groups were similar in age, marital status, and education, and with regard to baseline scores on key outcomes, such as self-esteem and loneliness. The appropriate statistical tests for comparing the two groups at baseline would be t-tests (for comparing differences in means) and chi-square tests (comparing differences in percentages).

b. As shown in the flow chart in Figure 1, there was a higher rate of attrition in the intervention group than in the control group (23.9% and 14.3%, respectively), and this difference was statistically significant, $p = .024$. The researchers explained (in the subsection called "Sensitivity Analysis") that they did examine differences in the baseline characteristics of participants who stayed in or dropped out of the study. In most respects, dropouts and completers were similar, but divorcees and homemakers were more likely to drop out of the study, regardless of treatment group. Women with higher levels of social support were more likely to drop out of the intervention group, while those with high scores on the loneliness scale were more likely to stay in the intervention group. Thus, different factors appear to have played a role in dropping out of the study in the two groups.

c. The authors used logistic regression to assess factors affecting the risk of dropping out of the study. In this case, their dependent variable was drop out status (either the participant dropped out or not), and characteristics of the women were used as predictors (independent variables).

d. The main analysis used to compare the efficacy of the computer intervention was analysis of covariance. The researchers used treatment group status as the independent variable, the 6-month scores on the six primary outcomes as the dependent variables, and the baseline scores for each outcome as the covariate. In other words, in addition to controlling confounding variables through randomization, the researchers further strengthened the internal validity of the study by controlling baseline traits through statistical procedures.

e. Yes, in Figure 3, the researchers plotted the mean values of the six outcome variables separately for each group for the three points of data collection, shown as dots. The vertical lines extending from the dots represent the 95% confidence intervals. These are most clearly seen in the graph for depression. At baseline, the two groups had similar levels of depression, and the overlapping CI lines indicate that the two groups were not significantly different (as noted in our comments for question a). At the 12-week point, the means for the two groups are quite different, and the 95% CI lines do not overlap, indicating a significant difference. The group difference in depression diminishes somewhat at 24 weeks, but again the nonoverlapping 95% CI bands indicate a significant difference.

f. Referring to Table 3:
   • The mean scores for the two groups were significantly different (at the conventional .05 level) for all outcomes except social support. For this outcome, the p value, as shown in the far-right column, was .097. This means that nearly once out of 10 times, a mean difference as large as that observed could occur by chance alone, which is an unacceptable risk

of a Type I error. All other p values are less than .05, and several of them were considerably less than .05.

- The significance level for the group differences was most pronounced for the outcome acceptance of illness: $p = .001$, only 1 chance in 1,000 that a group difference of the magnitude observed was spurious.
- For the Loneliness scale, the mean score for those in the intervention group was 43.2, compared to 44.6 for the control group. The difference between the two mean scores was −1.8, i.e., those in the intervention group scored nearly 2 points lower than those in the control group on loneliness.
- The 95% CI around the mean difference of 1.2 on the self-esteem scale was from 0.2 to 2.1. Because this interval does not include the value of 0.0, this indicates that the group means were significantly different at the .05 level. The *actual p* value, shown in the far right column, is .018: only 18 times out of 1,000 would a mean difference this large be the result of chance alone.

g. The report did not indicate that a power analysis was done to estimate sample size needs. However, the report also indicates that a fuller description of the project was provided in an earlier publication, and it is possible that information about a power analysis was included there.

CHAPTER 13

A. FILL IN THE BLANKS

1. interpretation
2. correlation
3. Effect
4. CONSORT
5. mixed
6. limitations
7. hypothesis
8. precision
9. discussion
10. significant

B. MATCHING EXERCISES

1. b   2. a   3. e   4. d   5. c
6. a, d   7. a   8. e

D. APPLICATION EXERCISES

Exercise D.1: Questions of Fact (Appendix A)

a. Yes, Figure 1 was a CONSORT-type flow chart that showed that 327 women were screened for the study and 309 were randomized. The chart then shows, for both the intervention and control groups, the numbers that were allocated to each group, the number followed-up at the end of the intervention, and the number that completed the final assessment at 6 months.

b. Baseline values on the key demographic and outcome variables were presented in Table 2 for both experimental and control group members, but neither the table nor the text specifically discussed the baseline comparability of the two groups. As noted in Chapter 12, however, we can see from the six graphs in Figure 3 that the two groups were comparable on all six outcome variables at baseline, because the vertical lines for the 95% CI for the two groups overlap.

c. There was attrition, and there were significantly different rates of attrition in the two groups (24% in the intervention group and 14% in the control group). The researchers did do an analysis to identify potential attrition biases. Moreover, they did a *sensitivity analysis* to assess whether the beneficial effects in the intervention group might have been a consequence of differential attrition. Although their procedure is too complex to discuss in detail here, suffice it to say that their sensitivity analysis suggested that the positive intervention effects did not reflect group differences in attrition.

d. Hypotheses with regard to the effects of the intervention were not formally stated, although they were clearly implied. Results were mixed—there were intervention effects for five outcomes but not for social support. There were, however, group differences on the social support scale in the predicted direction (and differences *were* significant at the first follow-up.) It is possible that the differences would have been significant at 24 weeks with a larger sample, but it is also possible that the beneficial effects deteriorated over time.

e. Yes, there was information about the precision of estimates of group differences; confidence intervals around the group differences for the six outcomes were presented in Table 3.

f. Conventional effect size estimates summarizing the magnitude of the intervention effects were not presented in the report. Table 3 has a column that is labeled *Intervention Effect*, but the information in this column is not the Cohen's *d* statistic that is widely used as the standardized measure of an effect size. The researchers reported the effect as the difference in mean group scores, after adjusting for baseline scores. Cohen's *d* is calculated by dividing the mean difference by the pooled standard deviation. Doing this makes it possible to compare effect sizes for outcomes with different measurement units—for example, an effect size for a body mass index can be compared to an effect size for blood pressure, heart rate, or scores on a depression scale.

g. There was no explicit discussion about internal validity in the Discussion section.

h. There was no explicit discussion about external validity or generalizability in the Discussion section. However, at the end of the Discussion, they noted that they have made many modifications to the intervention over the 15 years of the overall project, and that they expect the intervention to be adaptable clinically, implying their belief that the intervention can be used in other contexts.

i. There was no explicit discussion about statistical conclusion validity in the Discussion section. The researchers did not comment on factors that could affect statistical conclusion validity,

such as the adequacy of the sample size or intervention fidelity. However, given that significant effects were observed for almost all outcomes, we can be reasonably confident that the researchers attained statistical conclusion validity.

j. No, the findings were not discussed vis-à-vis findings from earlier research.

k. No, limitations of the study were not discussed.

Exercise D.2: Questions of Fact (Appendix D)

a. Attrition is not an issue in studies that collect data only at one point in time—except when there is a time lag between when people agree to participate and when they actually provide the study data. In this case, it appears that recruitment, informed consent, and actual completion of the questionnaires occurred virtually simultaneously.

b. Yes, the authors did an analysis for response bias. They compared the demographic and clinical characteristics of the 77 patients who participated in the study and the 19 who declined. The two groups did not differ significantly on any characteristic examined. The authors also mentioned the possibility of recall bias with regard to their method of obtaining data for their outcome, time to respond to their heart failure symptoms. They noted that with careful questioning and probing, recall bias can be minimized.

c. Hypotheses were not formally stated in the introduction of this article, and yet hypotheses were implied (by virtue of their conceptual model) and tested statistically. The study, however, is described as descriptive and exploratory, and so the results were not discussed as having supported or refuted the researchers' expectations.

d. Precision was not addressed—i.e., there were no confidence intervals.

e. The researchers did not specifically use effect-size language in discussing their results. But the value of R^2 can be directly interpreted as an effect size. The value of R^2 (.29) would be considered moderate. That is, the five predictors shown in Table 5 (age, gender, symptom distress, seriousness, and anxiety) had a moderately strong relationship with duration of dyspnea before seeking help.

f. The article did not discuss internal validity. Although the conceptual model suggests a causal chain, the authors avoided using causal language.

g. The authors did mention that the generalizability of the findings was limited because the sample was small and predominantly white.

h. The researchers did note that the small sample size was a limitation of their study. Small samples lead to analyses that are not sufficiently powerful to detect true (but modest) relationships.

i. Yes, the researchers did tie their findings to findings from earlier research, discussed in the last two paragraphs of the main Discussion section.

j. Yes, some important limitations of the study were explicitly noted in the Discussion section, as well as some strengths.

CHAPTER 14

A. FILL IN THE BLANKS

1. action
2. Ethnonursing
3. narrative
4. Feminist
5. Glaser, Strauss
6. participant
7. basic
8. lived
9. historical
10. Interpretive, hermeneutics
11. essence
12. constant
13. informants
14. critical
15. case
16. bracketing

B. MATCHING EXERCISES

B.1. 1. b   2. a   3. d   4. c   5. b
         6. a   7. b   8. c   9. d   10. c
         11. a   12. d

C. STUDY QUESTIONS

C.1.
a. Grounded theory
b. Ethnography
c. Phenomenology
d. Hermeneutics (Phenomenology)

D. APPLICATION EXERCISES

Exercise D.1: Questions of Fact (Appendix E)

a. The research by Byrne and colleagues was a grounded theory study.

b. The researchers used the Charmaz approach to grounded theory, a constructivist approach, as described in the first paragraph under "Methodology." They cited two of Glaser's writings in the section on Data Analysis.

c. The central phenomenon studied in this project was the care transition experiences of spousal caregivers when their spouses moved from a geriatric rehabilitation unit to home.

d. the study was longitudinal. Byrne and colleagues collected data from most study participants (15 out of 18) at multiple points in time to better understand the transition experience. The intent was to interview participants three times: 48 hours after discharge from the geriatric unit, 2 weeks after discharge, and 4 to 6 weeks after discharge.

e. This study was conducted in Ontario, Canada. Families were recruited through a long-term care hospital. Data were collected in the participants' homes.

f. Yes, in the Analysis subsection, the researchers stated that they used "the constant comparative method with all units of data." They also elaborated: "Constant comparison entailed comparing incident to incident and comparing incidents over time between and within participants."

g. Yes, Byrne and colleagues identified the basic social process as *reconciling in response to fluctuating needs*. (The authors did not, however, specifically describe the basic problem that caregivers experience during the spouses' transition from the geriatric rehabilitation unit to home.)

h. The methods used in this study were congruent with a grounded theory approach. The researchers conducted lengthy conversational interviews at multiple points in time with 18 caregivers whose spouses were transitioning from a geriatric rehabilitation unit. In addition, the researchers made observations of the interactions between the spouses and care recipients prior to, during, and after the interviews. As noted previously, constant comparison was used in analyzing the rich data.

i. No, this study did not have an ideologic perspective. Even if all of the study participants had been female (which they were not), gender was not a key construct in helping the researchers interpret the data—although the authors did discuss gender differences in the Discussion section of their paper.

Exercise D.2: Questions of Fact (Appendix F)

a. The study by Cummings was a phenomenological study, based in the interpretive phenomenological school of inquiry.

b. The central phenomenon of this study was the actual experience of listeners and storytellers when a traumatic event is being communicated within the dyad.

c. This study was cross-sectional. Interviews were conducted at a single point in time with the storytellers and the listeners.

d. The context for the study was the crash landing of U.S. Airways Flight 1549 in the Hudson River on January 15, 2009.

The researcher conducted interviews with 12 people who were on the flight (storytellers) and 12 friends or family members to whom they told their stories, mostly face-to-face. The settings and locations of the interviews were not described.

e. Even though the study involves two groups of people, storytellers and listeners, the focus was not on comparing their experiences—the focus was on the *sharing* of a traumatic event.

f. The in-depth interviewing methods used in this study were well suited to answering the research questions and were congruent with interpretive phenomenology. The researcher noted that she reached saturation (obtained redundant information) after interviewing 9 dyads, but interviews with an additional 3 dyads helped to confirm saturation.

g. No, there was no ideological perspective in this study.

CHAPTER 15

A. FILL IN THE BLANKS

1. Snowball or network
2. Theoretical
3. purposive or purposeful
4. maximum
5. saturation
6. critical
7. Photo elicitation
8. topic
9. semi-structured
10. unstructured
11. Photovoice
12. field, log
13. focus group

B. MATCHING EXERCISES

B.1. 1. b   2. c   3. a   4. d   5. a
        6. c   7. a   8. a   9. d   10. b

B.2. 1. a   2. a   3. b   4. c   5. a
        6. c   7. b   8. c   9. c   10. a

D. APPLICATION EXERCISES

Exercise D.1: Questions of Fact (Appendix B)

a. Specific eligibility criteria were not stated in this report. All of the study participants were nurses who worked "in a level IV NICU in a freestanding children's hospital in the Northeastern United States."

b. The article stated that study information was provided to the nurses through staff meetings, the hospital's intranet, and individual encounters in the NICU. The article did not discuss specific recruitment procedures.

c. The article implied that maximum variation was used in sampling nurses: informants "were selected for maximal variety of infant feeding and NICU experiences." There is a further statement that nurses were "purposively selected to provide a wide angle view of breast-feeding promotion."

d. The sample included 114 nurses who were general informants, out of 250 nurses employed in the NICU. For this general sample, 18 key informants were chosen who were followed more intensively and interviewed in depth.

e. The article did not mention data saturation.

f. The article described background characteristics of the nurses in the sample. For example, of the 114 general informants, 96 were white, and all but one were female. Among the 18 key informants, the mean age was 33, with a range between 22 and 51 years of age. There was also diversity in terms of education (from diploma to a master's degree) and level of expertise, from novice to clinical expert.

g. Yes, the study involved in-depth unstructured interviews with the 18 key informants in this study, who were nurses working in the NICU. In addition to formal interviews, the key informants were informally interviewed several times over the course of the study.

h. The article did not describe the interviews in detail. The formal interviews involved "open-ended questions," which presumably means that a semi-structured format was used—that is, the interviewer asked a set of predetermined questions. It seems likely that for the informal interviews, an unstructured format was used—that is, questioning was probably more ad hoc and was triggered by an event or activity that the researcher had observed.

i. No, examples of the questions asked in the interviews were not provided.

j. The article stated that the formal interviews lasted 1 hour.

k. The interviews were tape-recorded and subsequently transcribed verbatim.

l. Yes, participant observation was an important source of data in this study. There were a total of 128 observation sessions that lasted between 1 and 2 hours. The observations focused on "the nurses' behaviors during interactions with babies, families, nurses, and other healthcare professionals throughout everyday NICU activities." Examples included infant feedings, shift reports, and nurse-led breast-feeding support groups.

m. The article stated that "all observational and informal interview data were documented immediately after each session," presumably onto a computer file or in a handwritten set of notes.

n. The researcher gathered additional data through documents, such as breast-feeding standards of care, teaching plans, and written policies and procedures.

o. Cricco-Lizza herself collected the study data. The article stated that "the investigator introduced herself as a nurse researcher" and that her role "evolved from observation to informal interviews over time."

Exercise D.2: Questions of Fact (Appendix E)

a. The article indicates that the spousal caregivers, who were the participants, had to be returning home from the geriatric rehabilitation unit (GRU) with a husband or wife who did not have cognitive impairment or dementia.

b. Participants were recruited at the long-term care hospital through a GRU team member who was not affiliated with the study. Then, those who were willing to participate were approached by Byrne.

c. The researchers referred to "initial" sampling (presumably convenience sampling) and theoretical sampling that was used to guide data collection. Byrne and colleagues provided the readers with a specific example of their theoretical sampling having to do with how and when caregivers shifted the boundaries.

d. The sample consisted of 18 caregivers, 9 men and 9 women.

e. The report mentioned saturation of theoretical categories. The authors noted, "In accordance with theoretical sampling, the categories noted to be relevant to the development of the emerging theoretical framework guided the sampling process rather than particular sample characteristics such as demographics."

f. There is no mention of sampling confirming or disconfirming cases.

g. Characteristics of the 18 couples were briefly described. The caregivers' mean age was 77.4 years, and they had been married for 47 years, on average. Care recipients, who were on average slightly older, had had a mean length of stay on the GRU of 41 days.

h. Yes, the primary form of data collection was via self-report. The questions focused on "sensitizing concepts" from prior related research (e.g., changes in the relationship since returning home, social supports available).

i. In-depth face-to-face interviews in the participants' homes were used to collect self-report data. The goal was to conduct interviews longitudinally, at three points in time, but not all participants were able to adhere to this schedule.

j. The researchers gave a couple of examples: "Participants were asked how they would describe their relationship with their spouse currently… in comparison to before they were admitted to the GRU, and about who had been especially helpful to them in caring for their spouse."

k. Interviews lasted between 35 and 120 minutes.

l. All interviews were audio-recorded and transcribed verbatim by an experienced transcriptionist.

m. Yes, the researcher also observed and recorded interactions between the spouses. The report noted that the researcher (the first author) was "'finely tuned in' to look for interactions that would help elucidate processes and categories emerging from the data."

CHAPTER 16

A. FILL IN THE BLANKS

1. content
2. statistics
3. domain
4. circle
5. constitutive
6. line-by-line
7. memo
8. coding
9. constructivist
10. selective
11. metaphor
12. emergent
13. core
14. exemplars
15. taxonomic
16. open
17. Paradigm

B. MATCHING EXERCISES

1. a, b, c   2. a   3. b   4. a, b, c   5. a
6. c   7. b   8. d

C. STUDY QUESTIONS

C.1.
a. A grounded theory analysis would not yield themes—a phenomenological study involves a thematic analysis.
b. Texts from poetry are used by interpretive phenomenologists, not by ethnographers (unless the poetry is a product of the culture under study, which it is not in this case).
c. Phenomenological studies do not focus on domains; ethnographies do.
d. Grounded theory studies do not yield taxonomies; ethnographies do.
e. A paradigm case is a strategy in a hermeneutic analysis, not in an ethnographic one.

D. APPLICATION EXERCISES

Exercise D.1: Questions of Fact (Appendix E)

a. Yes, Byrne and colleagues audiotaped the interviews with the 18 spousal caregivers. The audiotapes were transcribed by an experienced transcriptionist. The article did not indicate how many pages of transcription resulted, but it did say that interviews were between 35 and 120 minutes long. In total, there were 45 interviews. This likely resulted in a total of hundreds of pages in the dataset that had to be read and re-read, coded, and analyzed.
b. Yes, at the end of the sub-section labeled *Data Collection*, the authors indicated that "data generation and data analysis occurred simultaneously, which supported follow-ups with participants about emerging codes and categories."
c. It does not appear that computer software was used in the analysis of data for this study.
d. Byrne and colleagues did not use quasi-statistics, but it is important to note that they did engage in (as do most qualitative researchers) a kind of qualitative "accounting." Here are two examples: "While spouses were on the GRU, *most caregivers* took daily trips to the hospital as a means of maintaining normalcy…" and "Declines in their own health and function were a very real worry, because *many knew* that if something happened to them, their spouse would end up in long-term care."
e. No, Byrne and colleagues did not use metaphors, although they used rich and compelling language to describe features of their framework (e.g., Getting into it, Getting on with it).
f. Yes, the report indicated that Byrne (the first author) wrote memos during the analysis: "When a code was raised to the level of a category, the first author created a memo describing the category, the elements contained in the category, illustrative quotes that reflected the category, and further ideas on which to follow up to ensure theoretical saturation of the category. These memos were shared and discussed among authors."
g. The report stated that Byrne engaged in line-by-line coding, and then all authors contributed to focused and theoretical coding. The researchers noted that moving from line-by-line to focused coding was not a linear process. Excellent examples of the coding process were provided in the section labeled Analysis.

Exercise D.2: Questions of Fact (Appendix F)

a. Yes, Cummings' interviews were audiotaped and transcribed verbatim by a transcriptionist who had completed special training relating to the protection of the rights of study participants.
b. The report did not mention that Cummings used computer software to organize and manage her data. Her statement about making marginal notes using different color highlighters strongly suggests that she relied exclusively on manual methods of organization and coding.
c. Cummings does not appear to have used any quasi-statistics. Again, however, there are several statements

suggesting a kind of "accounting," as in the following examples: *"Many listeners* described experiencing a feeling of awe while listening" and *"Many participants* found themselves imagining what happened as well as what could have happened."

d. Cummings reported that she used van Manen's phenomenologic approach.

e. The article stated that Cummings maintained a journal "to record additional observations and personal reflections."

f. Cummings discussed the analytic process in terms of the steps she attributed to van Manen: holding preconceived beliefs in abeyance; undertaking a holistic reading of each transcript to get a sense of it as a whole; rereading the transcripts to identify statements or phrases that best represented participants' experiences; identifying categories; and dwelling with the data to identify key themes. (Cummings did not follow van Manen's approach strictly, however, perhaps because of the sensitive nature of the inquiry. In van Manen's interpretive approach, researchers typically go back and forth with participants to have them reflect on the experiences, typically using the transcript of the first interview as a starting point in a subsequent conversation).

g. Cummings' analysis revealed five essential themes: (1) The story has a purpose; (2) the story may continue to change as different parts are revealed; (3) the story is experienced physically, mentally, emotionally, and spiritually; (4) Imagining the "what" as well as the "what if"; and (5) the nature of the relationship colors the experience of the listener and storyteller.

h. Yes, Cummings provided rich supportive evidence for her themes, in the form of direct quotes from the interviews. For example, here is a quote from theme 4, from a listener: "There is no way you can understand; there's no way, even if you had a similar experience, that you can put yourself in their shoes."

CHAPTER 17

A. FILL IN THE BLANKS

1. Credibility
2. triangulation
3. dependability
4. transferability
5. decision
6. thick description
7. confirmability
8. internal
9. observation
10. negative
11. member
12. Investigator
13. Authenticity
14. peer
15. prolonged

B. MATCHING EXERCISES

1. a   2. c   3. b   4. d   5. a   6. b

D. APPLICATION EXERCISES

Exercise D.1: Questions of Fact (Appendix E)

a. Yes, Byrne and colleagues devoted an entire subsection of their report to describing their approach to quality enhancement, labeled "Criteria for Rigor."

b. The researchers used two types of triangulation. First, there was method triangulation. The primary source of data was interviews with the spouse caregivers, but these data were augmented with observations of the interactions between caregivers and their spouses. They noted that they "used triangulation not to confirm existing data but rather to enhance completeness." Another form of triangulation was investigator triangulation. Byrne did much of the preliminary coding and analysis but shared her work with her coauthors, and all researchers contributed to the final framework. Although the multiple points of data collection suggest time triangulation, the researchers were less interested in *verification* in later interviews than they were in understanding how the process of reconciliation evolved over time.

c. Many strategies were used to enhance rigor in this study.

- It could be said that both persistent observation (the researchers' very thorough and in-depth scrutiny of the reconciliation process) and prolonged engagement (continuing to gather data and observe participants over a 6-week period) were used as quality-enhancement strategies in this study.
- The report indicated that the preliminary theoretical framework was shared with five caregivers as a member-checking strategy. The authors noted, "Caregivers reported being able to 'see' their own experience of transition in the processes presented." Moreover, the authors stated that the framework was modified based on feedback from participants.
- The report did not discuss any efforts to search for disconfirming evidence (although this does not necessarily mean it did not occur).
- The report indicates that the researcher maintained a reflexive journal, and that entries were made on an electronic notebook for each interview.
- The report stated that an audit trail was maintained, although details were not provided, except to note that an electronic field notebook was used to record audit trail details.

Exercise D.1: Questions of Fact (Appendix F)

a. No, Cummings did not have a section of her report specifically describing quality-enhancement strategies. Her strategies were presented in the second paragraph of the "Data Analysis" section.

b. Triangulation was not a key part of Cummings' quality-enhancement strategies. It is true that she gathered data from both storytellers and listeners,

but this is not really data source triangulation because the experiences of listener and storyteller were considered separately (i.e., the point of including the listeners was not to triangulate information from the storytellers, but to understand the parallel experience of the listeners). Investigator triangulation was not really used either—that is, it was not a *team* of investigators who undertook the analysis.

c. Several strategies were used to enhance rigor in this study.

- Cummings does not appear to have used persistent observation in her research. Although she gathered data from both parties to storytelling episodes, she did not (for example) go back to participants and ask them to reflect on transcripts and co-interpret them.
- Cummings used peer debriefing. She "collaborated with two professional colleagues and expert qualitative researchers who reviewed transcripts and findings."
- Cummings noted that "findings were presented and clarified with participants to assess whether the transcripts were accurate and whether identified themes resonated with them". The report did not indicate whether both listeners and storytellers were involved in the member checks, nor how many participants were asked to help.
- There was no mention of searching for disconfirming evidence.
- The report indicated that a journal was kept to record observations and personal reflections. Cummings also noted that the first step in the analysis process was to put aside preconceived notions and beliefs about the phenomenon under study.
- The report did not state that an audit trail was maintained, although this does not mean that it did not happen.
- The researcher is a doctorally trained nurse practitioner. She noted in the introduction that the issue of listening to traumatic events is crucial for nurse

practitioners, and that little is known about the impact of listening to stories of traumatic events on nurses. The acknowledgments at the end of the story suggest that Cummings herself was a listener to the story about the crash landing—her brother was on board the United Airlines plane that crashed into the Hudson River.

CHAPTER 18

A. FILL IN THE BLANKS

1. method
2. sequencing, prioritization
3. qualitative
4. embedded
5. sequential
6. concurrent
7. pragmatism
8. survey
9. test
10. clinical trial
11. effectiveness
12. intervention theory
13. impact
14. process
15. Outcomes
16. structure
17. secondary
18. methodological
19. randomized

B. MATCHING EXERCISES

1. a, b, c,   2. e   3. d   4. c   5. a
6. b   7. e   8. f

D. APPLICATION EXERCISES

Exercise D.1: Questions of Fact

a. Clinical trial:
   • The Weinert et al. study in Appendix A could be described as a clinical trial— a randomized design was used to test an innovative intervention with clear clinical applications.

b. Economic analysis
   • None of the studies in the appendices involved an economic analysis (or, if they did, that part of the study was not presented in the reports).

c. Outcomes research
   • None of the studies in the appendices could be described as outcomes research.

d. Survey research
   • The Jurgens et al. study (Appendix D) is the closest thing to a survey in the appendices, although it is not truly an example of survey research. Surveys typically gather self-report data from a broad population of respondents—like in an opinion poll—rather than from patients with a particular health problem served at a particular institution.

e. Secondary analysis:
   • All of the reports in the appendices described studies in which researchers collected original data; there are no secondary analyses.

f. Methodological research
   • None of the studies in the appendices could be described as methodological research.

Exercise D.3: Questions of Fact (Appendix D)

a. Yes, this was a mixed methods study. The purpose of the quantitative strand was to describe the duration of heart failure symptoms and to identify factors that influenced symptom duration prior to help seeking. The purpose of the qualitative strand was to enrich the description of the patients' symptoms, their responses to the symptoms, and their help-seeking behavior.

b. The quantitative strand had priority in the study design.

c. The design was concurrent—data for both strands were collected at the same time.

d. The design used in this study could be described as an embedded design. Qualitative data were used primarily in a supportive capacity.

e. Using the Creswell-Plano design types, the study design would be

QUAN(qual). The researchers used a similar notation: QUAN/qual.

f. Jurgens and colleagues used a sampling approach called identical sampling to obtain both qualitative and quantitative data from the same study participants.

g. The report stated that a matrix was created in the analysis of the qualitative data and that "the final step in the data analysis was integration of the qualitative and quantitative data."

CHAPTER 19

A. FILL IN THE BLANKS

1. meta-analysis
2. heterogeneity
3. difference
4. sensitivity
5. subgroup
6. random
7. null
8. ratio
9. grey
10. fixed
11. forest
12. intensity
13. publication
14. frequency
15. meta-summary

B. MATCHING EXERCISES

1. c   2. d   3. b   4. a   5. b
6. a   7. d   8. b

D. APPLICATION EXERCISES

Exercise D.1: Questions of Fact (Appendix G)

a. The purpose of Nam and colleagues' meta-analysis was "to evaluate the effectiveness of a culturally tailored diabetes intervention (CTDEI) on glycemic control in ethnic minorities with type 2 diabetes." The independent variable was receipt versus non-receipt of a special intervention, and

the dependent (outcome) variable was glycemic control.

b. To be eligible for this meta-analysis, the primary study had to (a) be a randomized controlled trial; (b) involve an educational intervention (not a drug intervention) for ethnic minorities with type 2 diabetes; and (c) report both preintervention and postintervention values for glycosylated hemoglobin (HbA_{1c}). A total of 12 studies met these criteria.

c. According to the article, all 12 studies were randomized controlled trails (RCTs). The article specifically states that quasi-experimental studies were excluded. (Inasmuch as the study question involved the effects of an intervention, studies with a nonexperimental design would not have been appropriate.)

d. Study quality was assessed based on four quality criteria: description of randomization procedures, information on attrition, description of the intervention, and description of the eligibility criteria. Each criterion was assessed as being absent (scored 0), partially described (scored 1), and clearly described (scored 2). Thus, scores could range from 0 to 8. It should be noted that this quality assessment differs from what is typical—in this meta-analysis, quality was defined in terms of what was reported, not in terms of methodologic rigor. For example, the researchers did not code for whether blinding was used, whether attrition was low, whether intervention fidelity was monitored, and so on. The report does not indicate that the quality assessment was performed by multiple people and assessed for interrater reliability (which does not mean that this did not occur).

e. Studies with scores below 6 were considered low quality, but studies of low quality were not excluded—i.e., quality was not an exclusion criterion. Six primary studies were scored as low quality and six as high quality.

f. The effect size, which they labeled ED, was "defined as the difference in the change of a measurement from baseline to follow-up between control and treatment groups" for HbA$_{1c}$. This is the standardized mean difference, which we referred to in the textbook as *d*.

g. Yes, the researchers tested for heterogeneity. They opted to use a random effects model.

h. The total number of participants in the 12 primary studies was 1,495, as reported in the subsection labeled "Participant Demographics Across Studies."

i. The overall effect size comparing reductions in HbA$_{1c}$ for those in the intervention group compared to a control group was −.29. As shown in Table 2, the 95% confidence interval around this value was −.46 to −.13, and thus is significant because the interval does not include zero. We can be 95% confident that the true beneficial effect lies somewhere in the interval between −.13 and −.46.

j. With regard to Figure 2:
   - The effect size (ES) favoring patients in the treatment condition was largest for the Rosal study (ES = −1.02), and this was statistically significant.
   - The ES was nonsignificant for the six studies in Figure 2 for which the horizontal lines indicating the 95% confidence interval crossed the center line, which represented zero (no effect). These were the studies by Anderson, Gucciardi, Hawthorne, O'Hare, Skelly, and Vincent.
   - Yes, in the Anderson study, the ES of +.11 indicated that the control group had slightly better (but not significantly better) changes to their HbA$_{1c}$ levels than those in the intervention group.

k. Yes, subgroup analyses were undertaken to explore the heterogeneity of effects across studies. The dimensions included settings of the interventions (community-based vs. clinic or hospital), timing of the follow-up measurements (3, 6, or 12 months after baseline), value of the baseline HbA$_{1c}$ (<8.5% vs. >8.5%), and study quality (low vs. high). As shown in Table 2, many of the subgroup analyses resulted in effect size estimates favoring the intervention group that were statistically significant (i.e., the 95% CI did not include zero). The subgroups for which the intervention effects were not significant were interventions in community settings; studies with 3 or 12 months of follow-up; low-quality studies; and studies in which the baseline HbA$_{1c}$ was greater than 8.5%. In several of these cases, the lack of statistical significance likely reflects the very small sample size for the subgroup.

Exercise D.2: Questions of Fact (Appendix H)

a. Beck undertook a metasynthesis of six of her own studies in her program of research on traumatic births, and did not search for other qualitative studies on the same or a related topic. Beck's was, thus, a special type of metasynthesis. (Of course, as an expert in the area of traumatic birth, Beck is thoroughly familiar with the literature in her field).

b. Beck did not explicitly discuss this controversy, although her approach would have integrated any of her studies on the topic of traumatic births, regardless of tradition. Her metasynthesis combined five phenomenological studies and one narrative analysis.

c. The data in the primary studies were all derived from self-reports, exclusively from Internet-based self-reports.

d. A total of 175 mothers participated in Beck's six primary studies.

e. Beck used Noblit and Hare's approach for doing a metasynthesis, which they described as a meta-ethnography. Beck provided an excellent description of the seven phases of the approach.

f. No, a meta-summary is a strategy developed by Sandelowski and colleagues, and Beck did not follow this approach.

g. Beck identified three overarching themes in her studies of birth trauma: (1) stripped of protective layers; (2) invisible wounds; and (3) insidious repercussions. Beck also discovered that traumatic childbirth had a domino effect on various aspects of new motherhood, which she identified as *amplifying causal looping*.

h. Yes, Beck included some powerful verbatim quotes from the primary studies in support of her thematic integration.